T Cell Protocols

METHODS IN MOLECULAR BIOLOGY™

John M. Walker, SERIES EDITOR

METHODS IN MOLECULAR BIOLOGY™

T Cell Protocols
Development and Activation

Edited by

Kelly P. Kearse

*Department of Microbiology and Immunology,
East Carolina University School of Medicine, Greenville, NC*

Humana Press ✳ Totowa, New Jersey

Dedication

To Kathy, for her unconditional devotion and support

Cover design by Patricia F. Cleary

Cover illustrations: Fig. 3 from Chapter 7, "Intrathymic Delivery of MHC Genes Using Recombinant Adenoviruses," by Ronald Rooke, Christophe Benoist, and Diane Mathis. Fig. 4 from Chapter 13, "Flow Cytometric Analysis of Murine T Lymphocytes: *A Practical Guide,*" by Melanie S. Vacchio and Elizabeth W. Shores.

For additional copies, pricing for bulk purchases, and/or information about other Humana titles, contact Humana at the above address or at any of the following numbers: Tel.: 973-256-1699; Fax: 973-256-8341; E-mail: humana@humanapr.com or visit our Website: http://humanapress.com

Photocopy Authorization Policy:
Authorization to photocopy items for internal or personal use, or the internal or personal use of specific clients, is granted by Humana Press Inc., provided that the base fee of US $10.00 per copy, plus US $00.25 per page, is paid directly to the Copyright Clearance Center at 222 Rosewood Drive, Danvers, MA 01923. For those organizations that have been granted a photocopy license from the CCC, a separate system of payment has been arranged and is acceptable to Humana Press Inc. The fee code for users of the Transactional Reporting Service is: [0-89603-810-6/00 $10.00 + $00.25].

Printed in the United States of America. 10 9 8 7 6 5 4 3 2 1

Library of Congress Cataloging in Publication Data

T cell protocols : development and activation / edited by Kelly P. Kearse
     p. cm. -- (Methods in molecular biology ; 134)
   Includes index.
   ISBN 0-89603-810-6(alk. paper)
   1. T cells Laboratory manuals. I. Kearse, Kelly P. II. Series: Methods in molecular biology
(Clifton, N.J.) ; 134
    [DNLM: 1. T-Lymphocytes--cytology. 2. T-Lymphocytes--physiology.
  3. Immunologic Techniques. 4. Lymphocyte Transformation. W1 ME9616J v. 134 2000]
   QR185.8.T2T14 2000
   616.07'97--dc21
   DNLM/DLC   99-25100
   for Library of Congress   CIP

Preface

The purpose of *T Cell Protocols: Development and Activation* is to collect a series of protocols, particularly those that have been developed within the past few years, to help investigators master new techniques (or improve existing ones) for the study of T-cell biology.

Invariably, in putting together a book like this it is difficult to decide which methods to include and which to leave out. To this end methods were selected from a variety of disciplines, including cellular immunology, biochemistry, and molecular biology, to try to provide something of interest for everyone who works on T-cell development and activation.

I would like to mention that my primary reason for agreeing to put this book together is that, when I was a graduate student, I purchased a copy of *Selected Methods in Cellular Immunology* by Mishell and Shigii which proved a tremendous help in learning the basics of one- and two-dimensional gel techniques (and other methods). The cover has long since fallen off, but it still remains one of my most valued reference books for the laboratory. It is my hope that *T Cell Protocols: Development and Activation* will prove similarly useful to current and future scientists wishing to learn new methods for exploring the development and activation of T cells.

I would especially like to thank the many investigators who contributed to this volume and were willing to share their expertise with others. I would also like to thank Dr. John Walker and the staff at Humana Press, Inc. for their guidance in putting this volume together.

Kelly P. Kearse

Contents

Contents *ix*

Contributors

T. PRESCOTT ATKINSON • *Department of Pediatrics, Division of Clinical and Developmental Immunology, University of Alabama at Birmingham, Birmingham, AL*

M. ALBERT BASSON • *Division of Molecular Immunology, MRC National Institute for Medical Research, London, UK*

CHRISTOPHE BENOIST • *Institut de Genetique et de Biologie Moleculaire et Cellulaire, Strasbourg, France*

GIDEON BERKE • *Department of Immunology, Weizmann Institute of Science, Rehovot, Israel*

KARINE BERNARD • *Genome Structure and Immune Function Lab Centre d'Immunologie, INSERM CNRS Marseille-Luminy, Marseille, France*

SETH MARK BERNEY • *Division of Rheumatology, Center of Excellence for Arthritis and Rheumatology, Louisiana State University Medical Center, Shreveport, LA*

JAY A. BERZOFSKY • *Molecular Immunogenetics and Vaccine Section, Metabolism Branch, National Cancer Institute, Bethesda, MD*

GUNNEL BIBERFELD • *Swedish Institute for Infectious Disease Control, Karolinska Institute, Stockholm, Sweden*

CAROLINE D. V. A. BISHOP • *Department of Biology, Haverford College, Haverford, PA*

ROBERT CHERVENAK • *Department of Microbiology and Immunology, Louisiana State University Medical Center, Shreveport, LA*

KEITH A. CHING • *Department of Biology and Molecular Biology Institute, San Diego State University, San Diego, CA*

ELIZABETH CRANE • *Department of Biology, Haverford College, Haverford, PA*

MORDECHAI DEUTSCH • *Schottenstein Cellscan Center, Physics Department, Bar-Ilan University, Ramat-Gan, Israel*

RATKO DJUKANOVIĆ • *Southampton University, Southampton University General Hospital, Immunopharmacology Group, Southampton, England, UK*

DARIUSH FARAHI FAR • *Department of Cellular and Molecular Immunology, UNITE 364 INSERM, Nice, France*

JACKIE FELBERG • *Department of Microbiology and Immunology, University of British Columbia, Vancouver, British Columbia, Canada*

PATRICK E. FIELDS • *Department of Pathology, University of Chicago Medical Center, Chicago, IL*

KARL J. FRANEK • *Department of Microbiology and Immunology, Louisiana State University Medical Center, Shreveport, LA*

THOMAS F. GAJEWSKI • *Department of Pathology and Department of Medicine, Section of Hematology/Oncology, University of Chicago Medical Center, Chicago, IL*

HANS GAINES • *Swedish Institute for Infectious Disease Control, Karolinska, Institute, Stockholm, Sweden*

TERRENCE G. GARDNER • *Department of Microbiology and Immunology, East Carolina University School of Medicine, Greenville, NC*

SAMUEL GRANJEAUD • *Genome Structure and Immune Function Lab Centre d'Immunologie, INSERM CNRS Marseille-Luminy, Marseille, France*

SHOJI IWAGAMI • *Department of Immunology, Shionogi Institute for Medical Science, Shionogi and Co. Ltd., Osaka, Japan*

PAULINE JOHNSON • *Department of Microbiology and Immunology, University of British Columbia, Vancouver, British Columbia, Canada*

AMY JOST • *Department of Biology, Haverford College, Haverford, PA*

JOHN KAPPLER • *Department of Medicine, Howard Hughes Medical Institute, National Jewish Center, Denver, CO*

MENACHEM KAUFMAN • *Schottenstein Cellscan Center, Physics Department, Bar-Ilan University, Ramat-Gan, Israel*

KELLY P. KEARSE • *Department of Microbiology and Immunology, East Carolina University School of Medicine, Greenville, NC*

TOSHIO KITAMURA • *Department of Hematopoietic Factors, The Institute of Medical Sciences, University of Tokyo, Tokyo, Japan*

GRAHAM R. LEGGATT • *Centre for Immunology and Cancer Research, Department of Medicine, University of Queensland, Princess Alexandra Hospital, Brisbane, Australia*

PHILIPPA MARRACK • *Department of Medicine, Howard Hughes Medical Institute, National Jewish Center, Denver, CO*

DIANE MATHIS • *Institut de Genetique et de Biologie Moleculaire et Cellulaire, Strasbourg, France*

TAKAJI MATSUTANI • *Department of Immunology, Shionogi Institute for Medical Science, Shionogi and Co. Ltd., Osaka, Japan*

BRADLEY W. MCINTYRE • *Department of Immunology, University of Texas, M. D. Anderson Cancer Center, Houston, TX*

BRADFORD L. McRAE • *Department of Pathology, University of Chicago, Chicago, IL*

ALISON M. MICHIE • *Department of Immunology, University of Toronto, Toronto, Ontario, Canada*

YOSHIHIRO MORIKAWA • *Department of Anatomy and Neurobiology, Wakayama Medical School, Wakayama, Japan*

DAVID H. W. NG • *Department of Microbiology and Immunology, University of British Columbia, Vancouver, British Columbia, Canada*

CATHERINE NGUYEN • *Genome Structure and Immune Function Lab Centre d'Immunologie, INSERM CNRS Marseille-Luminy, Marseille, France*

JOHN J. O' SHEA • *Leukocyte Cell Biology Arthritis and Rheumatology Branch, NIAMS, NIH, Bethesda, MD*

ELLEN M. PALMER • *Department of Pathology, University of Chicago, Chicago, IL*

JENNIFER A. PUNT • *Department of Biology, Haverford College, Haverford, PA*

ELLEN R. RICHIE • *The University of Texas, M. D. Anderson Cancer Center, Science Park-Research Division, Smithfield, TX*

RONALD ROOKE • *Transgene S. A., Strasbourg, France*

BERNARD ROSSI • *Department of Cellular and Molecular Immunology, UNITE 364 INSERM, Nice, France*

ROSHANAK TOLOUEI SEMNANI • *Department of Pathology, University of Chicago, Chicago, IL*

ELIZABETH W. SHORES • *Division of Hematologic Products, Center for Biologics Evaluation and Research, Food and Drug Administration, Bethesda, MD*

KENNETH SHORTMAN • *The Walter and Eliza Hall Institute of Medical Research, PO Royal Melbourne Hospital, Melbourne, Victoria, Australia*

LUMINITA A. STANCIU • *Southampton University, Southampton University General Hospital, Immunopharmacology Group, Southampton, England, UK*

JACK STANNERS • *Department of Biology and Molecular Biology Institute, San Diego State University, San Diego, CA*

HARUMI SUZUKI • *Department of Immunology, Keio University School of Medicine, Tokyo, Japan*

RYUJI SUZUKI • *Department of Immunology, Shionogi Institute for Medical Science, Shionogi and Co. Ltd., Osaka, Japan*

YOUSUKE TAKAHAMA • *University of Tsukuba, PRESTO, TARA Center, Tsukuba, Japan*

T. KENT TEAGUE • *Department of Immunology, University of Texas, M. D. Anderson Cancer Center, Houston, TX*

TOMOKO TOYOSAKI-MAEDA • *Department of Immunology, Shionogi Institute for Medical Science, Shionogi and Co. Ltd., Osaka, Japan*

CONSTANTINE D. TSOUKAS • *Department of Biology and Molecular Biology Institute, San Diego State University, San Diego, CA*

YUJI TSURUTA • *Department of Immunology, Shionogi Institute for Medical Science, Shionogi and Co. Ltd., Osaka, Japan*

MELANIE S. VACCHIO • *Experimental Immunology Branch, National Cancer Institute, NIH, Bethesda, MD*

GIJS A. VAN SEVENTER • *Department of Pathology, University of Chicago, Chicago, IL*

JEAN MAGUIRE VAN SEVENTER • *Department of Pathology, University of Chicago, Chicago, IL*

GENEVIÈVE VICTORÉRO • *Genome Structure and Immune Function Lab Centre d'Immunologie, INSERM CNRS Marseille-Luminy, Marseille, France*

DAWN A. WALKER • *Laboratory of Receptor Biology and Gene Expression, NIH, Bethesda, MD*

ALLAN M. WEISSMAN • *Laboratory of Immune Cell Biology, Division of Basic Sciences, National Cancer Institute, NIH, Bethesda, MD*

JANICE WHITE • *Department of Medicine, Howard Hughes Medical Institute, National Jewish Center, Denver, CO*

DARREN G. WOODSIDE • *Department of Immunology, University of Texas, M. D. Anderson Cancer Center, Houston, TX*

DAVID K. WOOTEN • *Department of Immunology, University of Texas, M. D. Anderson Cancer Center, Houston, TX*

LI WU • *The Walter and Eliza Hall Institute of Medical Research, PO Royal Melbourne Hospital, Melbourne, Victoria, Australia*

TAKESHI YOSHIOKA • *Department of Immunology, Shionogi Institute for Medical Science, Shionogi and Co. Ltd., Osaka, Japan*

ROSE ZAMOYSKA • *Division of Molecular Immunology, MRC National Institute for Medical Research, London, UK*

JUAN CARLOS ZÚÑIGA-PFLÜCKER • *Department of Immunology, University of Toronto, Toronto, Ontario, Canada*

NAOMI ZURGIL • *Schottenstein Cellscan Center, Physics Department, Bar-Ilan University, Ramat-Gan, Israel*

I

OVERVIEW: FOR CHAPTERS 2–15

1

Insights into T-Cell Development
from Studies Using Transgenic and Knockout Mice

M. Albert Basson and Rose Zamoyska

1. Introduction

T-cell differentiation is a tightly controlled developmental program observed as the stepwise progression of immature thymocytes through several unique stages characterized by the expression of distinct combinations of cell surface markers. The advancement of thymocytes from one stage to the next requires the successful completion of one or more specific developmental processes, accompanied by the acquisition of receptors, which signal a cell to transit through certain critical checkpoints to a more mature stage. The techniques of transgenesis and germ-line targeting are particularly useful in the study of such complex developmental programs, in that specific players can be manipulated in the context of an otherwise unaltered environment. Such studies have been instrumental in our understanding not only of how a number of thymocyte surface receptors are involved in the developmental program, but also in identifying some of the intracellular signaling mediators that are involved in regulation of transcription factors which are ultimately responsible for orchestrating the differentiated phenotype.

It is clear that the investigation of the molecular details of T-cell development has benefited greatly from transgenic and knockout methodology and we shall discuss a few examples of some key experiments in the present chapter. We shall not attempt to provide a comprehensive overview of all the genes that have been targeted or expressed, as some excellent up-to-date reviews are available. Our aim is to illustrate how the role of a few of these molecular components was elucidated and discuss the interpretation of these experiments within the framework of what is now a fairly well established pathway of thymocyte differentiation.

From: *Methods in Molecular Biology, Vol. 134: T Cell Protocols: Development and Activation*
Edited by: K. P. Kearse © Humana Press Inc., Totowa, NJ

1.1. Transgenic and Knockout Methodology and Their Application

Transgenesis is the process by which the gene of interest is injected into a fertilized oocyte. Successful integration of the DNA into the genome and propagation through the germline, allows the establishment of a line of mice stably expressing the transgene. Typically a number of founder mice are produced which differ from one another both in the site of integration and the number of copies of the transgene integrated into the genome. By altering the promotor and/or genetic control regions linked to the gene of interest, the level, tissue specificity, and developmental stage of gene expression can be controlled, allowing the influence of a single molecular species on the differentiation process to be followed. A second transgenic approach which has also had wide application, is the construction of mice expressing a mutated form of the gene of interest. Typically these have been nonfunctional variants that behave in a dominant negative fashion, disrupting the function of the gene of interest and simulating a negative phenotype.

Despite the immense amount such transgenic approaches have taught us, there are several disadvantages of this technology, which are very important, particularly when studying genes and gene products that are developmentally controlled. The forced expression of transgenes undoubtedly influences the balance of a finely tuned network of developmentally regulated signaling molecules, which cannot always be taken into consideration when conclusions are drawn from such experiments. The level of expression of most genes is naturally tightly regulated and the forced over-expression of a gene product may disrupt the status quo in ways we do not understand. Thus it is not always possible to correctly interpret phenotypic consequences of transgene expression in terms of molecular mechanisms. This criticism extends particularly to analysis of mice expressing dominant negative transgenes in that such mutations may disrupt the action of several other signaling molecules in addition to their predicted targets. Other relevant considerations are that the differences in the timing of expression of a transgene compared to the endogenous gene, as a result of expression under the control of heterologous tissue-specific promotors, could short-circuit or elongate the normal developmental program. Furthermore, the site of integration of the transgene may critically influence expression as the recently described phenomenon of position effect variegation could occur more frequently in transgenic mice than previously realized *(1)*. This phenomenon, described in detail in Drosophila and yeast occurs when a transgene integrates in close proximity to heterochromatin and becomes randomly silenced in a proportion of cells, unless the transgene contains specific regulatory sequences which can maintain an open chromatin configuration.

The expression of developmentally important genes on only certain cells in an otherwise homogeneous population of developing cells may serve to endow them with an advantage or disadvantage over their neighbors, thus affecting the normal developmental outcome in a manner not directly related to the primary function of the transgene.

In addition to transgenic technology, the ability to specifically disrupt expression of a gene of interest by targeted homologous mutation or "gene knockouts" has been particularly informative for examining the relevance of specific gene products to the differentiation process. This technique involves insertion of DNA, generally coding for a drug resistance marker into the gene of interest by homologous recombination. The major advantage of this technique is that the role of a specific gene product can be assessed in the context of an otherwise intact genome. To its disadvantage is the fact that knockout experiments tend to give an "all-or-none" answer i.e., differentiation is blocked at the first stage at which the molecule is required and the role of that particular molecule during later stages in development cannot be assessed. Redundancy also creates problems in that a seemingly normal phenotype does not necessarily mean that the molecule of interest is not active at a particular stage, as it is always possible that other members of the same family have compensated for the missing protein.

More recently, "knock-in" techniques have been established *(2)* in which specific mutations are introduced by replacement of gene segments using homologous recombination, which allows the subtle modification of gene products while maintaining normal regulation of expression, thus resolving potential disadvantages of transgenesis. These mutations are likely to exhibit a less severe phenotype than complete knockouts. Furthermore, the establishment of inducible bacterial promotor systems which can be utilized in transgenic mice to regulate gene expression *(3)* combined with traditional transgenic and knockout methodology allows the generation of experimental systems that can potentially be manipulated at any point during the course of development. It may be possible to control the level and timing of expression of genes of immunological interest so that the functions of specific gene products can be evaluated at all stages of differentiation. Together these techniques provide an enormous potential for unraveling the key events which regulate thymocyte differentiation.

2. Transcription Factors and Commitment to the T-Cell Lineage

Transcription factors involved in lineage decisions have been described in many developmental systems, including T-cell development. Disruption of the gene encoding for the zinc finger DNA binding protein, Ikaros, illustrates, not only the general usefulness of gene targeting for the identification of genes crucial to developmental decisions, but also some complications that can arise in the interpretation of the resulting phenotype. The first reported germline disruption of the Ikaros gene led to a severely immunocompromized mouse which lacked all lymphoid cells *(4)*, suggesting that the Ikaros gene product is absolutely essential for commitment to the lymphoid lineage. However, subsequent studies indicated that a truncated portion of the protein was still being produced in these mice, and may in fact be behaving as a dominant negative mutation *(5)*. A complete Ikaros-null mouse was subsequently generated and the phenotype found to be less severe than the initial mutation *(6)*. Development of the lymphoid lineage was severely affected in the fetus, but normal in the adult, indicating that the original dominant negative protein interfered with the function of another factor during differentiation in the adult. These observations, although originally confusing, led to the identification of another lymphoid-specific homologue, Aiolos *(7)*, with which the Ikaros gene product interacts presumably forming a functional transcription factor complex required for development of hematopoetic stem cells into the lymphoid lineage in adults.

Several transcription factors are widely expressed and may be essential during early embryogenesis, making it impossible to assess their roles in the development of cells of the lymphoid lineage. An example is the GATA-3 transcription factor that is expressed in T cells, central nervous system, kidney, adrenal gland and fetal liver, the targeted disruption of which leads to embryonic lethality *(8)*. However, it was possible to look at the role of GATA-3 in lymphoid development using the technique of blastocyst complementation. This involves injecting ES cells with targeted disruption of GATA-3 into RAG-deficient blastocysts. Any lymphoid cells which develop in such chimaeras must derive from the injected ES cell, and it was observed that the embryonic stem (ES) cells lacking GATA-3 could indeed give rise to cells belonging to the lymphoid lineage. In the resulting chimaeras, all cells belonging to the T-cell lineage were absent suggesting that this gene is essential for their development *(9)*. The expression of genes such as GATA-3 under the control of inducible promotors would be useful for examining their function at later stages of T-cell development.

3. Thymocyte Differentiation

3.1. Early Thymocyte Differentiation

The progression of T-cell precursors can be followed through different stages of differentiation by the expression of a number of surface molecules (**Fig. 1**). Various key players involved during the early stages of thymocyte differentiation have been identified using transgenic and knockout technolo-

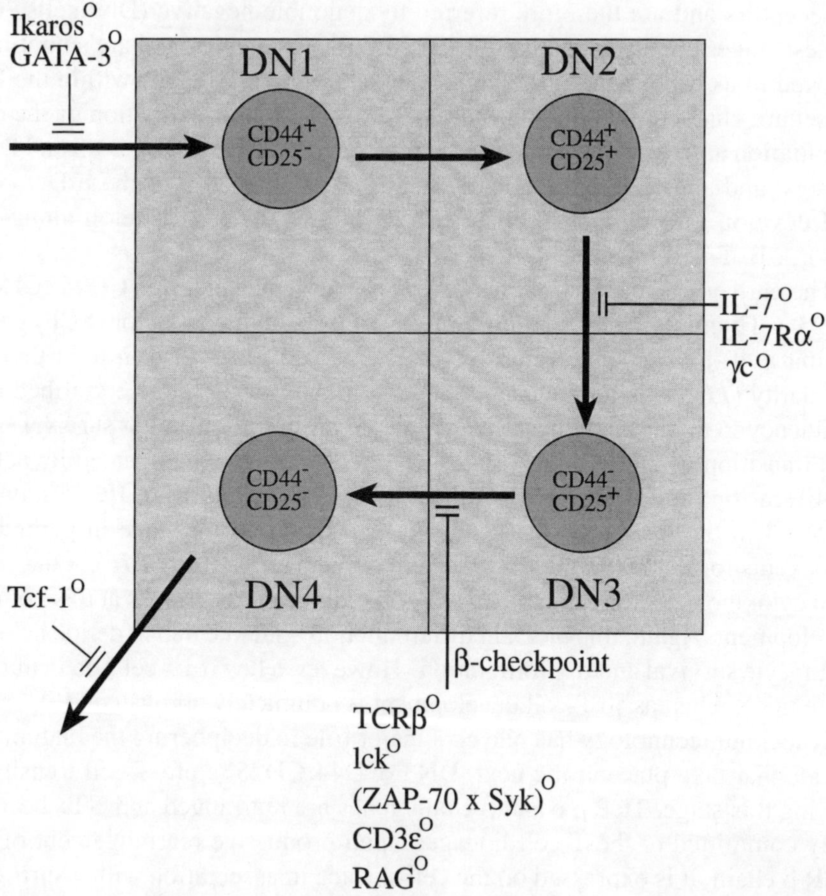

Fig. 1. Schematic representation of early events in thymocyte differentiation. Shown are examples of molecules that have been identified as important at specific points of this differentiation process using targeted gene disruption.

gies. In particular, the role of several cell surface receptors, intracellular signaling molecules, and transcription factors has been recognized which is essential for the transition of immature thymocytes through a major checkpoint in the early differentiation sequence (the β checkpoint).

Two T-cell lineages have been identified, αβ and γδ, characterized by the type of T-cell receptor (TCR) being expressed. The αβ lineage constitutes those cells that require the presentation of antigenic peptides on products of the classical major histocompatibility complex (MHC), whereas at least some γδ T cells seem capable of responding to antigen without any processing requirements *(10)*. The more immature thymocytes express neither CD4 nor CD8 co-receptors and are therefore referred to as double negative (DN) cells. The earliest stages are also negative for the CD3-TCR complex and are sometimes referred to as triple negatives (TN). The developmental stages within the DN subset are characterized by the successive expression or extinction of the differentiation antigens CD25 and CD44, referred to as DN1, DN2, DN3 and DN4 subsets, and shown diagramatically in **Fig. 1**. About 20% of these DN cells will develop into the $\gamma\delta$ T-cell lineage, whereas the rest develop along the major, $\alpha\beta$, T-cell lineage.

The earliest stage, DN1 expresses CD44 and is negative for CD25 ($CD44^+$ $CD25^-$). Thymi deficient for either of the c-kit or stem cell factor (SCF) genes exhibit a 40-fold reduction in DN1 cells and as a result also in total thymus cellularity *(11)*. This pronounced reduction in thymocytes can be ascribed to a deficiency in thymus colonization, thymocyte proliferation and/or survival *(12)*. The transition of DN1 to DN2 ($CD44^+CD25^+$) cells is accompanied by active proliferation and knockout studies have suggested that IL-7 may be involved in the regulation of thymocyte expansion at this stage in particular. Knockouts for IL-7 *(13)*, the IL-7 receptor α chain (IL-7Rα) *(14,15)* or the common cytokine receptor gamma chain (γc) *(16)* have partial blocks at this point in development. Again, this block in differentiation could be due to deficiencies in thymocyte survival and/or proliferation. However, a few $\alpha\beta$ T cells do mature in these mice, whereas $\gamma\delta$ T-cell development is completely abrogated *(17)*.

Knockout technology has played a major role in deciphering the maturation events that take place at the next, DN3 ($CD44^-CD25^+$), pre-T cell transition. During this stage, TCRγ, δ and β chain genes are rearranged and cells become fully committed to the T-cell lineage. Upon productive rearrangement of the TCR β chain, it is expressed on the cell surface in association with a surrogate light chain, pre-Tα (pTα) to form the pre-T cell receptor which associates with the CD3 complex, thus enabling it to transduce signals *(18)*. The development of cells which fail to express a functional β chain, and do not have the capacity to develop into the $\gamma\delta$ lineage, is arrested at this point, the β-checkpoint *(19)*. Emergence of the pre-TCR complex provides the signal for cells to undergo rapid expansion and turn on the CD4 and CD8 differentiation antigens, progressing to the double positive (DP) stage. It was initially supposed that TCRβ knockout mice, would have a complete block at the β-checkpoint, which would indicate that a successfully rearranged β chain provides the signal required for transition of DN thymocytes to the DP stage. However, as low numbers of DP thymocytes were found in TCRβ knockout mice, it was concluded that TCRβ rearrangement and expression is not essential for the expression of CD4 or CD8, but rather that the expansion of DN cells upon transition to the DP stage is dependent on TCRβ expression *(20)*. The development of $\gamma\delta$ T cells is not affected by the lack of TCRβ expression.

Further evidence that TCR gene rearrangement is required for the successful progression of thymocytes to the DP stage, came from mice deficient in either of the recombination activating genes, RAG-1 or RAG-2 *(21,22)*. The protein products of these genes are required for rearrangement of the TCR genes, by producing the double strand breaks associated with the recombination process, consequently these mice lack cells belonging to both $\alpha\beta$ and $\gamma\delta$ lineages. These thymi exhibit a complete developmental block at the CD4$^-$CD8$^-$CD44$^-$CD25$^+$ (DN3) stage. Expression of an already rearranged TCRβ transgene fully rescues the development of DP thymocytes in RAG-deficient thymi *(23)*. Transgenic mice expressing rearranged TCRβ chains fail to rearrange endogenous β chains, indicating that the expression of a rearranged TCRβ chain also provides the signal for shutting down any further rearrangement at the β locus *(24,25)*.

Although surface expression of the pre-TCR (TCRβ- pTα heterodimer) is apparently required for DN thymocytes to expand for progression to the DP stage, no extracellular ligand has been identified which interacts with this complex. Indeed, recent experiments have suggested that ligand engagement may not be required, as transgenic expression of TCRβ with pTα chains lacking extracellular domains permitted differentiation to the DP stage, indicating that assembly with the CD3 complex and transport to the cell surface sufficed *(26)*.

The role of components of the CD3 complex in the transduction of signals required for progression through the β-checkpoint has been examined in knockout mice for the individual CD3 polypeptides. For example, thymocytes deficient in the CD3ε subunit, fail to develop beyond the β-checkpoint *(27)*. The TCRα chain is not required for progression to the DP stage, as TCRα knockout mice have normal numbers of DP thymocytes and no effects are seen on the rearrangement of other TCR loci (β, γ or δ). No mature SP cells are observed in the thymi of these mice, although a few CD4$^+$ cells accumulate in the periphery of older mice *(19)*.

Intracellular tyrosine kinases, particularly those of the src-kinase family have been shown to be important for transducing signals for progression through the β-checkpoint. Two members of the src-family nonreceptor tyrosine kinases, p56^{lck} and p59^{fyn}, are expressed in the T-cell lineage. Biochemical evidence had suggested p56^{lck} to be the most proximal tyrosine kinase to become activated upon TCR-CD3 ligation. Mice deficient for the tyrosine kinase, p56^{lck}, were found to exhibit a similar phenotype to TCRβ and RAG gene knockout mice *(28)*. Very few DP and SP cells are present in the thymus, and some mature SP cells appear in the periphery. The importance of lck for transition through the TCRβ checkpoint can be demonstrated in RAG-deficient thymi by manipulations which induce lck activation. γ-irradiation or treatment of RAG-deficient thymi with CD3ε-specific antibodies promote the generation of DP thymocytes from DN precursors *(29)*, in a lck-dependent fashion *(30)*. Also, the forced expression of a constitutively active lck transgene leads to the production of normal numbers of DP thymocytes in RAG- *(31)* and pTα-deficient *(32)* thymi. In contrast, the absence of the other src family tyrosine kinase, p59[fyn], has no obvious effect on thymocyte differentiation *(33)*. However, double lck/fyn knockout animals exhibit a complete block at the DN stage, suggesting that fyn can in some cases compensate for the absence of lck *(34)*.

Currently we know little about the downstream signaling events which are involved at this stage, however, a role for the MAP kinase pathway in transition to the DP stage has been suggested in experiments in which a dominant negative MAPK/ERK kinase transgene was expressed *(35)*. Two closely related transcription factors, Tcf-1 and Lef-1 have also been implicated as being important at this stage of thymocyte differentiation. Tcf-1 is expressed in the T lineage only, whereas Lef-1 can be found in T cells and immature B cells. T-cell development in Tcf-1-deficient thymi is blocked at the immature CD8 SP stage *(36)*, at which DN precursors have initiated CD8 expression prior to becoming DP cells. These precursors do not proliferate and fail to develop any further. In contrast, T-cell development is apparently normal in Lef-1-deficient mice *(37)*, suggesting that there may be redundancy amongst these transcription factors such that Tcf-1 can substitute for Lef-1 in its absence.

3.2. DNA Damage Checkpoint in Early Thymopoiesis

Mutations in the tumor suppressor gene, p53, are found at high frequency in human cancers and p53-deficient mice or mice expressing a dominant negative p53 transgene are accordingly highly susceptible to the development of tumors, in particular thymic lymphoblastomas *(38,39)*. The action of p53 as a tumor suppressor is thought to occur either through the induction of G1 arrest in order to facilitate DNA repair or the induction of apoptosis. The murine *scid* mutation has been mapped to a deficiency in the DNA-dependent ser/thr protein kinase (DNA-PK), which is required for the repair of double-stranded DNA breaks *(40–42)*. As mentioned in the previous section, RAG-dependent double-stranded DNA breaks are intermediates during the rearrangement of TCR loci. V(D)J coding ends accumulate in *scid* thymocytes and differentiation is arrested at the β-checkpoint *(43,44)*. A deficiency in p53 was found to overcome this arrested development in *scid* thymi, and *scid* thymocytes on a p53-deficient background differentiated to the DP stage *(45,46)*. It was therefore proposed that p53 also acts as a checkpoint regulator during early thymopoesis and that the loss of this p53-dependent DNA damage checkpoint protects early thymocytes from apoptosis.

Several genes thought to be involved in the regulation of thymocyte apoptosis have been knocked out or transgenically expressed (*see* **Subheading**

3.3.). Probably the most familiar of these is bcl-2. The transgenic expression of bcl-2 could rescue thymocytes from high levels of apoptosis present in thymocytes deficient in the adenosine deaminase (ADA) enzyme, which also results in a severe combined immunodeficiency phenotype *(47)*. Interestingly, the apoptotic pathway operative in ADA-deficient thymocytes has been shown to be dependent upon p53. The regulation of DNA repair mechanisms, cell cycle control and apoptosis have to be tightly controlled in order to avoid the development of leukemia. Further investigation of gene products thought to be involved in any of these processes, using the technology described here, should lead to considerable insight into the molecular nature of T-cell development and tumorigenesis.

3.3. Positive Selection of the $\alpha\beta$ T-Cell Repertoire

Double positive thymocytes actively rearrange their TCRα loci and express low levels of surface TCR $\alpha\beta$ heterodimers which interact with the MHC-peptide complexes present on the thymic epithelium. Based on criteria we still do not fully understand, only a small proportion of cells receive signals for further differentiation, whereas more than 90% die by programmed cell death (reviewed in *48)*. Only those cells which express TCRs capable of interacting with self-MHC molecules are positively selected and progress to the next, and final stage of maturation. Thymocytes expressing TCRs that cannot interact with MHC molecules fail to undergo positive selection and die by neglect. On the other extreme, those cells expressing TCRs with high affinity for self-MHC are negatively selected. This process of negative selection, also referred to as deletion, is essential for the maintenance of self-tolerance, since T cells with high affinity receptors for self-MHC are potentially autoreactive and need to be eliminated. Some of the key molecules involved in these selection processes are illustrated in **Fig. 2**.

The first evidence for positive selection came from studies in which lethally irradiated mice were reconstituted with F_1 bone marrow. It was shown that T cells which matured in these chimaeras were restricted by the parental MHC type of the host and not the donor *(49,50)*. Transgenic mice expressing a specific T-cell receptor provided direct proof for the notion that the specificity of a given TCR determines the developmental program of thymocytes in which it is expressed. Teh et al. showed that transgenic mice expressing an MHC Class I-restricted $\alpha\beta$ T-cell receptor, specific for the H-Y peptide, which is presented in the context of H-2D^b in male mice only, directed the development of mature CD8 SP thymocytes in female mice of the H-2^b haplotype *(51)*. This observation not only established that an allele specific MHC-TCR interaction was required for positive selection of DP thymocytes, but also that the class of MHC molecule to which the TCR is restricted influences the choice of differ-

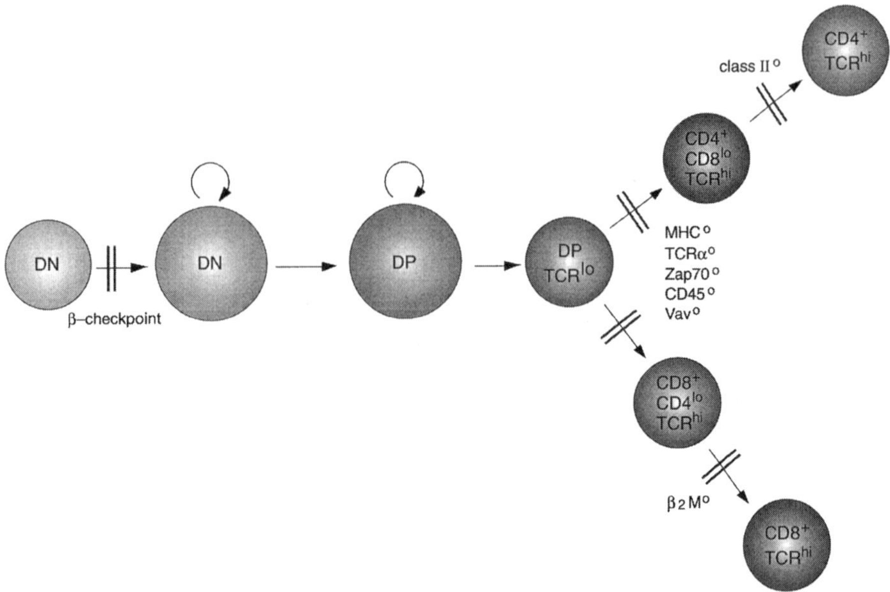

Fig. 2. Diagram of thymocyte maturation indicating some of the molecules whose function during the later stages of differentiation have been elucidated using gene knockout technology. Arrows indicate subpopulations in cycle. MHC° mice are generated by intercrossing class II° with b2M° mice.

entiation to the CD4 or CD8 lineage. Since these initial experiments, a number of other TCR transgenic mice have been described and shown to direct the development of thymocytes into the appropriate lineage, namely, CD8 for MHC class I-restricted TCRs and CD4 for MHC class II-restricted TCRs. However, expressing a rearranged transgenic TCR did not entirely prevent development of T cells into the other lineage in these mice, probably because rearrangement of endogenous TCR genes is not completely inhibited by the presence of a rearranged TCR transgene. Breeding of these TCR transgenic mice onto RAG-deficient backgrounds, resolves this issue and for most TCR transgenes results in expression of a single lineage only.

Studies in which MHC Class II or the Class I light chain (β2m) were knocked out, have confirmed that recognition of the appropriate class of MHC ligand is required for lineage commitment. Thus, MHC Class II knockout mice are deficient in CD4 SP cells *(52)* while β2m knockout mice lack mature, CD8 SP T cells *(53)* (**Fig. 2**). A set of elegant experiments utilized tissue-specific promotors for the expression of MHC Class II molecules on either thymic cortical or medullary cells to show that positive selection of CD4 SP cells required the expression of the positively selecting ligand on thymic cortical epithelium cells *(54,55)* whereas negative selection requires expression on the thymic medullary epithelium *(56)*.

Differentiation into the correct lineage requires not only interactions between the TCR and its selecting ligand, but also engagement of the correct coreceptor. Thus mutated MHC molecules which are unable to interact with their appropriate coreceptors, fail to direct selection of thymocytes into mature, single positive cells *(57,58)*. It was proposed that the coligation of a given TCR with the appropriate coreceptor upon binding its positively selecting MHC ligand (CD8 with MHC Class I and CD4 with MHC Class II), leads to the generation of distinct signals which directs the maturation into the correct lineage. This is known as the instructive model of thymocyte differentiation. An alternative model which has been put forward and is known as the stochastic/selective model, suggests that DP thymocytes randomly down-regulate either CD4 or CD8, coincidentally with commitment to either the cytotoxic or helper lineages, respectively. Unlike the instructive model, in the stochastic hypothesis this process is proposed to occur independently of the restriction specificity of the transgenic TCR. The resulting cells are subsequently screened for the expression of matched TCR-coreceptor specificities and the ones with mismatched TCR-coreceptors fail to differentiate further. Attempts to discriminate between these two models have been largely inconclusive and the mechanism of lineage choice remains to be elucidated *(59)*.

Several molecular cascades which have been described in the determination of lineage decisions in other experimental systems e.g., Drosophila and Xenopus, are also thought to play a role in T-cell differentiation. Recent experiments have implicated the Notch cascade to be involved in both $\alpha\beta$ vs $\gamma\delta$ *(60)* and CD4 vs CD8 *(61)* lineage decisions in the thymus.

Intracellular kinases have been implicated in transducing signals during the differentiation of DP thymocytes to mature SP thymocytes. Mice deficient in a member of the syk family of kinases, ZAP-70, one of the first downstream targets of lck, show a profound block at the DP stage and no mature T cells are present *(62)*. Interestingly, humans deficient in ZAP-70, lack CD8 SP T cells, but can still develop some CD4 SP cells *(63)*. It is probable that in human thymus the related kinase, Syk, can substitute for ZAP-70 during CD4 differentiation. This interpretation is supported by the observation that Syk is expressed at very low levels in mouse, compared to human DP thymocytes and that transgenic expression of Syk can rescue the block in positive selection in ZAP-70 knockout mice *(64)*. ZAP-70/Syk double knockout mice exhibit a complete developmental block at the DN3 stage *(65)*. Lck is also thought to be important for positive selection of DP thymocytes, as a dominant negative lck transgene expressed from the lck distal promoter which is turned on in late thymus differentiation blocked development of SP cells *(66)*. Furthermore, mice deficient in one of the key regulators of src kinase activity, the tyrosine phosphatase, CD45, also show a profound block in thymopoeisis at the double positive stage *(67,68)*. The basal signaling states and signaling capacity of these CD45$^{-/-}$ thymocytes are impaired, as expected of cells deficient in active lck. They contain lower levels of tyrosine-phosphorylated TCR-ζ proteins and TCR-induced CD3ϵ and ZAP-70 phosphorylation is impaired *(69)*. Deficiency in another interesting downstream kinase, p95^{vav} has been reported to affect both positive and negative selection, which seems to correlate with a greatly reduced TCR-induced Ca^{2+} flux *(70)*. Vav is a complex molecule containing not only src-homology 2 (SH2) and SH3 domains, but also a kinase and putative guanine nucleotide exchange domain, suggesting it to have a range of signaling capacities.

3.4. Apoptotic Signals and Negative Selection

Several candidate genes had been proposed to play a role during negative selection or deletion of double positive thymocytes. However, only a few proteins have so far been implicated directly as being important mediators of negative selection with the aid of knockout and transgenic mice. For example, CD30-deficient mice have been reported to exhibit impaired negative selection to anti-CD3 stimulation and antigen-induced programmed cell death *(71)*.

Recently, the influence of several members of the caspase family of proteins on thymocyte apoptosis has been investigated in a series of knockout mice. It was found that whereas thymocytes from caspase 9 deficient mice were resistant to cell death induced by treatment with anti-CD3, dexamethasone and γ-irradiation they remained sensitive to anti-CD95-induced cell death *(72,73)*. In contrast, caspase 1 and 11 knockout mice showed an opposite phenotype, with some resistance to anti-CD95 induced cell death but not to other apoptotic stimuli *(6)*. Finally, knockouts of two other family members, caspase 2 *(74)* and 3 *(75,76)*, had no apparent effect on the susceptibility of thymocytes to any of the inducers of apoptosis which were tested. Another protein family in which related members do not necessarily substitute for one another is the bcl-2/bax family. Overexpression of bcl-2 in transgenic mice protects thymocytes from apoptosis induced by dexamethasone, γ-irradiation and anti-CD3 *(77,78)*. More recently it has been shown that TCR transgenic thymocytes could be rescued from antigen-induced deletion by the transgenic expression of bcl-2, but not by its closely related family member, bax *(79)*.

Other gene families may be more likely to substitute for one another with respect to their influence on thymocyte apoptosis. For example, over-expression of a dominant negative transgene encoding the Nur77 transcription factor inhibited antigen-induced negative selection, whereas the expression of wild-type Nur77 was found to enhance apoptosis *(80)*. Interestingly, Nur77-deficient mice exhibit no gross abnormalities, implying functional redundancy of this gene product *(81)*. In this instance, other members of the same family, Nur1 and Nor-1 have been shown to behave in a similar fashion to Nur77 and further analyses of these gene products should prove extremely interesting *(82)*.

4. Mature T Cell Differentiation

The mechanisms of mature T cell survival in the absence of antigen and the functional differentiation of T cells upon activation are relatively new areas of research. A Krüppel-like zinc-finger, LKLF has recently been implicated in the survival of newly generated mature thymocytes and T cells *(83)*. There are suggestions that GATA-3 may also be involved in the decision between adopting a Th1 or Th2 phenotype in mature T cells and this issue will have to be resolved in conditional knockouts or inducible gene expression systems *(84)*.

5. Concluding Remarks

We have described but a few examples of experiments in which knockout and/or transgenic mice were instrumental in the elucidation of specific aspects relating to T-cell differentiation. What is striking about most of these experiments is the ability to pinpoint exactly where the gene product in question is first required and the wealth of information that can be gained by the analyses of mice deficient in various factors that all lead to developmental arrest at the same stage. This is particularly well illustrated in the case of genes whose absence leads to arrest at the β-checkpoint during early thymocyte differentiation. By discussing the role of some of the different factors that are involved at the β-checkpoint, we aimed to demonstrate how the analysis of several different players which act at the same stage, can provide information regarding molecular mechanism and regulation of differentiation.

Some of the genes referred to in the text, in particular intracellular signaling molecules and transcription factors, are likely to be required at several stages during differentiation, and the development of technology that allows the controlled expression of these factors at early stages of differentiation, with the ability to switch them off later-on in development, is one of the major challenges at present.

The discovery of new molecules involved in thymocyte differentiation will no doubt continue to improve our understanding of this complex process. The issue of redundancy as well as functional associations between different gene products can be addressed by examining a combination of intercrosses between knockout, mutant and transgenic mouse lines. Also, the continued reinterpretation of previous observations as new evidence comes to light may yet make significant contributions to the field.

Finally, advancements in technology, the generation of more knockouts, mutants and transgenic strains of mice, combined with sound scientific analyses and sober interpretation of the resulting phenotypes will no doubt continue to provide immunologists with some of the most powerful tools available for the dissection of the molecular basis underlying the differentiation of mature T cells from their bone marrow-derived progenitors.

References

1. Kioussis, D. and Festenstein, R. (1997) Locus control regions: overcoming heterochromatin-induced gene inactivation in mammals. *Current Opinion in Genetics and Development* **7,** 614–619.
2. Baudoin, C., Goumans, M. J., Mummery, C., and Sonnenberg, A. (1998) Knockout and knockin of the beta 1 exon D define distinct roles for integrin splice variants in heart function and embryonic development. *Genes Dev.* **12,** 1202–1216.
3. Kistner, A., Gossen, M., Zimmermann, F., Jerecic J., Ullmer, C., Lubbert, H., and Bujard, H. (1996) Doxycycline-mediated quantitative and tissue-specific control of gene expression in transgenic mice. *Proc. Natl. Acad. Sci. USA* **93,** 10,933–10,938.
4. Georgopoulos, K., Bigby, M., Wang, J.-H., Molnar A., Wu, P., Winandy, S., and Sharpe, A. (1994) The Ikaros gene is required for the development of all lymphoid lineages. *Cell* **79,** 143–156.
5. Sun L., Liu, A., and Georgopoulos, K. (1996) Zinc finger-mediated protein interactions modulate Ikaros activity, a molecular control of lymphocyte development. *EMBO J.* **15,** 5358–5369.
6. Wang, J. H., Nichogiannopoulou, A., Wu, L., Sun L., Sharpe, H., Bigby, M., and Georgopoulos, K. (1996) Selective defects in the development of the fetal and adult lymphoid system in mice with an Ikaros null mutation. *Immunity* **5,** 537–549.
7. Morgan, B., Sun, L., Avithal, N., Andrikopoulos, K., Ikeda, T., Gonzales E., Wu, P., Neben, S., and Georgopoulos, K. (197) Aiolos, a lymphoid restricted transcription factor that interacts with Ikaros to regulate lymphocyte differentiation. *EMBO J.* **16,** 2004–2013.
8. Pandolfi, P. P., Roth, M. E., Karis, A., Leonard, M. W., Dzierzak, E., Grosveld, F. G., Engel, J. D., and Lindenbaum, M. H. (1995) Targeted disruption of the GATA3 gene causes severe abnormalities in the nervous system and in fetal liver haematopoiesis. *Nature Genet.* **11,** 40–44.
9. Ting, C. N., Olson, M. C., Barton, K. P., and Leiden, J. M. (1996) Transcription factor GATA-3 is required for development of the T-cell lineage. *Nature* **384,** 474–478.
10. Chien, Y., Jores, R., and Crowley, M. P. (1996) Recognition by γ/δ T cells. *Annu. Rev. Immunol.* **14,** 511–532.
11. Rodewald, H.-R., Ogawa, M., Haller, C., Waskow, W., and DiSanto, J. P. (1997) Prothymocyte expansion by c-kit and the common cytokine receptor γ chain is essential for repertoire formation. *Immunity* **6,** 265–272.

12. Di Santo, J. P. and Rodewald H.-R. (1998) In vivo roles of receptor tyrosine kinases and cytokine receptors in early thymocyte development. *Curr. Opin. Immunol.* **10,** 196–207.
13. Von Freeden-Jeffry, U., Vieira, P., Lucian, L. A., McNeil, T., Burdach, S. E., and Murray, R. (1995) Lymphopenia in interleukin (IL)-7 gene-deleted mice identifies IL-7 as a nonredundant cytokine. *J. Exp. Med.* **181,** 1519–1526.
14. He, Y. W. and Malek, T. R. (1996) Interleukin-7 receptor a is essential for the development of $\gamma\delta^+$ T cells, but not natural killer cells. *J. Exp. Med.* **184,** 289–293.
15. Maki, K., Sunaga, S., Komagata, Y., Kodaira, Y., Mabuchi, A., Karasuyama, H., Yokomuro, K., Miyazaki, J. I., and Ikuta, K. (1996) Interleukin 7 receptor-deficient mice lack $\gamma\delta$ T cells. *Proc. Natl. Acad. Sci. USA* **93,** 7172–7177.
16. Cao, X., Shores, E. W., Hu-Li, J., Anver, M. R., Kelsall, B. L., Russell, S. M., Drago, J., Noguchi, M., Grinberg, A., Bloom, E. T., et al. (1995) Defective lymphoid development in mice lacking expression of the common cytokine receptor gamma chain. *Immunity* **2,** 223–238.
17. Moore, T. A., Von Freeden-Jeffry, U., Murray, R., and Zlotnik, A. (1996) Inhibition of gamma delta T cell development and early thymocyte maturation in IL 7$^{-/-}$ mice. *J. Immunol.* **157,** 2366–2373.
18. von Boehmer, H. and Fehling, H. J. (1997) Structure and function of the pre-T cell receptor. *Annu. Rev. Immunol.* **15,** 433–452.
19. Mombaerts, P., Clarke, A. R., Rudnicki, M. A., Iacomini, J., Itohara, S., Lafaille, J. J., Wang, L., Ichikawa, Y., Jaenisch, R., Hooper, M. L., and Tonegawa, S. (1992) Mutations in T-cell antigen receptor genes α and β block thymocyte development at different stages. *Nature* **360,** 225–231.
20. Hoffman, E. S., Passoni, L., Crompton, T., Leu, T. M. J., Schatz, D.G., Koff, A., Owen M. J., and Hayday, A. C. (1996) Productive T-cell receptor β-chain gene rearrangement: coincident regulation of cell cycle and clonality during development in vivo. *Genes Dev.* **10,** 948–962.
21. Mombaerts, P., Iacomini, J., Johnson, R. S., Herup, K., Tonegawa, S., and Papaioannou, V. E. (1992) RAG-1-deficient mice have no mature B and T lymphocytes. *Cell* **68,** 869–877.
22. Shinkai, Y., Rathbun, G., Lam, K.-P., Oltz, E. M., Stewart, V., Mendelsohn, M., Charron, J., Datta, M., Young, F., Stall, A. M., and Alt, F. W. (1992) RAG-2-deficient mice lack mature lymphocytes owing to inability to initiate V(D)J rearrangement. *Cell* **68,** 855–867.
23. Shinkai, Y., Koyasu, S., Nakayama, K., Murphy, K. M., Loh, D. Y., Reinherz, E. L., and Alt, F. W. (1993) Restoration of T cell development in RAG-2-deficient mice by functional TCR transgenes. *Science* **259,** 822–825.
24. Dudley, E. C., Petrie, H. T., Shah, L. M., Owen, M. J., and Hayday A. C. (1994) T cell receptor β chain rearrangement and selection during thymocyte development in adult mice. *Immunity* **1,** 83–93.
25. Uematsu, Y., Ryser, S., Dembic, S. Z., Borgulya, P., Krimpenfort, P., Berns, A., Von Boehmer, H., and Steinmetz, M. (1998) In transgenic mice the introduced functional T cell receptor β gene prevents expression of endogenous β genes. *Cell* **52,** 831–841.

26. Irving, B. A., Alt, F. W., and Killeen, N. (1998) Thymocyte development in the absence of pre-T cell receptor extracellular immunoglobulin domains. *Science* **280,** 905–908.
27. Malissen, M., Gillet, A., Ardouin, L., Bouvier, G., Trucy, J., Ferrier, P., Vivier, E., and Malissen, B. (1995) Altered T cell development in mice with a targeted mutation of the CD3ε gene. *EMBO J.* **14,** 4641–4653.
28. Molina, T. J., Kishihara, K., Siderovski, D. P., Van Ewijk, W., Narendran, A., Timms, E., Wakeman, A., Paige, C. J., Hartmann, K.-U., Veilette, A., Davidson, D., and Mak, T. W. (1992) Profound block in thymocyte development in mice lacking p56^{lck}. *Nature* **357,** 161–164.
29. Wu, G., Danska, J. S., and Guidos, C. J. (1996) Lck dependence of signaling pathways activated by gamma-irradiation and CD3 epsilon engagement in RAG-1$^{(-/-)}$-immature thymocytes. *Int. Immunol.* **8,** 1159–1164.
30. Levelt, C. N., Mombaerts, P., Wang, B., Kohler, H., Tonegawa, S., Eichmann, K., and Terhorst, C. (1995) Regulation of thymocyte development through CD3: functional dissociation between p56^{lck} and CD3ζ in early thymic selection. *Immunity* **3,** 215–222.
31. Mombaerts, P., Anderson, S. J., Perlmutter, R. M., Mak, T. W., and Tonegawa, S. (1994) An activated lck transgene promotes thymocyte development in RAG-1 mutant mice. *Immunity* **1,** 261–267.
32. Fehling, H. J. and von Boehmer H. (1997) Early αβ T cell development in the thymus of normal and genetically altered mice. *Curr. Opin. Immunol.* **9,** 263–275.
33. Appleby, M. W., Gross, J. A., Cooke, M. P., Levin, S. D., Qian, X., and Perlmutter, R. M. (1992) Defective T cell receptor signaling in mice lacking the thymic isoform of p59^{fyn}. *Cell* **70,** 751–763.
34. Van Oers, N .S. C., Lowen-Kropf, B., Finlay, D., Conolly, K., and Weiss, A. (1996) αβ T cell development is abolished in mice lacking both lck and fyn protein tyrosine kinases. *Immunity* **5,** 429–436.
35. Crompton, T., Gilmour, K. C., and Owen, M. J. (1996) The MAP kinase pathway controls differentiation from double-negative to double-positive thymocyte. *Cell* **86,** 243–251.
36. Verbeek, S., Izon D., Hofhuis, F., Robanus-Maandag, E., Te Riele, H., van de Wetering, M., Oosterwegel, M., Wilson, A., MacDonald, H. R., and Clevers, H. C. (1995) An HMG-box-containing T-cell factor required for thymocyte differentiation. *Nature* **374,** 70–74.
37. Van Genderen, C., Okamura, R. M., Farinas, I., Quo, R., Parslow, T. G., Bruhn, L., and Grosschedl, R. (1994) Development of several organs that require inductive epithelial-mesenchymal interactions is impaired in LEF-1-deficient mice. *Genes Dev.* **8,** 2691–2703.
38. Lavignueur, A., Maltby, V., Mock, D., Rossant, J., Pawson, T., and Bernstein, A. (1989) High incidence of lung, bone and mymphoid tumors in transgenic mice overexpressing mutant alleles of the p53 oncogene. *Mol. Cell. Biol.* **9,** 3982–3991.
39. Donehower, L., Harvey, M., Slagle, B., McArthur, C., Montgomery, C., Butel, J., and Bradley, A. (1992) Mice deficient for p53 are developmentally normal but susceptible to spontaneous tumours. *Nature* **356,** 215–221.

40. Blunt, T., Finnie, N. J., Taccioli, G. E., Smith, G. C. M., Demengeot, J., Gottlieb, T. M., Mizuta, R., Varghese, A. J., Alt, F. W., Jeggo, P. A., and Jackson, S. P. (1995) Defective DNA-dependent protein kinase activity is linked to V(D)J recombination and DNA repair defects associated with the murine *scid* mutation. *Cell* **80,** 813–823.

41. Kirchgessner, C. U., Patil, C. K., Evans, J. W., Cuomo, C. A., Fried, L. M., Carter, T., Oettinger, M. A., and Brown, J. M. (1995) DNA-dependent kinase (p350) as a candidate for the murine SCID defect. *Science* **267,** 1178–1182.

42. Peterson, S. R., Kurimasa, A., Oshimura, M., Dynan, W. S., Bradbury, E. M., and Chen, D. J. (1995) Loss of catalytic subunit of the DNA-dependent protein kinase in DNA double-strand break repair mutant mammalian cells. *Proc. Natl. Acad. Sci. USA* **92,** 3171–3174.

43. Bosma, G. C., Custer, R. P., and Bosma, M. J.(1983) A severe combined immunodeficiency mutation in the mouse. *Nature* **301,** 527–530.

44. Schuler, W., Weiler, I., Schuler, A., Phillips, R. A., Rosenberg, N., Mak, T. W., Kearny, J. F., Perry, R. P., and Bosma, M. J. (1986) Rearrangement of antigen receptor genes is defective in mice with severe combined immune deficiency. *Cell* **68,** 855–899.

45. Guidos, C. J., Williams, C. J., Grandal, I., Knowles, G., Huang, M. T. F., and Danska, J. S. (1996) V(D)J recombination activates a p53-dependent DNA damage checkpoint in *scid* lymphocyte precursors. *Genes Dev.* **10,** 2038–2054.

46. Nacht, M., Strasser, A., Chan, Y. R., Harris, A. W., Schlissel, M., Bronson, R. T., and Jacks, T. (1996) Mutations in the p53 and SCID genes cooperate in tumorigenesis. *Genes Dev.* **10,** 2055–2066.

47. Benveniste, P. and Cohen, A. (1995) p53 expression is required for thymocyte apoptosis induced by adenosine deaminase deficiency. *Proc. Natl. Acad. Sci. USA* **92,** 8373–8377.

48. Page, D. M., Kane, L. P., Onami, T. M., and Hedrick, S. M. (1996) Cellular and biochemical requirements for thymocyte negative selection. *Sem. Immunol.* **8,** 69–82.

49. Bevan, M. J. (1977) In a radiation chimaera, host H-2 antigens determine immune responsiveness of donor cytotoxic cells. *Nature* **269,** 417–418.

50. Zinkernagel, R. M., Callahan, G. N., Althage, A., Cooper, S., Klein, P. A., and Klein, J. (1878) On the thymus in the differentiation of "H-2 self-recognition" by T cells: Evidence for dual recognition? *J. Exp. Med.* **147,** 882–896.

51. Teh, H. S., Kisielow, P., Scott, B., Kishi, H., Uematsu, Y., Bluthmann, H., and von Boehmer, H. (1988) Thymic major histocompatibility complex antigens and the ab T-cell receptor determine the CD4/CD8 phenotype of T cells. *Nature* **335,** 229–233.

52. Cosgrove, D., Grey, D., Dierich, A., Kaufman, J., Lemeur, M., Benoist, C., and Mathis, D. (1991) Mice lacking MHC class II molecules. *Cell* **66,** 1051–1066.

53. Zijlstra, M., Bix, M., Simister, N., Loring, J., Raulet, D., and Jaenisch, R. (1990) β2–Microglobulin deficient mice lack CD4$^-$8$^+$ cytolytic T cells. *Nature* **344,** 742–746.

54. Berg, L. J., Pullen, A. M., Fazekas de St. Groth, B., Mathis, D., Benoist, C., and Davis, M. M. (1989) Antigen/MHC-specific T cells are preferentially exported from the thymus in the presence of their MHC ligands. *Cell* **58,** 1035–1046.

55. Cosgrove, D., Chan, S. H., Waltzinger, C., Benoist, C., and Mathis, D. (1992) The thymic compartment responsible for positive selection of CD4[+] T cells. *Int. Immunol.* **4,** 707–710.
56. Laufer, T. M., DeKoning, J., Markowitz, J. S., Lo, D., and Glimcher, L. H. (1996) Unopposed positive selection and autoreactivity in mice expressing class II MHC only on thymic cortex. *Nature* **383,** 81–85.
57. Aldrich, C. J., Hammer, R. E., Jones-Youngblood, S., Koszinowski, U., Hood, L., Stroynowski, I., and Forman, J. (1991) Negative and positive selection of antigen-specific cytotoxic T lymphocytes affected by the $\alpha 3$ domain of MHC I molecules. *Nature* **352,** 718–720.
58. Riberdy, J. M., Mostaghel, E., and Doyle, C. (1998) Disruption of the CD4-major histocompatibility complex class II interaction blocks the development of CD4[+] T cells in vivo. *J. Immunol.* **95,** 4493–4498.
59. von Boehmer, H. (1996) CD4/CD8 lineage commitment: Basic Instruction. *J. Exp. Med.* **183,** 713–715.
60. Robey, E. and Fowlkes, B. J. (1998) The ab versus $\gamma\delta$ T-cell lineage choice. *Curr. Opin. Immunol.* **10,** 181–187.
61. Robey, E., Chang, D., Itano, A., Cado, D., Alexander, H., Lans, D., Weinmaster, G., and Salmon P. (1996) An activated form of Notch influences the choice between CD4 and CD8 T cell lineages. *Cell* **87,** 483–492.
62. Negishi, I., Motoyama, N., Nakayama, K., Senju, S., Hatakeyama, S., Zhang, Q., Chan, A. C., and Loh, D. Y. (1995) Essential role for ZAP-70 in both positive and negative selection of thymocytes. *Nature* **376,** 435–438.
63. Arpaia, E., Shahar, M., Dadi, H., Cohen, A., and Roifman, C. M. (1996) Defective T cell receptor signaling and CD8[+] thymic selection in humans lacking ZAP-70 kinase. *Cell* **76,** 947–958.
64. Gong, Q., White, L., Johnson, R., White, M., Negishi, I., Thomas, M., and Chan, A. C. (1997) Restoration of thymocyte development and function in ZAP-70$^{-/-}$ mice by the Syk protein tyrosine kinase. *Immunity* **7,** 369–377.
65. Cheng, A. M., Negishi, I., Anderson, S. J., Chan, A. C., Bolen, J., Loh, D. Y., and Pawson, T. (1997) The Syk and ZAP-70 SH2-containing tyrosine kinases are implicated in pre-T cell receptor signaling. *Proc. Natl. Acad. Sci. USA* **94,** 9797–9801.
66. Hashimoto, K., Sohn, S. J., Levin, S. D., Tada, T., Perlmutter, R. M., and Nakayama, T. (1996) Requirement for p56lck tyrosine kinase activation in T cell receptormediated thymic selection. *J. Exp. Med.* **184,** 931–943.
67. Kishihara, K., Penninger, J., Wallace, V. A., Kundig, T. M., Kawai, K., Wakeham, A., Timms, E., Pfeffer, K., Ohashi, P. S., Thomas, M. L., et al. (1993) Normal B lymphocyte development but impaired T cell maturation in CD45-exon6 protein tyrosine phosphatase-deficient mice. *Cell* **74,** 143–156.
68. Byth, K. F., Conroy, L. A., Howlett, S., Smith, A. J., May, J., Alexander, D. R., and Holmes, N. (1996) CD45-null transgenic mice reveal a positive regulatory role for CD45 in early thymocyte development, in the selection of CD4+CD8+ thymocytes, and B cell maturation. *J. Experiment. Med.* **183,** 1707–1718.

69. Stone, J. D., Conroy, L. A., Byth, K. F., Hederer, R. A., Howlett, S., Takemoto, Y., Holmes, N., and Alexander, D. R. (1997) Aberrant TCR-mediated signaling in CD45-null thymocytes involves dysfunctional regulation of Lck, Fyn, TCR-ζ, and ZAP-70. *J. Immunol.* **158,** 5773–5782.

70. Turner, M., Mee, P. J., Walters, A. E., Quinn, M. E., Mellor, A. L., Zamoyska, R., and Tybulewicz, V. L. (1997) A requirement for the Rho-family GTPase exchange factor Vav in positive and negative selection of thymocytes. *Immunity* **7,** 451–460.

71. Amakawa, R., Hakem, A., Kundig, T. M., Matsuyama, T., Simard, J. J., Timms, E., Wakeham, A., Mittruecker, H. W., Grieser, H., Takimoto, H., Schmitts, R., Shahinian, A., Ohashi, P., Penninger, J. M., and Mak, T. W. (1996) Impaired negative selection of T cells in Hodgkin's disease antigen CD30-deficient mice. *Cell* **84,** 551–562.

72. Kuida, K., Haydar, T. F., Kuan, C.-Y., Gu, Y., Taya, C., Karasuyama, H., Su, M.S.-S., Rakic, P., and Flavell, R. A. (1998) Reduced apoptosis and cytochrome c-mediated caspase activation in mice lacking caspase 9. *Cell* **94,** 325–337.

73. Hakem, R., Hakem, A., Duncan, G. S., Henderson J. T., Woo, M., Soengas, M. S., Elia A., de la Pompa, J. L., Kagi, D., Khoo, W., Potter, J., Yoshida, R., Kaufman, S. A., Lowe, S. W., Penninger, J. M., and Mak, T. W. (1998) Differential requirement for caspase 9 in apoptotic pathways in vivo. *Cell* **94,** 339–352.

74. Bergeron, L., Perez, G., Macdonald, G., Shi, L., Sun, Y., Jurisicova, A., Varmuza, S., Latham, K., Flaws, J., Salter, J., et al. (1998) Defects in regulation of apoptosis in caspase-2-deficient mice. *Genes Dev.* **12,** 1304–1314.

75. Kuida, K., Zheng, T., Na, S., Kuan, C., Yang, D., Karasuyama, H., Rakic, P., and Flavell, R. (1996) Decreased apoptosis in the brain and premature lethality in CPP32-deficient mice. *Nature* **384,** 368–372.

76. Woo, M., Hakem, R., Soengas, M., Duncan, G., Shahinian, A., Kagi, D., Hakem, A., McCurrach, M., Khoo, W., Kaufman, S., et al. (1998) Essential contribution of caspase 3/CPP32 to apoptosis and its associated nuclear changes. *Genes Dev.* **12,** 806–819.

77. Strasser, A., Harris, A., and Cory, S. (1991) bcl-2 transgene inhibits T cell death and perturbs thymic self-sensorship. *Cell* **67,** 889–899.

78. Sentman, C., Shutter, J., Hockenberry, D., Kanagawa, O., and Korsemeyer, S. (1991) bcl-2 inhibits mutliple forms of apoptosis but not negative selection in thymocytes. *Cell* **67,** 879–888.

79. Williams, O., Norton, T., Halligey, M., Kioussis, D., and Brady, H. J. M. (1998) The action of Bax and Bcl-2 on T cell selection. *J. Exp. Med.* **188,** 1125–1133.

80. Calnan, B., Szychowski, S., Chan, F. K. M., Cado, D., and Winoto, A. (1995) A role of the orphan steroid receptor Nur77 in antigen-induced negative selection. *Immunity* **3,** 273–282.

81. Lee, S. L., Wesselschmidt, R. L., Linette, G. P., Kanagawa, O., Russell, J. H., and Milbrandt, J. (1995) Unimpaired thymic and peripheral T cell death in mice lacking the nuclear receptor NGFI-B (Nur77). *Science* **269,** 532–535.

82. Cheng, L. E., Chan, F. K., Cado, D., and Winoto, A. (1997) Functional redundancy of the Nur 77 and Nor-1 orphan steroid receptors in T-cell apoptosis. *EMBO J.* **16,** 1865–1875.

83. Kuo, C. T., Veselits, M. L., and Leiden, J. M. (1997) LKLF: A transcriptional regulator of single- positive T cell quiescence and survival. *Science* **277,** 1986–1990.
84. Murphy, K. T (1998) lymphocyte differentiation in the periphery. *Curr. Opin. Immunol.* **10,** 226–232.

II

T Cell Development

2

Isolation and Characterization
of Murine Early Intrathymic Precursor Populations

Li Wu and Ken Shortman

1. Introduction

The earliest steps along the pathway leading to mature T cells in mouse thymus have been defined *(1,2)*. Within the thymus, several minute but discrete populations of T cell precursors develop in sequence, preceding the stage of $CD4^+8^+$ thymocytes (**Fig. 1**). The earliest identifiable intrathymic precursors in the adult mouse, termed "low CD4" precursors, express low levels of CD4 and Thy-1, and are positive for Sca-1, Sca-2, CD44 and c-kit but negative for CD25 *(3)*. This precursor population represents only 0.03–0.05% of total thymocytes. It is not exclusively T-lineage committed and retains the potential to form NK cells, B cells and dendritic cells (DC) *(4–6)*. The low CD4 precursor population then loses surface CD4 and develops into $CD3^-4^-8^-$ triple negative (TN) precursors. Among the TN precursors, four subpopulations, representing 2–3% of total thymocytes, can be characterized by the early expression of CD44 and c-kit, and by transient expression of CD25. The developmental progression, deduced from precursor activities, is $c\text{-}kit^+CD44^+CD25^-$ -> $c\text{-}kit^+CD44^+CD25^+$ -> $c\text{-}kit^-CD44^-CD25^+$ -> $c\text{-}kit^-CD44^-CD25^-$ *(7–10)*. The earliest $c\text{-}kit^+CD44^+CD25^-$ TN subpopulation, although believed to be more mature than the low CD4 precursors, has many features overlapping those of the low CD4 precursors. It also retains the potential to develop into NK cells, B cells and DC (L. Wu, unpublished observations). The next step involves the $c\text{-}kit^+CD44^+CD25^+$ subpopulation, which has lost the potential to form NK cells and B cells, but still retains a capacity to form DC *(9)*. It is not until the $c\text{-}kit^-CD44^-CD25^+$ stage that the precursors are completely committed to T lineage development *(9)*. Both $c\text{-}kit^-CD44^-CD25^+$ and $c\text{-}kit^-CD44^-CD25^-$ subpopulations are committed T cell precursors.

From: *Methods in Molecular Biology, Vol. 134: T Cell Protocols: Development and Activation*
Edited by: K. P. Kearse © Humana Press Inc., Totowa, NJ

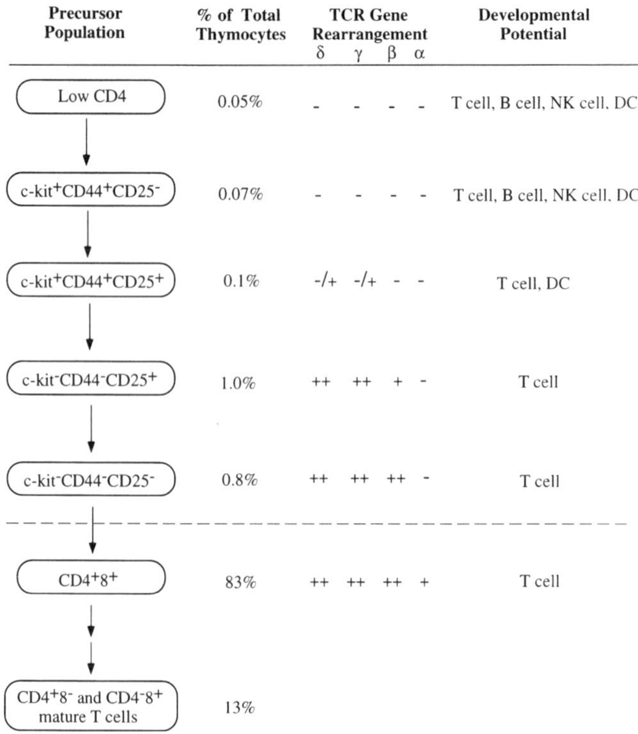

Fig. 1. A summary of the pathway of intrathymic T cell development. The precursor sequence was deduced based on the state of TCR gene rearrangement, the precursor activity and developmental kinetics of each precursor population *(3,5,6,8,9)*. The proportion of each precursor population amongst all thymocytes is an average value for C57BL/6 mice.

The intrathymic precursors are rare cells in adult thymus, about 97% thymocytes being either immature CD4$^+$8$^+$ or mature CD4$^+$8$^-$, CD4$^-$8$^+$, or CD3$^+$CD4$^-$8$^-$ cells. Accordingly, the principle for isolating these minute precursor populations is to maximally enrich for them prior to fluorescence activated cell sorting, in order to reduce the cost and maximize purity. This can be achieved by a large scale depletion of the mature and immature thymocytes, as well as other non-T lineage cells, using a combination of density centrifugation and immuno-magnetic bead depletion. Note that it is important to deplete non-T lineage cells, including erythrocytes, macrophages and DC, which may otherwise contaminate the precursor preparation, especially if CD44 is a sorting parameter. Although the phenotype of the low CD4 precursors and the TN c-kit$^+$CD44$^+$CD25$^-$ subpopulation overlaps, the low CD4 precursor population will be partially lost if anti-CD4 antibody is included in the depletion procedure, as normally used for isolating TN precursors. We therefore developed two separate procedures for purifying either the low CD4 precursors or the four TN precursor populations.

2. Materials

2.1. Mice

C57BL/6J (Ly 5.2) mice at 5–6 wk of age have been used for thymic precursor cell isolation and as donors in precursor transfer experiments. C57BL/6 Ly 5.1-Pep[3b] mice at age of 8–12 wk have been used as recipients in precursor transfer experiments.

2.2. Media for Single Cell Suspension and for Immuno-Fluorescent Staining

1. Balanced Salt Solution (BSS): A mouse tonicity (308m. osmolar or equivalent to 0.168M NaCl), HEPES buffered balanced salt solution at pH 7.2 and supplemented with 3% fetal calf serum (FCS) is used for single-cell suspension and immunofluorescent staining.
2. RPMI-1640-HEPES-FCS: RPMI-1640 culture medium adjusted to mouse tonicity, buffered with HEPES at pH 6.8–7.0 and supplemented with 10% FCS is used for adhesion depletion for macrophages.
3. Fetal Calf Serum: FCS is filtered through a 0.22 micron membrane and heat-inactivated at 56°C for 30 min.
4. Density Separation Medium: Nycodenz is purchased from Nycomed Pharma AS, Oslo, Norway as analytical grade powder, 50 g bottles, MW 821. Make a stock 0.372M (30.55 g per 100 mL final) and mix well before adjusting to final volume. Store frozen and protect from light. This stock should be close to 308m osmolar (adjust if not) and have a density about 1.16g/cm^3 at 4°C. Dilute this stock with BSS, mix thoroughly, to density 1.086g/cm^3 at 4°C. Use a weighing bottle to get precise density. To calculate stock dilution for the approximate density use the following formula:

$$100 \times 1.16 \text{ (stock density)} + 1.0 \times a = (100 + a) \times 1.086 \text{ (required density)}$$

   where a = additional volume of BSS to be added to 100 mL stock. Note that the (100 + a) final volume is measured after thorough mixing. Store frozen in sealed tubes or bottles. Mix thoroughly on thawing and before use. During separation maintain a temperature around 4°C to avoid density changes.

2.3. Monoclonal Antibodies for Depletion

Cocktails of monoclonal antibodies (MAb) for depletion are prepared and stored in small aliquots at –70°C (for details of each MAb, *see* **Table 1**). Each MAb is pretitrated using immunofluorescent staining with anti-Ig second stage, then is used at near saturating concentration in the final mix. The cocktail of MAb is used at 10 µL per 10^6 cells. Two different MAb cocktails are employed.

Table 1
mAbs Used in this Procedure

Specificity	Clone name	Reference
anti-CD3	KT3-1.1	*(11)*
anti-CD4	GK1.5	*(12)*
anti-CD8	53.6.7	*(13)*
anti-CD25	PC61	*(14)*
anti-Thy-1.2	30H-12	*(15)*
anti-B220	RA3-6B2	*(16)*
anti-Mac-1(CD11b)	M1/70	*(17)*
anti-Gr-1	RB6-8C5	*(18)*
anti-erythrocyte antigen	TER-119	From Dr T Kina, Dept Immunology, Chest Disease Research Institute, Kyoto University, Japan
anti-MHC Class II	M5/114	*(19)*
anti-c-kit	Ack-2	*(20)*
anti-NK1.1	DX5	Pharmingen, San Diego, CA
anti-Ly5.2	ALI-4A2	*(21)*

Most of these mAbs are available as purified antibody or fluorescent-conjugated antibodies from Pharmingen (San Diego, CA) or Caltag (Burlingame, CA).

1. For isolation of low CD4 precursors: anti-CD3, KT3-1.1; anti-CD8, 53.6.7; anti-CD2, RM2-1; anti-CD25, PC61; anti-B220, RA3-6B2; anti-Mac-1, M1/70; anti-Gr-1, RB6-8C5; anti-erythrocyte antigen, TER-119; anti-MHC class-II, M5/114.
2. For isolation of TN precursors: anti-CD3, KT3-1.1; anti-CD4, GK1.5; anti-CD8, 53.6.7; anti-B220, RA3-6B2; anti-Mac-1, M1/70; anti-Gr-1, RB6-8C5; anti-erythrocyte antigen, TER-119; anti-MHC class-II, M5/114.

2.4. Immunomagnetic Beads for Depletion

1. Paesel and Lorei beads: Goat anti-rat IgG coated magnetic beads are purchased from Paesel and Lorei (GMBH & Co, Frankfurt, Germany). For reasons of economy these beads are used for the first round magnetic bead depletion at a bead:cell ratio of 3:1. The beads are washed three times in 3–5 mL BSS-FCS before use, to remove the preservative which is toxic to cells. A Dynal magnet is used to recover the beads. Note that Paesel and Lorei beads are very small and therefore migrate slowly in the magnetic field. To avoid losing beads, leave the tube on the magnet for at least 3–5 min when washing the beads or recovering depleted cells.
2. Dynabeads: Sheep anti-rat Ig coated beads M450 Dynabeads (Dynal, Oslo, Norway) are used for the second round magnetic bead depletion at a bead: cell ratio of 5:1. The beads are washed three times in 3–5 mL BSS-FCS before use to remove the preservative. A Dynal magnet is used to recover the beads.

2.5. Antibodies for Immunofluorescent Staining

Fluorescent conjugated antibodies for immunofluorescent staining are either purchased from Caltag (Burlingame, CA), or Pharmingen (San Diego, CA), or are made in our laboratory. The following are used:

1. FITC-conjugated antibodies: FITC-anti-Thy-1.2 (30H-12); FITC-anti-c-kit (Ack-2); FITC-anti-Ly 5.2 (ALI-4A2).
2. PE- or Cy-3-conjugated antibodies: These can be used interchangeably in the same fluorescent channel (excitation at 488nm and emission at 570–575nm). These conjugates are: PE-anti-CD4 (GK1.5); PE-anti-B220 (RA3-6B2); Cy3-anti-CD25 (PC61).
3. APC- or Cy-5-conjugated antibodies: These can be used interchangeably in the same fluorescent channel (excitation at 605nm and emission at 660–670 nm). The conjugated antibodies are: APC-anti-c-kit (Ack-2); Cy5-anti-Mac-1 (M1/70); Cy5-anti-Gr-1 (RB6-8C5); Cy5-anti-CD8 (YTS 169.4).
4. Biotinylated antibodies: biotin-anti-Thy-1.2 (30H-12); biotin-anti-CD3 (KT3-1.1); biotin-anti-NK1.1 (DX5). Texas-Red-avidin is used as the second stage reagent.

Sorting and analysis is performed on a FACStar-Plus instrument (Becton Dickinson) or equivalent instrument permitting at least three fluorescent channel operation.

2.6. Miscellaneous Equipment

Spiral Mixer: The type with a series horizontal rollers, used for equilibrium dialysis, is set up in cold room. Fit 5 mL round-bottom Falcon tubes with a "collar" (cut from thick tubber tubing) around the lid, so the tubes will rotate slowly at an angle of ~30° when placed on the rollers.

3. Methods

3.1. Isolation of the Earliest Intrathymic Precursor Population– the "Low CD4 Precursors"

1. Single-cell suspension: A thymocyte suspension from 16 thymuses is prepared by gently forcing thymus lobes through a stainless steel sieve in BSS-3%FCS. The cell suspension is transferred into four 10 mL conical tubes (~4 thymuses per tube), underlaid with 0.5 mL FCS and centrifuged at $580 \times g$ for 7 min at 4°C, in a benchtop centrifuge.
2. Density centrifugation: This step selects the 15–20% of thymocytes with a density less than $1.086 g/cm^3$, including the low CD4 precursors, and removes dead cells and higher density cells, including some mature $CD4^+8^-$ and $CD4^-8^+$ thymocytes, small $CD4^+8^+$ thymocytes and erythrocytes. Transfer 5 mL of well mixed $1.086 g/cm^3$ Nycodenz medium to four 14 mL round bottom polypropylene Falcon tubes. Resuspend the cell pellet in each conical tube in an additional 5 mL Nycodenz

medium and overlay this cell/Nycodenz suspension onto the 5 mL Nycodenz medium in the Falcon tube (i.e., cells from 4 thymuses per tube). Then layer 2 mL of FCS above the cells. Slightly mix the interface bands with a Pasteur pipet to make a gentle density gradient. Centrifuge in a swing-out rotor refrigerated centrifuge (4°C) for 10 min at 1700 g. Using a Pasteur pipet, collect the light density fraction as all upper zones down to a little below the lower interface, leaving behind the pellet and 2 mL or so of medium above it. Dilute the collected fraction with BSS to 30–40 mL, mix well, take a small sample to count cell yield at this stage, then centrifuge the cells to a pellet at 580 g for 7 min.

3. Adhesion depletion of macrophages: This step removes macrophages by adhesion to a plastic surface. Resuspend the cell pellet in 10 mL RPMI-1640-10%FCS. Transfer the cell suspension into a 10 cm plastic Petri dish and ensure even distribution over the whole area of the dish. Incubate in a 37°C CO_2-in-air incubator for 60 min. After incubation, the nonadherent cells are collected by gently washing the dish twice with 10 mL prewarmed (37°C) RPMI-1640–10% FCS (*see* **Note 1**). Take a small sample for a cell count, then collect the cells by centrifugation.

4. Immunomagnetic bead depletion: This step is to remove most cells bearing markers of mature thymocytes, of more mature precursor cells and other non-T lineage cells. Add to the cell pellet 10 µL/10^6 cells of the depletion MAb cocktail for low CD4 precursor isolation (*see* **Materials**) and mix well. Incubate at 4°C for 30–40 min. Dilute cells in 9 mL of BSS-3%FCS, underlayer with 1 mL of FCS, then spin down cells through the FCS underlay at 580 g for 7 min. Remove the supernatant carefully from the top. Washing using a serum underlay removes residual antibody with only one washing step.

5. The antibody-coated cells are then removed using two rounds of treatment with anti-Ig coated beads. For the first round of depletion, the Paesel and Lorei beads are used for economic reasons, since large amount of beads are required at this stage. Prewash the required amount (beads : cells = 3 : 1) of anti-rat IgG coated beads in a 5 mL round bottom Falcon tube with BSS-3%FCS three times to remove the preservative. Separate the beads from the washing fluid with a Dynal magnet. Resuspend the MAb coated cells in 300–500 µL BSS-3% FCS, then transfer the suspension into a 5 mL Falcon tube containing washed beads. Mix the slurry of cells and beads, seal the tube with a cap and place a "collar" around the cap. Mix continuously for 20 min at 4°C, by rotating at a 30° angle on a spiral mixer. To recover the undepleted cells, dilute the bead-cell mix in 5 mL BSS-3%FCS, then remove beads and attached cells with Dynal magnet. Recover the bead-free cell suspension with a Pasteur pipet and once again treat with the magnet to remove any residual beads. Take a small sample of cells to count, then recover the cells by centrifugation (580 g, 7 min).

6. The second round depletion is to remove the residual antibody-coated cells, in order to obtain the maximum enrichment. Resuspend cell pellet again in 300–500 µL BSS-3%FCS, and add cells to prewashed anti-rat Ig coated Dynabeads at a ratio of bead : cell = 5 : 1. Mix the bead and cell slurry for 20 min. Dilute with

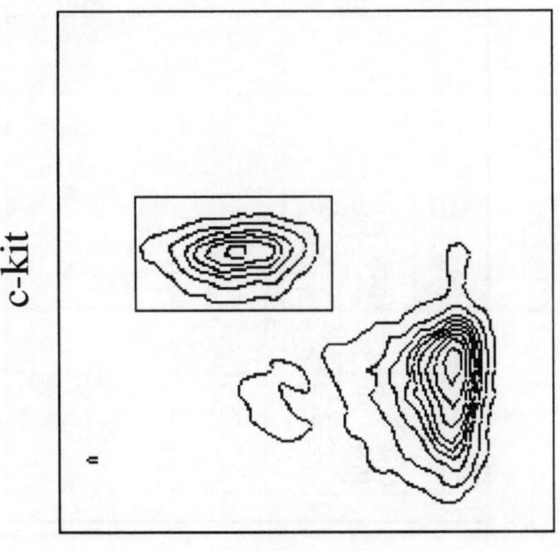

Fig. 2. A typical flow cytometric analysis of the depleted preparation, enriched for the low CD4 precursors. The preparation was immunofluorescent stained with FITC-anti-c-kit and PE anti-Thy-1.2. The low CD4 precursor population is represented by the Thy-1^{lo}c-kit$^+$ cells. The box shows the sorting gates for this population.

2 mL BSS-3%FCS, and remove beads and attached cells with Dynal magnet. Recover the bead-free cell supernatant with a Pasteur pipet and again remove residual beads with the magnet. Recover the nondepleted cells by centrifugation at 580 g for 7 min. At this stage, the precursor cells are enriched about 500-fold, and make up ~10–20% of the cells.

7. Immunofluorescent staining and flowcytometric sorting: To obtain pure low CD4 precursors, the depleted preparation is stained in two fluorescent colors with FITC-anti-c-kit and PE-anti-Thy-1.2 (*see* **Note 2**). Propidium iodide (PI) is added to the final wash at 0.5–1.0 µg/mL. Stained cells are then analyzed on a FACStar-Plus, a file of 10,000 cells being collected. The low CD4 precursor population is represented by the Thy-1^{lo}c-kit$^+$ subpopulation, which usually equals 10–20% of stained cells (*see* **Fig. 2**). The precursor population is sorted, setting up the live gates for Thy-1^{lo}c-kit$^+$ cells and excluding dead cells are on the basis of very low forward scatter and positivity for PI. The purity of the sorted precursor population is determined by reanalysis on FACStar Plus and is usually >98%. The number of low CD4 precursors recovered is usually 2–3 × 10^4 cells per thymus.

3.2. Isolation of CD3⁻4⁻8⁻ Triple Negative Precursor Populations

A procedure similar to that described above is used for isolation of the TN thymic precursor populations, except that a different depletion MAb cocktail is used. After adhesion depletion of macrophages, cells are incubated with the

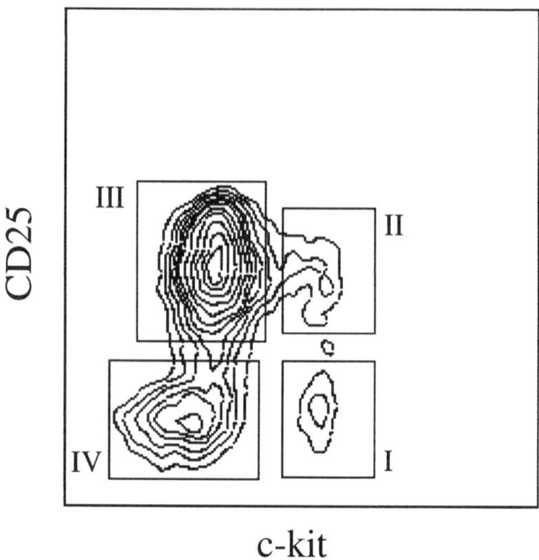

Fig. 3. A typical flow cytometric analysis of the depleted preparation enriched for the TN precursors. The preparation was immunofluorescent stained with FITC-anti-c-kit and Cy3-anti-CD25. Four subpopulations of precursor cells are shown, namely c-kit$^+$CD25$^-$(I),c-kit$^+$CD25$^+$(II),c-kit$^-$CD25$^+$(III) and c-kit$^-$CD25-(IV). The boxes represent sorting gates for each precursor population.

depletion MAb cocktail for TN precursors (*see* **Materials**). This is then followed by two rounds of immunomagnetic bead depletion, as above. At this stage, the TN precursor populations are enriched 50–200-fold.

To obtain pure cells of each TN subpopulation, the depleted preparation is stained in two fluorescent colors with FITC-anti-c-kit and Cy3-anti-CD25, together with PI (*see* **Note 3**). The stained cells are analyzed on a FACStar-Plus and a file of 10,000 cells is collected. Four TN subpopulations can be segregated as seen in the contour plot (**Fig. 3**), namely: c-kit$^+$CD25$^-$ (I), c-kit$^+$CD25$^+$ (II), c-kit$^-$CD25$^+$ (III) and c-kit$^-$CD25$^-$ (IV), representing 3–4%, 6%, 50% and 40% of stained cells respectively. Each precursor population is sorted by setting up live gates as shown in **Fig. 3**. Dead cells are excluded by gating out cells with very low forward scatter and staining with PI. Purity of the sorted precursor populations is determined by reanalysis on FACStar Plus and is generally around 98–99%. The number of TN precursors recovered per initial thymus is generally: I,~3 ×10^4; II, ~5×10^4; III, ~5×10^5 and IV, ~4×10^5.

3.3. Precursor Activity Analysis

1. Intrathymic transfer of isolated precursor populations: The developmental potential of each precursor population can be determined by their capability to recon-

stitute T cell development in an irradiated recipient thymus lobe. Ly 5 disparate mice are used in this analysis. Eight to twelve week old C57BL/6 Ly 5.1-Pep[3b] recipient mice are irradiated (750 Rad, 1 Rad = 0.01 Gy) and used 1–3 h later. The irradiated mice are anesthetized by intraperitoneal injection of a mixture of Ketavet 100 (Ketamine hydrochloride 0.05mg/g body weight; Delta Veterinary Laboratories Pty.Ltd. NSW Australia) and Rompun (a muscle relaxant, Xylazine hydrochloride 0.01mg/g body weight; Bayer AG, Germany). The intrathymic injection procedure described by Goldschneider et al. *(22)* is used. A midline incision is made in the skin overlying the lower cervical and upper thoracic region, and the upper third of the sternum is bisected longitudinally with fine scissors to expose the thymus. A suspension (10 µL) containing the appropriate number of purified precursor cells from C57BL/6 (Ly 5.2) mice is injected directly into the anterior upper portion of each thymus lobe using a 50-µL Hamilton syringe with a 30-gauge needle (PrecisionGlide Needle 30G1, Becton Dickinson, Franklin Lakes, NJ). The incision is then closed with wound clips (MikRon Precision. Inc., NJ). The mice are kept under a warm lamp until they recover.

2. Intravenous transfer of isolated precursor populations: The potential of the precursors to develop into other hemopoietic lineages can be determined by intravenous injection into lethally irradiated Ly 5.1 recipients. Eight to twelve week old Ly 5.1 recipient mice are irradiated with two doses of 550 rads with a 3 hr interval. A suspension (200 µL) containing the appropriate number of purified precursor cells together with 5×10^4 recipient-type bone marrow cells is injected into the tail vein (*see* **Note 4**). Antibiotics are added to the drinking water (Polymyxin B sulfate 10^6u/L and Neomycin sulfate 1.1g/L) for two weeks after irradiation.

3. Analysis of progeny of transferred precursor populations: At various times after precursor transfer, the recipients are sacrificed and the thymus, spleen, lymph nodes and bone marrow are removed. Cell suspensions are prepared, and the percentage of donor and host origin cells are quantified by immunofluorescent staining and flowcytometric analysis. Cell suspensions are stained with FITC-anti-Ly 5.2 in combination with differenat lineage markers. For T-lineage cell reconstitution, cells are stained with FITC-anti-Ly 5.2, PE-anti-CD4, Cy5-anti-CD8 and biotin-anti-CD3 or biotin-anti-Thy-1, followed by Texas-red-avidin as second stage reagent. For reconstitution of other lineages, cells are stained with FITC-anti-Ly 5.2 together with PE-anti-B220, Cy5-anti-Mac-1 or Cy5-anti-Gr-1, and biotin-anti-NK1.1, followed by Texas-red-avidin as a second stage reagent. Donor-derived cells are revealed by gating for Ly 5.2^+ cells, then analyzing their lineage marker expression (*see* **Note 5**).

4. Notes

1. It is important to use warm but not cold medium to wash the dish, otherwise adherent cells will be released.
2. Despite the name, CD4 is generally not used in the staining and sorting to produce low CD4 precursors, since staining with a combination of Thy-1 and c-kit gives the best separation of this population.

3. CD44 expression by each precursor population is tightly correlated with the expression of c-kit, so CD44 antibody staining can be used as a sorting parameter. However, it is generally not used in order to avoid the blocking effect of anti-CD44 antibody on precursor homing in the precursor transfer analysis.
4. The recipient-type bone marrow cells are injected to ensure long-term survival of the irradiated recipients.
5. The erythroid lineage, which does not express Ly 5, cannot be monitored by this approach. Alternative approaches, such as spleen colony assay or in vitro colony formation assay, can be used.

References

1. Shortman, K. and Wu, L. (1996) Early T lymphocyte progenitors. *Ann. Rev. Immunol.* **14,** 29–47.
2. Godfrey, D. I. and Zlotnik, A. (1993) Control points in early T-cell development. *Immunol. Today* **14,** 547–553.
3. Wu, L., Scollay, R., Egerton, M., Pearse, M., Spangrude, G. J., and Shortman, K. (1991) CD4 expressed on earliest T-lineage precursor cells in the adult murine thymus. *Nature* **349,** 71–74.
4. Wu, L., Antica, M., Johnson, G. R., Scollay, R., and Shortman, K. (1991) Developmental potential of the earliest precursor cells from the adult thymus. *J. Exp. Med.* **174,** 1617–1627.
5. Matsuzaki, Y., Gyotoku, J., Ogawa, M., Nishikawa, S., Katsura, Y., Gachelin, G., and Nakauchi, H. (1993) Characterization of c-kit positive intrathymic stem cells that are restricted to lymphoid differentiation. *J. Exp. Med.* **178,** 1283–1291.
6. Ardavin, C., Wu, L., Li, C.-L., and Shortman, K. (1993) Thymic dendritic cells and T cells develop simultaneously within the thymus from a common precursor population. *Nature* **362,** 761–763.
7. Godfrey, D. I., Zlotnik, A., and Suda, T. (1992) Phenotypic and functional characterization of c-kit expression during intrathymic T cell development. *J. Immunol.* **149,** 2281–2285.
8. Godfrey, D. I., Kennedy, J., Suda, T., and Zlotnik, A. (1993) A developmental pathway involving four phenotypically and functionally distinct subsets of CD3$^-$CD4$^-$CD8$^-$ triple-negative adult mouse thymocytes defined by CD44 and CD25. *J. Immunol.* **150,** 4244–4252.
9. Wu, L., Li, C.-L., and Shortman, K. (1996) Thymic dendritic cell precursors: relationship to the T-lymphocyte lineage and phenotype of the dendritic cell progeny. *J. Exp. Med.* **184,** 903–911.
10. Tourigny, M. R., Mazel, S., Burtrum, D. B., and Petrie, H. T. (1997) T cell receptor (TCR)-beta gene recombination: dissociation from cell cycle regulation and developmental progression during T cell ontogeny. *Journal of Experimental Medicine* **185,** 1549–56.
22. Goldschneider, I., Komschlies, K. L., and Greiner, D. L. (1986) Studies of thymocytopoiesis in rats and mice. I. Kinetics of appearance of thymocytes using a direct intrathymic adoptive transfer assay for thymocyte precursors. *Journal of Experimental Medicine* **163,** 1–17.

11. Tomonari, K. (1988) A rat antibody against a structure functionally related to the mouse T-cell receptor/T3 complex. *Immunogenetics* **28,** 455–458.

12. Dialynas, D., Quan, Z., Wall, K., Pierres, A., Quintans, J., Loken, M., Pierres, M., and Fitch, F. (1983) Characterization of the murine T cell surface molecule, designated L3T4, identified by monoclonal antibody GK1.5: similarity of L3T4 to the human Leu-3/T4 molecule. *J. Immunol.* **131,** 2445–2451.

13. Ledbetter, J. A. and Herzenberg, L. A. (1979) Xenogeneic monoclonal antibodies to mouse lymphoid differentiation antigens. *Immunol. Rev.* **47,** 63–90.

14. Ceredig, R., Lowenthal, J., Nabholz, M., and MacDonald, R. (1985) Expression of interleukin-2 receptors as a differentiation marker on intrathymic stem cells. *Nature* **314,** 98–100.

15. Sarmiento, M., Dialynas, D., Lancki, D., Wall, K., Lorber, M., Loken, M., and Fitch, F. (1982) Cloned T lymphocytes and monoclonal antibodies as probes for cell surface molecules active in T cell mediated cytolytis. *Immunol. Rev.* **68,** 135–169.

16. Coffman, R. L. (1982) Surface antigen expression and immunoglobulin gene rearrangement during mouse pre-B cell development. *Immunol. Rev.,* **69,** 5–23.

17. Springer, T., Galfre, G., Secher, D. S., and Milstein, C. (1979) Mac-1: A macrophage differentiation antigen identified by monoclonal antibody. *Eur. J. Immunol.* **9,** 301–306.

18. Holmes, K. L., Langdon, W. Y., Fredrickson, T. N., Coffman, R. L., Hoffman, P. M., Hartley, J. W., and Morse, H. C. (1986) Analysis of neoplasms induced by CAS-BR-M MULV tumour extracts. *J. Immunol.* **137,** 679–688.

19. Bhattacharya, A., Dorf, M. E., and Springer, T. A. (1981) A shared alloantigenic determinant on Ia antigens encoded by the IA and IE subregions: evidence of I region gene duplication. *J. Immunol.* **127,** 2488–2495.

20. Ogawa, M., Matsuzaki, Y., Nishikawa, S., Hayashi, S.-I., Kunisada, T., Sudo, T., Kina, T., Nakauchi, H., and Nishikawa, S.-I. (1991) Expression and function of c-kit in hemopoietic progenitor cells. *J. Exp. Med.* **174,** 63–71.

21. Spangrude, G. J. and Scollay, R. (1990) A simplified method for enrichment of mouse hematopoietic stem cells. *Exp. Hematol.* **18,** 920–926.

23. Pearse, M., Wu, L., Egerton, M., Wilson, A., Shortman, K., and Scollay, R. (1989) An early thymocyte development sequence marked by transient expression of the IL-2 receptor. *Proc. Natl. Acad. Sci. USA* **86,** 1614–1618.

3

Differentiation of Mouse Thymocytes in Fetal Thymus Organ Culture

Yousuke Takahama

1. Introduction

Most T cells develop in the thymus. Thymic development of T cells offers an excellent experimental system to pursue many issues of developmental biology, including

1. lineage decisions, e.g., CD4[+] T cells vs CD8[+] T cells, and TCR-$\alpha\beta^+$ T cells vs TCR-$\gamma\delta^+$ T cells,
2. clonal selection, e.g., positive selection of useful T-cell clones and negative selection of harmful T-cell clones, and
3. cell migration, e.g., entry into and emigration from the thymus.

In addition, better understanding of T-cell differentiation and selection is crucial for aiding many clinical situations, such as immune deficiencies, autoimmune diseases, and various infectious diseases.

Consequently, the research field of thymocyte development has attracted many scientists since Miller first described the immunological function of the thymus in 1961 *(1)*.

The experimental approach for analysis of T-cell development in organ culture of mouse fetal thymus lobes was first established in the early seventies by Owen *(2,3)* and by Mandel *(4,5)* and later refined mostly by Owen's group *(6–9)*. The fetal thymus organ culture (FTOC) technique serves a unique in vitro cell culture system in that functional T cells are differentiated from immature progenitor cells *(10,11)*. T-cell development in FTOC very well represents T-cell development during fetal life, even in time course (**Fig. 1**; also *see* **ref**. *11–13*). FTOC allows in vitro T-cell development isolated from any further cellular or humoral supplies by other organs; thus, it is suitable for the addition of any reagents, such as drugs and antibodies to the culture, for examining their effects

From: *Methods in Molecular Biology, Vol. 134: T Cell Protocols: Development and Activation*
Edited by: K. P. Kearse © Humana Press Inc., Totowa, NJ

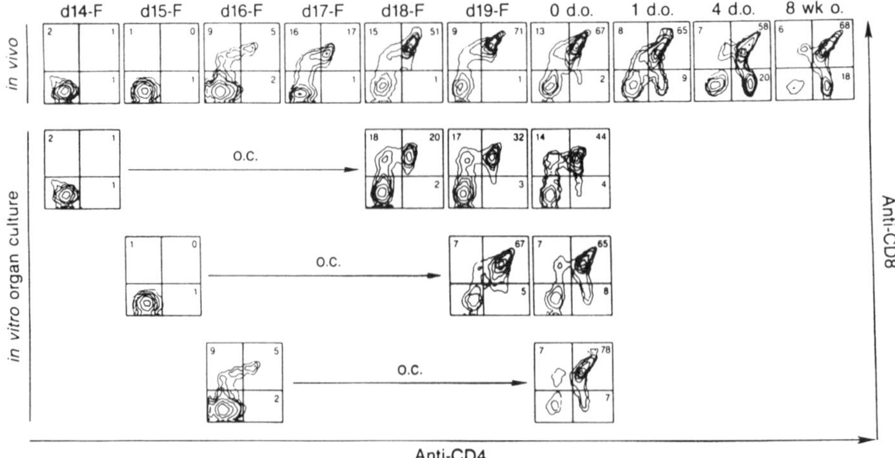

Fig. 1. Ontogeny of mouse thymocytes in vivo and in vitro. Contour histograms indicate CD4/CD8 two-color immunofluorescence profiles of in vivo generated (top panels) or in vitro FTOC-generated thymocytes (lower panels). Day 14 fetal thymus lobes were organ-cultured (O.C.) for 4, 5, or 6 d; day 15 fetal thymus lobes for 4 or 5 d; and day 16 fetal thymus lobes for 4 d. Numbers indicate frequency of the cells within the box.

on T-cell development. Recent advances in retroviral gene transfer techniques further enable gene manipulation of developing T cells in FTOC *(14–17)*. FTOC is also useful for the analysis of T-lymphopoietic capability by hematopoietic progenitor cells *(7,8,18–20)*.

This chapter describes a basic method for FTOC (**Subheading 3.1–3.4**) and several related techniques, including the reconstitution of thymus lobes with progenitor cells (**Subheading 3.5**), high-oxygen submersion culture (**Subheading 3.6**), and retrovirus-mediated gene transfer in FTOC (**Subheading 3.7**).

2. Materials

2.1. Equipment and Supplies

1. Dissecting microscope with zoom, e.g., 7×–42× magnification, preferably equipped with fiber lights. The microscope should be placed in a clean hood.
2. Clean hood for sterile procedures. Basic techniques for cell culture procedures are essential.
3. CO_2-incubator (set at 5% CO_2 concentration).
4. Type 7 forceps, Biology grade (e.g., Dumont, Switzerland). Stored sterile in 70% ethanol.
5. Regular dissecting forceps and scissors. At least 1 set for nonsterile use to dissect skins, and 2–3 autoclaved sets for sterile use.

6. Polycarbonate filter membranes: Costar, Nucleopore Corp. PC membrane, #110409, 13-mm diameter. Autoclave to sterilize and store dry at room temperature.
7. Sterile Helistat collagen sponges (Colla-Tec, Inc., Plainsboro, NJ 08536). Small pieces (e.g., 1-inch square) are stored dry at room temperature.
8. Gauze sponges (e.g., Johnson and Johnson, 2×2-inch square, 6–8ply, sterile)
9. 100-mm plastic dishes (sterile)
10. 24-well plates (16-mm diameter, sterile)
11. 1-mL syringes
12. 26-gauge needles
13. 30-mm plastic dishes
14. Nylon mesh (~300 meshes/square inch). Cut into small pieces of approx 5-mm square.
15. For the reconstitution experiments only: Terasaki 60-well plates (sterile).
16. For high-oxygen submersion cultures only: 96-well round-bottom plates (sterile).
17. For high-oxygen submersion cultures only: plastic 3–5L air bags and a heat-sealer.
18. For retrovirus infection experiments only: 96-well flat-bottom plates (sterile).

2.2. Mice and Reagents

1. Timed pregnant mice: Mice may be mated in the animal facility of the laboratory. We usually mix female and male mice in a cage in the evening (7–8 pm), and separate them in the morning (8–9 am). Gestational days are tentatively designated by assigning the day at which mice are separated as day 0, and are confirmed on the day of experiment according to the size and many developmental features of fetuses *(21–23)*. Timed pregnant mice may be purchased from animal breeding farms.
2. Culture Medium: RPMI1640 supplemented with 10% fetal calf serum (FCS), 50μM 2-mercaptoethanol, 10mM HEPES, 2mM L-glutamine, 1x nonessential amino acids, 1mM sodium pyruvate, 100U/mL penicillin, and 100μg/mL streptomycin. All medium components except 2- mercaptoethanol are purchased from Gibco-BRL, Gaithersburg, MD. 2-mercaptoethanol is purchased from Sigma Chemicals, (St. Louis, MO). FCS is pretreated for 30 min at 56°C, and stored frozen in 50-mL aliquots. Screening of FCS is essential (*see* **Note 1**).
3. 70% Ethanol.
4. Staining buffer: PBS, pH 7.2 supplemented with 0.2% BSA and 0.1% NaN_3.
5. For the reconstitution experiments only: 2-deoxyguanosine (Yamasa, Chiba, Japan). Aliquots of a stock solution at 13.5 mM in PBS are stored frozen at –20°C, and can be thawed at 42°C.
6. For high-oxygen submersion cultures only: gas consisting of 70% O_2, 25% N_2 and 5% CO_2.
7. For retrovirus infection experiments only: recombinant mouse IL-7 (Genzyme, Cambridge, MA).

3. Methods

3.1. Isolation of Fetuses from Pregnant Mice

1. All of the procedures should be performed under clean conditions in a clean hood.
2. Prepare 100-mm sterile dishes containing 20–30 mls of medium each (3 dishes/group).

3. Kill timed-pregnant mice by cervical dislocation.
4. Wipe the abdomens of the mice with 70% ethanol, and open them with nonsterile set of scissors and forceps.
5. Take out fetus-filled uteri with a sterile set of scissors and forceps. About 8 fetuses are expected from a pregnant C57BL/6 mouse.
6. Transfer uteri to an empty 100-mm plastic dish.
7. Using a sterile set of sharp scissors and forceps, take out fetuses from uteri, and transfer fetuses to a new dish containing medium.
8. Ascertain gestation age of fetuses, omitting fetuses with deviated developmental features as judged by size and other developmental signs such as the formation of hair follicles and crests in the limbs (*see* **Subheading 2.2.1** and **ref.** *21–23*).
9. Wash out blood by transferring fetuses to new a dish containing fresh medium.
10. Repeat washing 2–3 times to remove blood. Gentle swirling of the dishes helps in removing the blood and debris.
11. Count the number of fetuses and plan the experiment. For flow cytometry analysis, 4–6 fetal thymuses are usually used for one group. Fetuses may be stored in a refrigerator or on ice while preparing culture wells as below.

3.2. Preparation of Culture Wells

1. Cut Helistat sponge into ~1-cm^2 pieces using a clean set of sterile scissors and forceps.
2. Place one piece of the sponge in a culture well of a 24-well plate.
3. Fill a culture well with 1 mL of culture medium.
4. Flip the sponge with forceps, so that the smooth side of the sponge faces up.
5. Place a sterile PC membrane on a sponge. Flip the membrane with forceps, so that both sides of the membrane are completely wet with culture medium.
6. Gently remove 0.5 mL of the medium from a well using a 1-mL pipet. The final volume of the culture medium is 0.5 mL per well.

3.3. Isolation and Organ Culture of Fetal Thymus Lobes

1. Place a dissecting microscope in a clean hood. If appropriate, wear a mask.
2. Prepare a surgery dish by wetting ~5 mL medium to a 2" × 2" gauge in a 100-mm dish.
3. Wash two sterile #7 forceps with culture medium. Removal of ethanol from the forceps is important to prevent exposure of the thymus organ to ethanol.
4. The following procedures are done using #7 forceps under the microscope.
5. Place a fetus under the microscope and turn the abdomen up (**Fig. 2A, B**).
6. Flip up the head (**Fig. 2C**)
7. Gently open the chest and locate the two lobes of the thymus (**Fig. 2D**).
8. Take thymus lobes out of the body and place them on the gauze to remove blood.
9. Place thymus lobes onto the filter membrane in a culture well. Usually, 4–6 lobes are placed on a membrane. Try to randomize the way the lobes are placed; 2 lobes from one fetus should be divided into different groups when multiple experimental groups are set up.

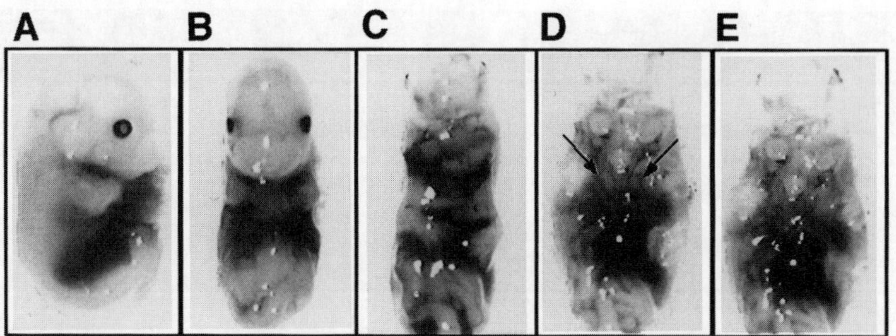

Fig. 2. Isolation of thymus lobes from fetal mice. (**A**) A fetus at day 14 gestational age from C57BL/6 mice is placed under dissecting microscope. (**B**) The fetus is turned so that the abdomen faces up. (**C**) The neck is flipped up to expose the chest. (**D**) The chest is opened to expose two thymus lobes as shown by arrows. (**E**) The fetus after removal of the thymus.

10. Ascertain that the lobes are placed at the interface between the membrane and air. The lobes should not be sunk in culture medium.
11. When reagents are added, first remove 50 µL of culture medium. Then, add 50 µL of 10× concentrated reagents slowly onto the lobes. Do the same treatment to the medium-alone group.
12. Add 1–2mls of fresh culture medium to an empty well of the 24-well plate to minimize evaporation from the culture wells.
13. Place the culture plate in a CO_2 incubator (**Fig. 3**).

3.4. Isolation of Single-Cell Suspension from Fetal Thymus Organ Culture

1. Make a drop of 100µL of the Staining buffer at the center of the reverse side of the lid of a 30-mm dish.
2. Transfer thymus lobes into the drop using #7 forceps. Count the number of lobes.
3. Place a small (~5-mm^2) piece of nylon mesh on the drop.
4. Attach 26-gauge needles to 1-mL syringes. Bend the tip (top 5-mm, 90° angle) of needles, using forceps. You need two needle/syringe sets per group.
5. Gently tease thymus lobes with the needles, pushing under the filter mesh. If needed, use a dissecting microscope.
6. Transfer the cell suspension to a plastic tube, and count cell numbers. Use the cell suspensions for further examination of T-cell development; e.g., immunofluorescence and flow cytometry analysis.

3.5. Optional Technique: Reconstitution of Deoxyguanosine-Treated Thymus Lobes with T-Precursor Cells

1. Thymus lobes from fetal mice at day 14 or day 15 of gestation are cultured in the presence of 1.35mM of 2-deoxyguanosine (dGuo) for 5–7 d. In a typical experiment, 10–20 thymus lobes are treated with dGuo (*see* **Note 5**).

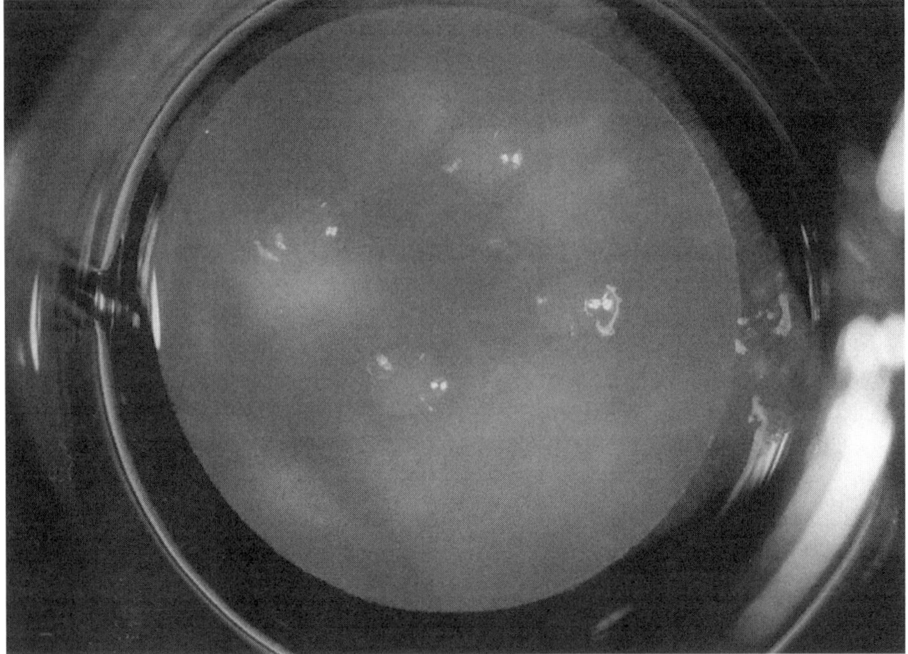

Fig. 3. Organ-cultured thymus lobes. Shown are four lobes of day 14 fetal thymus from C57BL/6 mice cultured for 5 d in FTOC. FTOC was carried out in a culture well of a 24-well-plate.

2. Fill 30-mm sterile dish with 3–4mL of culture medium. Detach individual thymus lobes from the filter membrane into the medium, by sterile forceps and a micropipet. Swirl the thymus lobes in the medium.
3. Change to fresh medium by transferring with a micopipet.
4. Diffuse away dGuo at room temperature for about 1 h.
5. Change twice to fresh medium by transferring with a micopipet.
6. Transfer 15 µL of culture medium containing one of the dGuo-treated thymus lobes into a well of a Terasaki plate.
7. Add 20 mL of culture medium containing T-precursor cells, e.g., 100–1,000 fetal thymocytes or 1,000–10,000 fetal liver cells.
8. Place the lid on the plate and gently invert.
9. Ascertain that thymus lobes are located at the bottom of the drop. If not, then gently pipet the well.
10. Culture in CO_2 incubator for 1 d.
11. Transfer the thymus lobes to a freshly prepared filter/sponge for regular thymus organ culture conditions.
12. Culture in CO_2 incubator, typically for 1–2 wk.

3.6. Optional Technique: High Oxygen Submersion Culture of Fetal Thymus Lobes

1. Fetal thymus lobes are placed in round-bottom wells of a 96-well plate (1 lobe/ well). For the reconstitution of deoxyguanosine-treated thymus lobes, cells for the reconstitution are also included in the culture (*see* **Note 6**).
2. Spin the plate at 150 *g* for 30 s, to settle the thymus lobes at the very bottom of the well.
3. Place the culture wells in a plastic bag (3–5L), and heat-seal the bag.
4. Fill the bag with a gas consisting of 70% O_2, 25% N_2 and 5% CO_2, and heat-seal the bag.
5. Place the bag in a CO_2 incubator. Culture typically for 5–10 days.

3.7. Optional Technique: Retroviral Gene Transfer into Developing Thymocytes In Fetal Thymus Organ Cultures

1. Make single-cell suspension of day 14 or 15 mouse fetal thymocytes.
2. Set up suspension culture in 96-flat wells. Usually $0.5–2\times10^5$ fetal thymocytes and $2–5\times10^3$ virus producer cells are mixed in a well. Culture cells in the presence of 1–5 ng of recombinant mouse IL-7 for 1–2 days (*see* **Note 7**).
3. Collect cells by gentle pipeting.
4. Purify gene-transferred cells. Our virus constructs produce green fluorescence protein in addition to a gene of interest, so that gene-transferred cells can be enriched by sorting for GFP^+CD45^+ cells on a flow cytometric cell sorter. CD45 is used to distinguish thymocytes from fibroblast-derived virus-producing cells.
5. Transfer the virus-infected cells (usually 1,000–2,000 cells) to a deoxyguanosine-treated fetal thymus lobe in a hanging drop in Terasaki wells. Use of Ly5-allele-congenic mice is recommended for thymus lobes, to distinguish donor cells from residual cells.
6. Next day, transfer lobes to regular organ culture filters.

4. Notes

1. It is important to screen the FCS for FTOC. We usually prescreen 10–20 independent lots of FCS by suspension culture of adult thymocytes for overnight and by counting cell numbers recovered. Five to six best FCS lots that allow cell recovery close to 100% are selected for further screening in an actual test of T-cell development in FTOC. Progression along the CD4/CD8 developmental pathway as shown in **Fig. 1** and increase in cell number as listed in **Table 1** would be a good indication of T cell development in culture.
2. The advantages of using FTOC for analyzing T-cell development include the reproducibility of cellular behavior and convenient handling in vitro, whereas disadvantages include the limitation of cell numbers obtained (**Table 1**) and the limitation in microscopic observations of opaque organs (**Fig. 3**).
3. If FTOC is an unfamiliar technique, preliminary organ-cultures of day 15 fetal thymus lobes for 4–5 d are recommended. The fetuses and fetal thymuses are easiest to handle at day 15.

**Table 1
Cell Numbers Recovered
from Fetal Thymus Organ Cultures**

Fetal Thymus	Fresh	FTOC
day 13	$<10^4$	$\sim5\times10^4$
day 14	$\sim10^4$	$1\sim2\times10^5$
day 15	$\sim5\times10^4$	$5\sim8\times10^5$
day 16	$\sim10^5$	$\sim10^6$
day 17	$\sim5\times10^5$	$\sim10^6$
day 18	1×10^6	$2\sim3\times10^6$
day19	$2\sim5\times10^6$	$0.5\sim1\times10^6$

Approximate cell numbers (viable cells per lobe) obtained from fresh or 5-d organ-cultured fetal thymus lobes are listed. Fetal thymus lobes were obtained from normal C57BL/6 mice at indicated gestational ages. Day 19 fetal age usually correspond to 0-day-old of new born mice.

4. Neonatal thymus organ culture (NTOC) has been used for the analysis of positive selection signals inducing the generation of 'single-positive' thymocytes *(24–26)*. NTOC of 0 day old newborn thymus lobes is useful for in vitro stimulation of in vivo generated $CD4^+CD8^+$ thymocytes. However, it should be noted that, unlike FTOC, total cell numbers decrease during 4–5-d cultures in the NTOC condition (**Table 1**), which may complicate the interpretation of obtained results.
5. For the dGuo-treatment, fetal thymus lobes should be cultured with dGuo at least for 5 d. Otherwise, residual T-cell precursors retain their developmental potential and undergo T-cell development. Thymus lobes cultured for 7–8 d with dGuo are still capable of supporting T-cell development of reconstituted precursor cells.
6. High oxygen submersion cultures of FTOC *(17,27)* are useful for the reconstitution of limited numbers of progenitor cells, since the cultures of thymus lobes can be done at the bottom of round or V-shaped culture wells. However, it should be noted that T-cell development in this high-oxygen condition seems to occur more rapidly than T-cell development in vivo or in the regular FTOC condition.
7. For retroviral gene transfer of immature thymocytes, including IL-7 in the suspension cultures is essential in order to retain the developmental potential of T-precursor cells *(17)*.
8. Another critical factor for the successful retroviral gene transfer is the frequent monitoring of virus titers. We have obtained efficient gene-transfer using virus-producer clones exhibiting virus-titers of more than 10^6 cfu/mL *(17)*. The titers may drop suddenly; therefore, frozen stocks of multiple vials for good virus-producer clones are recommended.

Acknowledgments

This work was supported by PRESTO Research Project 'Unit Process and Combined Circuit', Inamori Foundation, Kowa Foundation, and the Ministry of Education, Science, Sports and Culture of Japan. I thank Dr. A. Singer for kind permission of the use of **Fig. 1** which was made in his laboratory.

References

1. Miller, J. F. A. P. (1961) Immunological function of the thymus. *Lancet*, 748–749.
2. Owen, J. J. T. and Ritter, M. A. (1969) Tissue interaction in the development of thymus lymphocytes. *J. Exp. Med.* **129,** 431–442.
3. Owen, J. J. T. (1974) Ontogeny of the immune system. *Prog. in Immunol.* **2,** 163–173.
4. Mandel, T. and Russel, P. J. (1971) Differentiation of foetal mouse thymus. ultrastructure of organ cultures and of subcapsular grafts. *Immunology* **21,** 659–674.
5. Mandel, T. E. and Kennedy, M. M. (1978) The differentiation of murine thymocytes in vivo and in vitro. *Immunology* **35,** 317–331.
6. Jenkinson, E. J., van Ewijk, W., and Owen, J. J. T. (1981) Major histocompatibility complex antigen expression on the epithelium of the developing thymus in normal and nude mice. *J. Exp. Med.* **153,** 280–292.
7. Jenkinson, E. J., Franchi, L. L., Kingston, R., and Owen, J. J. T. (1982) Effect of deoxyguanosine on lymphopoiesis in the developing thymus rudiment in vitro: application in the production of chimeric thymus rudiments. *Eur. J. Immunol.* **12,** 583–587.
8. Kingston, R., Jenkinson, E. J., and Owen, J. J. T. (1985) A single stem cell can recolonize an embryonic thymus, producing phenotypically distinct T-cell populations. *Nature* **317,** 811–813.
9. Anderson, G., Jenkinson, E. J., Moore, N. C., and Owen, J. J. T. (1993) MHC class II-positive epithelium and mesenchyme cells are both required for T-cell development in the thymus. *Nature* **362,** 70–73.
10. Kisielow, P., Leiserson, W., and von Boehmer, H. (1984) Differentiation of thymocytes in fetal organ culture: analysis of phenotypic changes accompanying the appearance of cytolytic and interleukin-2-producing cells. *J. Immunol.* **133,** 1117–1123.
11. Ceredig, R. (1988) Differentiation potential of 14-day fetal mouse thymocytes in organ culture. Analysis of CD4-CD8-defined single-positive and double-negative cells. *J. Immunol.* **141,** 355–362.
12. Husmann, L. A., Shimonkevitz, R. P., Crispe, I. N., and Bevan, M. J. (1988) Thymocyte subpopulations during early fetal development in the BALB/c mouse. *J. Immunol.* **141,** 736–740.
13. Takahama, Y., Hasegawa, T., Itohara, S., Ball, E. L., Sheard, M. A., and Hashimoto, Y. (1994) Entry of CD4⁻CD8⁻ immature thymocytes into the CD4/CD8 developmental pathway is controlled by tyrosine kinase signals that can be provided through T cell receptor components. *Int. Immunol.* **6,** 1505–1514.
14. Crompton, T., Gilmour, K. C., and Owen, M. J. (1996) The MAP kinase pathway controls differentiation from double-negative to double positive thymocyte. *Cell* **86,** 243–251.
15. Heemskerk, M. H. M., Blom, B., Nolan, G., Stegmann, A. P. A., Bakker, A. Q., Weijer, K., Res, P. C. M., and Spits, H. (1997) Inhibition of T cell and promotion of natural killer cell development by the dominant negative helix loop helix factor Id3. *J. Exp. Med.* **186,** 1597–1602.

16. Spain, L. M., Law, L. L., and Takahama, Y. (1998) Retroviral infection of T cell precursors in thymic organ culture, in *Developmental Biology Protocols* (Tuan, R. S. and Lo, C. W., eds.), Humana Press, Totowa, NJ, in press.

17. Sugawara, T., Di Bartolo, V., Miyazaki, T., Nakauchi, H., Acuto, O., and Takahama, Y. (1998) An improved retroviral transfer technique demonstrates inhibition of CD4⁻CD8⁻ thymocyte development by kinase-inactive ZAP-70. *J. Immunol.* **161,** 2888–2894.

18. Ikuta, K., Kina, T., MacNeil, I., Uchida, N., Peault, B., Chien, Y. H., and Weissman, I. L. (1990) A developmental switch in thymic lymphocyte maturation potential occurs at the level of hematopoietic stem cells. *Cell* **62,** 863–874.

19. Tsuda, S., Rieke, S., Hashimoto, Y., Nakauchi, H., and Takahama, Y. (1996) IL-7 supports D-J but not V-DJ rearrangement of T cell receptor β gene in fetal liver progenitor cells. *J. Immunol.* **156,** 3233–3242.

20. Sagara, S., Sugaya, K., Tokoro, Y., Tanaka, S., Takano, H., Kodama, H., Nakauchi, H., and Takahama, Y. (1997) B220 expression by T lymphoid progenitor cells in mouse fetal liver. *J. Immunol.* **158,** 666–676.

21. Theiler, K. (1989) *The House Mouse.* Springer-Verlag, New York, NY.

22. Kaufman, M. H. (1992) *The Atlas of Mouse Development.* Academic, San Diego, CA.

23. Butler, H. and Juurlink, B. H. (1987) A*n Atlas for Staging Mammalian and Chick Embryos.* CRC, Boca Raton, FL.

24. Takahama, Y., Suzuki, H., Katz, K. S., Grusby, M. J., and Singer, A. (1994) Positive selection of CD4+ T cells by TCR ligation without aggregation even in the absence of MHC. *Nature* **371,** 67–70.

25. Takahama, Y. and Nakauchi, H. (1996) Phorbol ester and calcium ionophore can replace TCR signals that induce positive selection of CD4 T cells. *J. Immunol.* **157,** 1508–1513.

26. Tokoro, Y., Tsuda, S., Tanaka, S., Nakauchi, H., and Takahama, Y. (1996) CD3-induced apoptosis of CD4+CD8+ thymocytes in the absence of clonotypic T-cell antigen receptor. *Eur. J. Immunol.* **26,** 1012–1017.

27. Watanabe, Y. and Katsura, Y. (1993) Development of T cell receptor αβ-bearing T cells in the submersion organ culture of murine fetal thymus at high oxygen concentration. *Eur. J. Immunol.* **23,** 200–205.

4

Purification of Immature CD4⁺CD8⁺ Thymocytes by Panning with Anti-CD8 Antibody

Terrence G. Gardner and Kelly P. Kearse

1. Introduction

Most T lymphocytes of the immune system differentiate within the thymus along the CD4/CD8 developmental pathway by a highly ordered process termed thymic selection *(1,2)*. The maturation status of thymocytes is commonly assessed by their expression of the coreceptor proteins CD4 and CD8 and their surface density of $\alpha\beta$ T cell receptors ($\alpha\beta$ TCR), *(1)*. Three major subpopulations of T cells exist within the thymus that exemplify the progression of thymocytes along the CD4/CD8 developmental pathway:

1. CD4⁻CD8⁻ (double-negative) thymocytes which express no $\alpha\beta$ TCR;
2. CD4⁺CD8⁺ (double-positive) thymocytes, which express no/low $\alpha\beta$ TCR; and
3. CD4⁺CD8⁻ and CD4⁻CD8⁺ (single positive) thymocytes, both of which express high surface density of $\alpha\beta$ TCR *(1–4)*, (**Fig. 1**).

Immature double-positive thymocytes are the predominant T lymphocyte subset in the thymus, accounting for approx 85% of T cells within the thymus *(1,2)*. Other thymocyte subsets constitute 3–8% each of remaining T cells in these approximate ratios: CD4⁻CD8⁻ thymocytes (3%); CD4⁺CD8⁻ thymocytes (7%); and CD4⁻CD8⁺ thymocytes (5%).

This chapter describes a simple procedure for the purification of murine CD4⁺CD8⁺ thymocytes by panning with anti-CD8 antibody (Ab). Briefly, a single-cell suspension of thymocytes is added to tissue culture plates that have been coated with anti-CD8 Ab, nonadherent cells are removed by washing, and CD8⁺ cells are recovered (**Fig. 2**). Because mature CD4⁻CD8⁺ (single-positive) thymocytes constitute a only small portion of total thymocytes, resultant cell populations are highly enriched for CD4⁺CD8⁺ (double-positive) thymocytes (approx 94–98% of purified cells).

From: *Methods in Molecular Biology, Vol. 134: T Cell Protocols: Development and Activation*
Edited by: K. P. Kearse © Humana Press Inc., Totowa, NJ

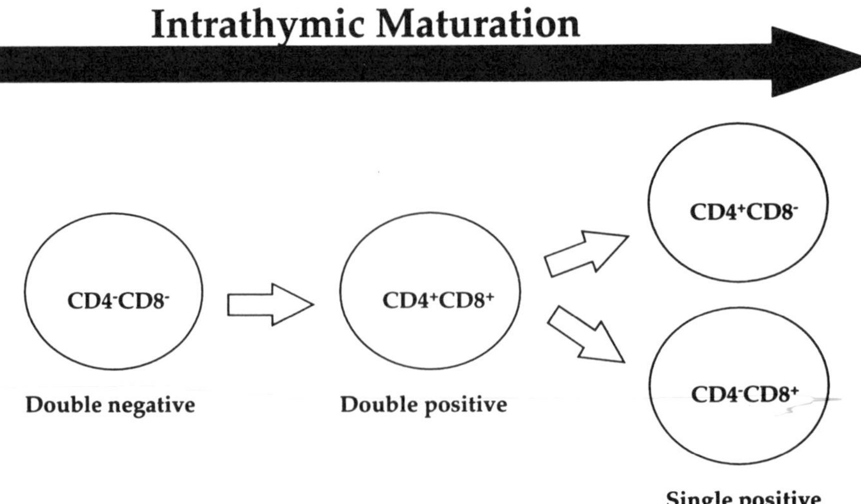

Fig. 1. Intrathymic development of thymocytes along the CD4/CD8 developmental pathway. Immature CD4⁻CD8⁻ thymocytes develop into progeny CD4⁺CD8⁺ thymocytes which maintain low expression of $\alpha\beta$TCR. Immature CD4⁺CD8⁺ thymocytes expressing $\alpha\beta$TCR of appropriate specificities are selected for further differentiation into mature T cells that express either CD4 (CD4⁺CD8⁻) or CD8 (CD4⁻CD8⁺) coreceptor molecules, but not both. Mature CD4⁺CD8⁻ and CD4⁻CD8⁺ thymocytes emigrate from the thymus to the periphery where they may localize in lymphoid organs (for example, lymph node or spleen).

2. Materials

2.1. Preparation of Anti-CD8 Antibody (Ab)

1. 83-12-5 anti-CD8 antibody (Ab), *(5)*; B hybridoma cells producing 83-12-5 Ab are commercially available from ATCC (ATCC # CRL-1971). In this procedure, 83-12-5 is collected as ascites fluid and purified by $NH_4(SO_4)_2$ precipitation (*see* **Note 2**).
2. $(NH_4)_2SO_4.$
3. Borate buffered saline (BBS), pH 8.5.
4. BBS, pH 8.5 containing 0.02% NaN_3.
5. Dialysis tubing (molecular weight cutoff ~ 6,000–8,000 kDa).
6. 0.45 µm membrane filters.

2.2. Purification of CD4⁺CD8⁺ (Double-Positive) Thymocytes by Panning

1. Phosphate buffered saline (PBS), pH 7.2.
2. 1 *M* $NaHCO_3$, pH 8.5 (filtered sterilized through 0.45 µm membrane and stored at room temperature; pH should be measured each time before use and adjusted if necessary).

Thymocyte single cell suspension

Anti-CD8 coated plates

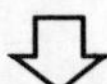

Incubate @ 4°C

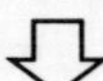

**Nonadherent cells
removed by washing**

**Adherent cells
detached by pipetting**

94-98% CD4+CD8+ thymocytes

Fig. 2. Purification of CD4+CD8+ thymocytes by panning with anti-CD8 Ab. Summary flow diagram of the procedure described in this protocol.

3. Panning solution: PBS, pH 7.2 containing 100 mM NaHCO$_3$.
4. RPMI medium containing 10% heat inactivated fetal calf serum (FCS), glutamine, penstrep, β-mercaptoethanol.
5. Tissue culture plates (Falcon # 1029).
6. 12cc syringe and 18g needles.
7. Nylon mesh.
8. Cotton gauze.

2.3. Analysis of Purified Populations

1. Hank's buffered saline solution (HBSS) without phenol red (Gibco-BRL, Gaithersburg, MD) containing 5% Bovine Serum Albumin (BSA-fraction V, Sigma Chemical Co., St. Louis, MO).
2. FITC-conjugated anti-CD4 and biotin (or rhodamine)-conjugated anti-CD8 monoclonal antibodies (MAb).

3. Methods

3.1. Preparation of Anti-CD8 Antibody (Ab)

1. Collect approx 40 mls of 83-12-5 ascites fluid and filter through gauze by gravity.
2. Add in (NH$_4$)$_2$SO$_4$ to give 50% saturation [40 mls × 0.305 g/mL = 12.2g (NH$_4$)$_2$SO$_4$].

3. Stir to dissolve and incubate for 5 h at 4°C.
4. Centrifuge at 10,000 *g* for 20 min.
5. Remove supernatant and resuspend pellet in 3 mls of BBS, pH 8.5.
6. Dialyze against 1L of BBS pH 8.5, 0.02% NaN_3 for approx 12 h at 4°C.
7. Repeat **step 6** twice.
8. Remove the solution from the dialysis tubing and centrifuge at 1,500 *g* for 10 min.
9. Remove the supernatant and filter this through a 0.45 µm membrane.
10. Varying dilutions of Ab solution are tested for their effectiveness (typically 1:20,000, 1:40,000, 1: 60,000 and 1:80,000). The working dilution of Ab should allow the cells to be washed off of the plate with moderate ease and give good purity. If the cells are difficult to remove from the plate (the cells should come off relatively easily with pipeting), the Ab solution is too concentrated; if the cells do not readily stick to the plate, the Ab solution is too dilute (*see* **Note 2**).
11. Stock Ab solution may be stored in the refrigerator for at least one year without loss of activity; for longer storage times, keep at –20°C (in small aliquots to avoid repeated freeze-thawing).

3.2. Purification of CD4⁺CD8⁺ (Double Positive) Thymocytes by Panning

1. The panning solution is made the day before cell purification. For 100 mls, combine 90 mls PBS, pH 7.2 with 10 mls 1 *M* $NaHCO_3$, pH 8.5. The pH of the $NaHCO_3$ solution should be checked before use (paper pH strips are ideal for this—because the stock solution is sterile, test only the portion that you need); adjust the pH with concentrated HCl if necessary.
2. The amount of panning solution that is needed is calculated as follows: 15 mls of solution are added to each tissue culture plate. The number of plates required is equal to the number of thymuses × 1.5 (two rounds of panning are performed, the second round requires only 1/2 the number of plates used in the first round). If you have an odd number of thymuses, round up to the nearest whole number (i.e., 3 thymuses = 3 × 1.5 = 4.5 = 5 plates; in this case use 3 plates for the first round of panning and 2 for the second). You should expect approx 40% total cell recovery or ~ 6–8 × 10^7 cells from each thymus used (*see* **Note 1**).
3. Filter the panning solution through a 0.45 µm membrane (*see* **Note 3**).
4. Add the Ab to the panning solution at the appropriate dilution (typically 1:40,000–1:60,000).
5. Add 15 mls of panning solution containing Ab to each tissue culture plate (Falcon#1029).
6. Swirl the plates gently to evenly distribute the solution (make sure all areas are covered).
7. Incubate the plates overnight at 37°C (in incubator); recheck the plates after placing them in the incubator to ensure that the solution remains evenly distributed.
8. The next day, prepare a single-cell suspension of thymocytes by first gently rolling the thymus back and forth across gauze (sterile if cells are to be used for

culture experiments); this will remove much of the blood and debris that may adhere to the thymus during its removal.

9. Place 1–3 thymuses in a Petri dish containing 2–3 mls of medium and gently tease the organ into a single-cell suspension. Two 18g needles (one straight, the other bent at a 90° angle) work well for this—hold the thymus down with the straight needle and use the bent needle to release the cells.

10. Add 10 mls of medium to the dish, pipet up the thymocytes, and filter this through a small square of nylon mesh (to remove debris) which is overlaid across a 50 mL centrifuge tube.

11. Tease the thymus organ again and pipet the cells as described in **step 10**.

12. Centrifuge cells at 300 g for 10 min at 4°C.

13. While cells are spinning, remove the Ab-coated plates from incubator.

14. Remove the Ab solution and discard.

15. Wash the plates 3× with 10 mls each of RPMI media (10% FCS); allow the media to flow gently down the side of the dish. On the last wash step, leave the media on the plate to prevent plates from drying; remove media immediately prior to adding cells (*see* **Note 4**).

16. Resuspend the thymocytes in 10 mls RPMI medium (10% FCS). Remove a small aliquot of unseparated (total) thymocytes for purity analysis (only 2×10^6 cells are needed—*see* **Subheading 3.3.**). Adjust the volume such that 10 mls of cell suspension will be added to each plate (1 plate/thymus).

17. Add the thymocyte cell suspension to plates.

18. Place plates on a level surface in the refrigerator and incubate for 1 h.

19. Remove the plates from the refrigerator. Tilt the plates toward you and remove the media by pipeting (aspiration of media by vaccum should be avoided as this tends to pull the cells off of the plate).

20. Carefully add 10 mls of media down the side of the plate, swirl plates (gently) in a circular motion, and remove the media. Repeat this step twice. The bottom of the plate should have a "frosted" appearance at this stage due to the adherence of cells.

21. Add 10 mls of media directly to the center of the plate (forcefully is okay); the plate should become clear in this region due to the removal of cells. Continue rinsing the plate until it becomes completely clear and all of the cells have been removed.

22. Centrifuge cells at 300 g for 10 min at 4°C.

23. While cells are spinning, remove the remaining Ab-coated plates from the incubator.

24. Wash the plates as described in **steps 14–15**.

25. Resuspend the thymocytes in RPMI medium (10% FCS) at 10 mls for each plate (this volume should be approx half of the original volume).

26. Add the thymocyte cell suspension to the plates.

27. Repeat **steps 18–21**.

28. Centrifuge the cells at 300 g for 10 min at 4°C; resuspend in 10 mls of media and count the cells. The cell yield should be approx 40% of the starting cell number; purity is analyzed as described in **Subheading 3.3.** below.

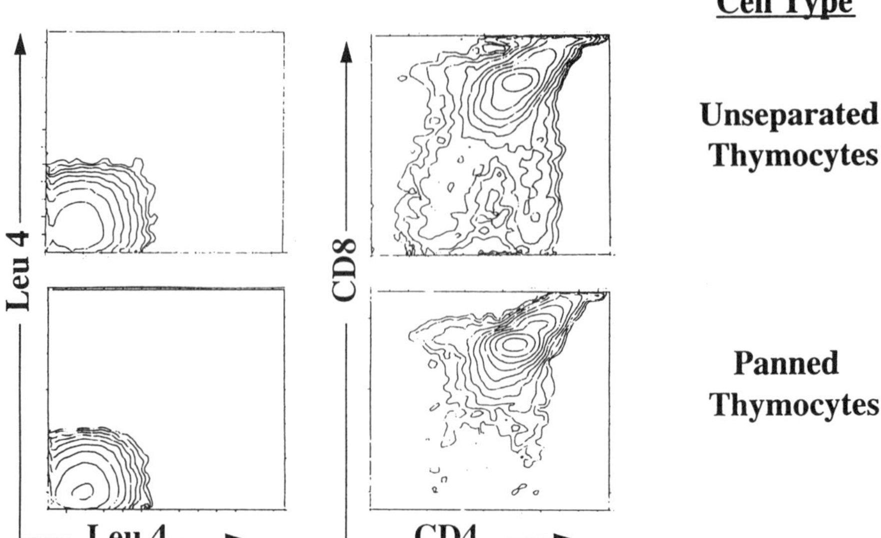

Fig. 3. Analysis of purified CD4+CD8+ thymocytes by flow cytometry. Two color analysis of CD4 and CD8 expression. Unseparated or anti-CD8 panned thymocytes were stained with FITC-conjugated anti-CD4 mAb and biotin-conjugated anti-CD8 mAb; Leu4 mAbs were used as negative controls. Note the enrichment of the CD4+CD8+ thymocytes in panned groups.

3.3. Analysis of Purified Populations

1. The cell purity is determined by standard flow cytometry methods, analyzing both unseparated (total) thymocytes and Ab-purified thymocytes for their surface expression of CD4 and CD8, using two color analysis.
2. In the example shown here, FITC- and Biotin-conjugated Leu4 MAbs (specific for human CD3 proteins) were used as negative controls.

   The cells were stained as follows (approx 1×10^6 cells/group):

Cell population	FITC Ab	Biotin Ab
a. Unseparated thymocytes	Leu4	Leu4
b. Unseparated thymocytes	CD4	CD8
c. Panned thymocytes	Leu4	Leu4
d. Panned thymocytes	CD4	CD8

3. A representative analysis is shown in **Fig. 3**. Note that the relative proportion of CD4+CD8+ thymocytes is enriched upon panning (**Fig. 3**).

4. Notes

1. The cellularity of the thymus is age-dependent; in general, the younger the mouse, the larger the thymus and the greater the cell yield. Mice 4–6 wk of age contain

$\sim$1.5–2.0 $\times$ 10^8 cells/thymus, which may vary somewhat according to strain. Additionally, CD4$^+$CD8$^+$ thymocytes are particularly susceptible to environmental stress. Therefore, it is advisable to allow mice a few days to recover from potentially traumatic events, e.g., shipping, before use.

2. Several forms of murine CD8 exist, i.e. Lyt 2.1 and Lyt 2.2. The anti-CD8 described in this procedure recognizes Lyt 2.2 (CD8 alpha 2.2) and is therefore not compatible with certain mouse strains, for example C3H/HeJ.

3. Do not add the 83-12-5 Ab to the panning solution before filtering—it will stick to the membrane and dramatically decrease the panning efficiency. The Ab solution contains NaN$_3$ and should therefore not require filtering for sterilization.

4. Much of the success of this technique relies on the appropriate rigor of swirling and washing. In starting out, it would be best to go easy and if the purity is less than desired, increase as necessary.

References

1. Fowlkes B. J. and Pardoll, D. M. (1989) Molecular and cellular events of T cell development. *Adv. Immunol.* **44,** 207–265.
2. von Boehmer, H. (1994) Positive selection of lymphocytes. *Cell* **76,** 219–227.
3. Blackman, M., Kappler, J., and Marrack, P. (1990) The role of the T cell receptor in positive and negative selection of developing T cells. *Science* **248,** 1335–1341.
4. Weissman, I. L. (1994) Developmental switches in the immune system. *Cell* **76,** 207–218.
5. Leo, O., Sachs, D., Samelson, L. E., Foo, M., Quinones, R., Gress, R., and Bluestone, J. A. (1986) Identification of monoclonal antibodies specific for the T cell receptor complex by Fc receptor-mediated CTL lysis. *J. Immunol.* **137,** 3874–3880.

5

Transfection and Transcription of Genes in Developing Thymocytes

Alison M. Michie and Juan Carlos Zúñiga-Pflücker

1. Introduction

Thymocyte development is characterized by the stage-specific expression of CD4 and CD8 surface molecules *(1)*. The earliest thymic immigrants, arriving from the fetal liver or bone marrow, lack CD4 and CD8 expression (CD4⁻ CD8⁻, double negative (DN)) *(2)*. This population can be further subdivided into four discrete subsets defined by the differential expression of CD117 (stem cell factor, SCF, receptor; c-kit) and CD25 (IL-2Rα) *(3)*. The earliest population is identified as CD117$^+$ CD25$^-$, and contains precursors for T, B, and natural killer (NK) lymphocyte lineages. Induction of CD25 expression on progenitor CD117$^+$ thymocytes characterizes commitment to the T cell lineage *(4)*. The CD117$^+$ CD25$^+$ stage is also accompanied by an increased rate of cellular proliferation *(5)*. Loss of CD117 expression correlates with the initiation of TCR-β gene rearrangement *(6)*. Only thymocytes that successfully rearrange their TCR-β locus expand and differentiate to the next stage; this important developmental checkpoint is known as β-selection *(7,8)*. Expression of CD25 ends with the generation of a functionally rearranged TCR-β chain, which together with the pre-TCR-α (pre-Tα) chain forms the pre-TCR complex *(9)*.

Pre-TCR-mediated signals induce a burst of proliferation and differentiation to the CD4$^+$ CD8$^+$ (double positive, DP) stage, at which point initiation of TCR-α gene rearrangement occurs *(8)*. DP thymocytes expressing a complete αβ-TCR/CD3 complex undergo positive and negative selection *(10,11)*, which results in the generation of mature CD4$^+$ CD8$^-$ and CD4$^-$ CD8$^+$ thymocytes.

T cell development is regulated by two key stage-specific checkpoints *(1)*. The first, β-selection, allows DN thymocytes with a functionally rearranged T cell receptor (TCR)-β chain gene to proliferate and differentiate to the DP stage

From: *Methods in Molecular Biology, Vol. 134: T Cell Protocols: Development and Activation*
Edited by: K. P. Kearse © Humana Press Inc., Totowa, NJ

of thymocyte differentiation; failure to generate a proper TCR-β chain results in thymocyte apoptosis. The second checkpoint allows DP thymocytes that have generated an α/β-TCR complex with the proper affinity/avidity for self-MHC to become positively selected and differentiate to the mature CD4 or CD8 single positive T cell stage *(12)*. Thymocytes that fail to rearrange a functional TCR-α chain gene or generate a TCR-α/β complex with high affinity/avidity for self-MHC die by apoptosis, either due to neglect or negative selection, respectively.

To study the regulation of gene expression or cellular signaling events during thymocyte development several experimental strategies are available. These approaches rely on the introduction of foreign DNA into thymocytes *(13)*. A wide variety of DNA transfection protocols have been developed, such as the use of retroviruses, liposomes, adenoviruses, gene-gun, and electroporation *(13–16)*. Each of these approaches has its own merits and drawbacks, depending on the stage of development being studied and the type of assay system employed for analytical readout. In the current chapter, a method is described for the transfection of thymocytes by electroporation.

1.1. Electroporation as One Option for the Transfection of Thymocytes

As pointed out in the Introduction, several experimental approaches are available for the transfection of thymocytes. This chapter will detail electroporation as the most effective method for DNA transfection of thymocytes, for the transient analysis of gene expression or for cellular signal transduction studies of a particular subset of developing thymocytes. This approach can be used in combination with different types of reporter-gene plasmids, such as luciferase, β-galactosidase, and chloramphenicol acetyl transferase (CAT).

Transfection of thymocytes by means other than electroporation have been reported. Retroviral infection of early fetal thymocytes allowed for stable expression of transduced genes during thymocyte differentiation *(14)*. This was achieved by incubating day 13 fetal thymus lobes in Terasaki wells, as a hanging drop, for 40 h with a confluent monolayer of adherent retroviral packaging cells. Thereafter the lobes are allowed to differentiate using a standard fetal thymic organ culture (FTOC). A second method of transfecting thymocytes *in situ* employs the use of a gene-gun, used to bombard fetal thymic lobes with DNA-coated gold microspheres *(13)*. This approach allows for the transient transfection of thymuses to assay for gene expression or cellular signaling events.

One key advantage of electroporation over those approaches mentioned in the Introduction is its reproducibility and the fact that it is easily applicable to thymocytes in cell suspension *(17)*. Thus, one can isolate by flow cytometry cell sorting or magnetic bead separation, a particular target population of thymocytes to be assayed.

2. Materials

2.1. Source of Developing Thymocytes

1. The basis of this protocol is the transfection of developing thymocytes, therefore it is necessary to use freshly isolated thymuses as a source of developing thymocytes (*see* **Note 1**).
2. Fetal thymuses isolated from gestational day 14–16 timed-pregnant mice (*see* **Note 1**).
3. Thymuses from recombination activating gene-2-deficient (RAG-2$^{-/-}$) mice *(18)* can be used as an alternative source of early developing thymocytes (*see* **Note 2**).
4. Nylon mesh filters, 70 µm pore size (BioDesign, Carmel, NY) (*see* **Note 3**).

2.2. Solutions and Media

1. All solutions and reagents for the luciferase and β-galactosidase assays are included with the purchase of the Dual-Light reporter gene assay system (Tropix, Perkin Elmer-Applied Biosystems, Norwalk, CT).
2. Media for growing thymocytes: DMEM-high glucose (Gibco-BRL, Gaithersburg, MD), plus 10% fetal calf serum (FCS), and antibiotics (Pen/Strep; Gibco-BRL).
3. Media for electroporation: RPMI-1640 (Gibco-BRL), plus 20% FCS.
4. Phosphate-buffered saline (PBS) (Gibco-BRL).

2.3. Plasmids

1. All plasmids to be used for electroporation should be purified by CsCl-gradient centrifugation, or by anion-exchange chromatography, such as Qiagen columns (Valencia, CA).
2. TE: 10 m*M* Tris-HCl, pH 7.4, 1 m*M* EDTA pH 8.0
3. All plasmids used were obtained from Stratagene (La Jolla, CA) (*see* **Note 4**). Plasmids were purified using Qiagen columns and resuspended in TE, at a concentration range of 2–5 µg/µL.

2.4. Electroporator and Electroporation Supplies

1. There are several electroporators available, we have optimized our protocol using a BTX-Electro Cell Manipulator 600 (BTX, San Diego). This unit provides several features, which makes it a great choice for this particular protocol.
2. Electroporation cuvets, 4 mm-gap (BTX).
3. 1 mL pipets (Falcon Labware, Franklin Lakes, NJ), these pipets allow for easy transfer of electroporated cells from the cuvets to tissue culture plates.
4. Tissue culture plates, 96 well round-bottom (Falcon Labware).
5. Dual-Light reporter gene assay system (Tropix, Perkin Elmer-Applied Biosystems).

3. Methods

3.1. Isolation of Developing Thymocytes

1. Prepare a single-cell suspension, in PBS, from thymuses obtained from a day 14–15 fetal mouse or young-adult RAG-2$^{-/-}$ mouse (*see* **Notes 1** and **2**). If cell sorting is desired prior to electroporation, *see* **Note 3**.

2. Pass the thymus cell suspension through a 70-µm nylon mesh filter and count the number of cells.
3. Wash the cells in RPMI with 20% FCS.
4. Resuspend the thymocytes in RPMI with 20% FCS using the appropriate volume to obtain a cell concentration of $1–4 \times 10^7$ cells/mL, depending on the number of cells to be used per electroporation condition.
5. Place the thymocyte suspension on ice.

3.2. Electroporation and Culture Conditions

1. To a dry and sterile electroporation cuvet add 10–20 µg of each DNA-plasmid. The volume of the plasmid solution should not be greater than 25 µL or 10% of the total electroporation volume (250 µL) (*see* **Note 5**).
2. Place the DNA-containing cuvets on ice for 5 min.
3. To the cold DNA-containing cuvets add 250 µL of thymocytes ($1–4 \times 10^7$ cells/mL).
4. Place on ice for 10 min. Gently shake the cuvet prior to electroporation.
5. Transfer the cuvet to the electroporator, using the following settings: 260 V, 186 Ω, and 1,700 µF. Apply the electrical current. The time constant should read 80–90 msec.
6. Place the cuvet on ice for 10 min.
7. Transfer the electroporated cells, using a 1 mL pipet, into two wells of a 96-well round-bottom plate.
8. Rinse the cuvet with 200 µL of DMEM with 10% FCS, and transfer 100 µL of the remaining cells to the same wells as before.
9. Place the 96-well plate in an incubator (37°C, 5% CO_2) for 8–24 h, depending on the readout system used for the analysis (*see* **Note 6**). Alternatively, if a treatment is desired, incubate the electroporated thymocytes for 4–6 h prior to the addition of antibody, cytokine, or pharmacological reagents. Thereafter, continue incubating for 12–18 h prior to analysis.

3.3. Preparation of Cell Extracts
and Reporter-Gene Detection Assay

1. Resuspend the electroporated thymocytes and follow the manufacturer's instructions for the preparation of the cell extracts and luciferase and/or β-galactosidase analysis, *see* **Note 7**.
2. Detailed instructions and all necessary reagents are provided with the purchase of the Dual-Light reporter gene assay system (Tropix, PE-Applied Biosystems).

4. Notes

1. As this protocol is specifically aimed at transfecting developing thymocytes, the best source of these cells comes from freshly isolated day 14 to 15 fetal thymuses. Mate mice to obtain timed-pregnant females for the desired day of gestation. Breeding pairs should be set up in the late afternoon. Examine female mice the next morning. The day on which a vaginal plug is detected is designated as day 0.

2. As an alternative to using fetal thymic lobes as a source of developing thymocytes, one can dissect thymuses from 3-week-old RAG$^{-/-}$ mice. Thymocytes from these mice are unable to complete T cell development and become arrested at the CD117$^-$CD25$^+$ stage. Therefore, the thymus phenotype of adult RAG$^{-/-}$ mice resembles that of immature day 15 fetal mice. The age of the mice is important, as the thymic cellularity of these mice decreases with age ($\sim$3 $\times$ 10^6 thymocytes in a 3-week-old mouse to $\sim$1 $\times$ 10^6 cells in adult mice).

3. To carry out electroporations of specific cell populations from the thymus, flow cytometric cell sorting of total thymocytes is required. Single-cell suspensions can be stained with the desired antibodies (e.g., CD117 and CD25 or CD3, CD4, and CD8) in Hank's balanced salt solution (without phenol red) containing 1% BSA (staining buffer) in a volume of 300 µL. Incubate on ice for 20 min, wash twice in staining buffer, and pass the cell suspension through a 70 µm nylon filter prior to sorting. Please note that it is essential to obtain at least 2.5 $\times$ 10^6 sorted cells for each electroporation condition.

4. In this protocol we have made use of novel reporter-plasmids (commercially-available from Stratagene) for in vivo analysis of the mitogen-activating protein kinase (MAPK) signaling pathway. Moreover, plasmids are also available for the study of other signaling pathways such as; c-Jun N-terminal kinase (JNK) and cyclic AMP-dependent protein kinase (PKA). This approach takes advantage of three plasmids: the first one encodes for a fusion protein containing an activation domain derived from the specific substrate recognition site for each kinase (pFA-Elk) and a DNA binding protein domain derived from the yeast DNA transcriptional activator GAL4; the second plasmid encodes for the luciferase gene controlled by five repeats of GAL4 binding element followed by a basic transcriptional promoter (TATATA) (pFR-Luc); the third plasmid provides a positive control, encoding for constitutively active versions of the MAP kinase to be tested, which is under the transcriptional control of strong enhancer/promoter elements. When the fusion-activator and luciferase-reporter plasmids are cotransfected into mammalian cells, with or without the positive control plasmid (pFC-MEK1), direct or indirect phosphorylation of the fusion-activator protein, results in the induced transcription of the luciferase gene from the reporter plasmid. The intensity of signal can be measured by carrying out a standard luciferase assay. To control for transfection efficiency and cell viability during the experiment, the thymocytes are cotransfected with a plasmid encoding β-galactosidase, which is under the transcriptional control of the CMV promoter/enhancer. The β-galactosidase activity is used to index the luciferase signal detected, as assays for luciferase and β-galactosidase activity can be performed within the same sample tube. This is accomplished using a novel detection system, in which both enzymatic reactions are measured in the form of light emission; i.e., luciferase upon catalytic breakdown of the substrate luciferin, and β-galactosidase upon catalysis of a novel substrate, Galacton-Plus (Tropix, Bedford, MA).

5. This procedure has been applied to the activation of the MAPK signaling cascade upon stimulation of thymocytes with the phorbol ester, phorbol-12-myristate-13-acetate (PMA) and the calcium ionophore, ionomycin (*see* **Fig. 1**). This was

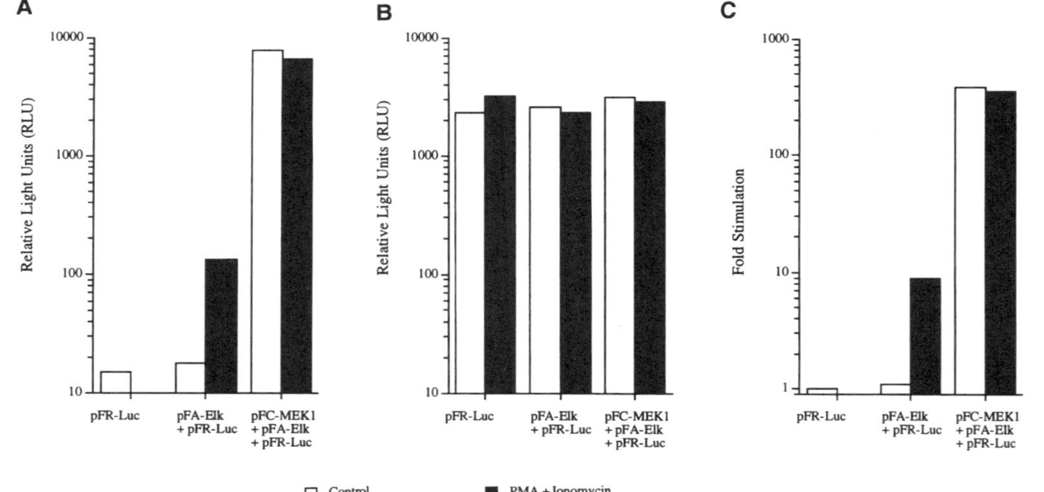

Fig. 1. Transfection of RAG-deficient thymocytes by electroporation for the detection of MAPK signaling activity following mitogenic stimulation. Thymocytes from RAG$^{-/-}$ mice were electroporated and stimulated with PMA and ionomycin, see text and **Notes 5–7** for details. (a) Analysis of luciferase activity assayed from cell lysates of RAG$^{-/-}$ thymocytes, data are presented as relative light units (RLU) detected from each sample. Thymocytes were transfected by electroporation as indicated, using a combination of the following plasmids: pFR-Luc, pFA-Elk and pFC-MEK1. Data are shown for control-unstimulated (open bars) and PMA/ionomycin-stimulated (filled bars) thymocytes. (b) Analysis of β-galactosidase activity assayed from the same cell lysate sample tube used in part (a), data are presented as RLU detected from each sample. All thymocyte groups, shown in part (a), were cotransfected with the CMV-βgal plasmid. (c) Fold stimulation of luciferase activity of RAG$^{-/-}$ thymocytes following mitogenic stimulation, determined by setting the luciferase activity of the control pFR-Luc sample as the denominator. The data are also indexed according to level of β-galactosidase activity detected for each sample, as shown in part (b). Background RLU readings (empty tube) were subtracted from all of the data points. The data analyses shown are all derived from assays carried out in duplicate, with a numerical range of < 5% RLU.

achieved by using the in vivo 'pathdetect' signaling reporter plasmids from Stratagene (*see* **Note 4**). The reporter plasmids (pFR-Luc, pFA-Elk and pFC-MEK1) were each utilized at a concentration of 20 µg, and 10 µg of CMV-βgal was used. Plasmid concentrations of 2–5 µg/µL allowed for the addition of no more than 25 µL of plasmid DNA solution per cuvet.

6. Electroporated cells were incubated in a 96-well round bottom plate for 12–18 h, and just prior to stimulation the thymocytes from each well were transferred to one well of a 12-well plate with 2 mL of DMEM with 10% FCS. PMA (10 ng/mL) and ionomycin (1 ng/mL) were added to the cells and incubated at 37°C for a further 4–6 h.

7. To increase the sensitivity for luciferase and β-galactosidase activity, lyse the thymocytes in the minimum volume required, and not as outlined in the instructions for the Dual Light Kit. Therefore, if the experiment is carried out in duplicate, lyse the cells with 50 µL of lysis buffer, and use 25 µL/assay. The rest of the procedure is performed as indicated in the kit's instructions.

References

1. Godfrey, D. I. and Zlotnik, A. (1993) Control points in early T-cell development. *Immunol. Today* **14,** 547–553.
2. Godfrey, D. I., Kennedy, J., Suda, T., and Zlotnik, A. (1993) A developmental pathway involving four phenotypically and functionally distinct subsets of CD3⁻CD4⁻CD8⁻ triple negative adult mouse thymocytes defined by CD44 and CD25 expression. *J. Immunol.* **150,** 4244–4252.
3. Zúñiga-Pflücker, J. C. and Lenardo, M. J. (1996) Regulation of thymocyte development from immature progenitors. *Curr. Opin. Immunol.* **8,** 215–224.
4. Zúñiga-Pflücker, J. C., Jiang, D., and Lenardo, M. J. (1995) Requirement for TNF-α and IL-1α in fetal thymocyte commitment and differentiation. *Science* **268,** 1906–1909.
5. Pénit, C., Lucas, B., and Vasseur, F. (1995) Cell expansion and growth arrest phases during the transition from precursor (CD4⁻8⁻) to immature (CD4⁺8⁺) thymocytes in normal and genetically modified mice. *J. Immunol.* **154,** 5103–5113.
6. Godfrey, D. I., Kennedy, J., Monbaerts, P., Tonegawa, S., and Zlotnik, A. (1994) Onset of TCR-β rearrangement and role of TCR-β expression during CD3⁻CD4⁻CD8⁻ thymocyte differentiation. *J. Immunol.* **152,** 4783–4792.
7. Hoffman, E. S., Passoni, L., Crompton, T., Leu, T. M., Schatz, D. G., Koff, A., Owen, M. J., and Hayday, A. C. (1996) Productive T-cell receptor beta-chain gene rearrangement: coincident regulation of cell cycle and clonality during development in vivo. *Genes. Dev.* **10,** 948–962.
8. von Boehmer, H. and Fehling, H. J. (1997) Structure and function of the pre-T cell receptor. *Annu. Rev. Immunol.* **15,** 433–452.
9. Saint-Ruf, C., Ungewiss, K., Groettrup, M., Bruno, L., Fehling, H. J., and von Boehmer, H. (1994) Analysis and expression of a cloned pre-T cell receptor gene. *Science* **266,** 1208–1212.
10. Fowlkes, B. J. and Schweighoffer, E. (1995) Positive selection of T cells. *Curr. Opin. Immunol.* **7,** 188–195.

11. Kisielow, P. and von Boehmer, H. (1990) Negative and positive selection on immature thymocytes: timing and the role of ligand for α/β T cell receptor. *Semm. Immunol.* **2,** 35–44.
12. Allen, P. M. (1994) Peptides in positive and negative selection: a delicate balance. *Cell* **76,** 593–596.
13. Zúñiga-Pflücker, J. C., Schwartz, H. L., and Lenardo, M. J. (1993) Gene transcription in differentiating immature T cell receptor[neg] thymocytes resembles antigen-activated mature T cells. *J. Exp. Med.* **178,** 1139–1149.
14. Crompton, T., Gilmour, K. C., and Owen, M. J. (1996) The MAP kinase pathway controls differentiation from double-negative to double positive thymocyte. *Cell* **86,** 243–251.
15. Suzuki, H., Zelphati, O., Hildebrand, G., and Leserman, L. (1991) CD4 and CD7 molecules as targets for drug delivery from antibody bearing liposomes. *Exp. Cell Res.* **193,** 112–119.
16. Rooke, R., Waltzinger, C., Benoist, C., and Mathis, D. (1997) Targeted complementation of MHC class II deficiency by intrathymic delivery of recombinant adenoviruses. *Immunity* **7,** 123–134.
17. Nickoloff, J. A., editor (1995) *Animal Cell Electroporation and Electrofusion Protocols.* Vol. 48. Methods in Molecular Biology. Humana Press Inc., Totowa, NJ.
18. Shinkai, Y., Rathbun, G., Lam, K.-P., Oltz, E. M., Stewart, V., Mendelsohn, M., Charron, J., Datta, M., Young, F., Stall, A. M., and Alt, F. W. (1992) RAG-2-deficient mice lack mature lymphocytes owing to inability to initiate V(D)J rearrangement. *Cell* **68,** 855–867.

6

Analysis of CD4/CD8 Lineage Commitment by Pronase Treatment and Reexpression Assay

Harumi Suzuki

1. Introduction

During the developmental process of T cells in the thymus, immature CD4CD8 double positive thymocytes (DP) are subject to undergo positive selection process to become either CD4 single positive (SP) or CD8-SP mature cells *(1–3)*. Since both CD4-SP and CD8-SP mature T cells are the progeny of immature DP thymocytes, positive selection requires a lineage commitment step in which synthesis of one or the other coreceptor molecule is terminated. The mechanism of CD4/8 lineage commitment process, i.e., how does thymocyte stop one or the other coreceptor synthesis, is still unclear although many types of models have been presented *(4–10)*.

The assay termed "coreceptor reexpression assay" *(7)* was developed in order to study CD4/8 lineage committed cells. To detect CD4/8 lineage commitment, i.e., status of internal CD4/8 synthesis of individual cell regardless of its surface CD4/8 phenotype, sorted thymocytes are subjected to pronase digestion to remove existing CD4/8 coreceptor on the cell surface, and then let them reexpress CD4 and/or CD8 during overnight suspension culture at 37°C. If a cell reexpresses CD4 but not CD8 after incubation, this indicates commitment to the CD4 lineage and that the cell is synthesizing only CD4. (**Fig. 1**). Both CD4 and CD8 are susceptible to pronase digestion *(11)*, and most of the surface CD4/8 molecules can be removed by pronase treatment even in the presence of antibodies bound to CD4/8 (**Fig. 2**). Reexpression of coreceptors requires *de novo* mRNA and protein synthesis because inhibitors of protein synthesis and mRNA synthesis block coreceptor reexpression (**Fig. 2**). A reexpressed CD4/8 phenotype therefore represents the CD4/8 transcription status inside the cell, i.e., CD4/8 lineage commitment. A great advantage of this method is detection of CD4/CD8 lineage commitment of cells of any surface

From: *Methods in Molecular Biology, Vol. 134: T Cell Protocols: Development and Activation*
Edited by: K. P. Kearse © Humana Press Inc., Totowa, NJ

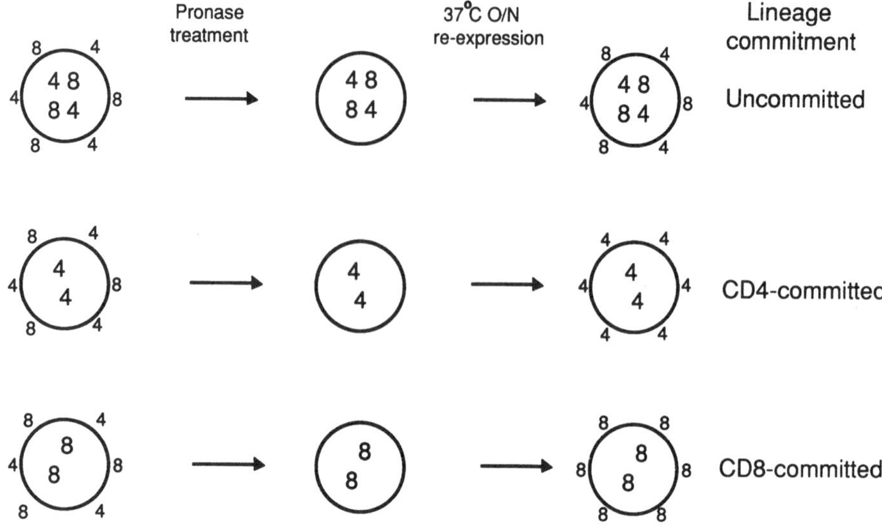

Coreceptor Re-expression Assay

Fig. 1. Principle of coreceptor reexpression assay DP thymocytes committed to the CD4 lineage should synthesize CD4 but not CD8, regardless of their surface CD4/8 phenotype. In order to evaluate the CD4/8 transcription status, preexisting surface CD4/8 are first removed by pronase digestion. Pronase-treated cells are then placed in suspension culture which will allow them to reexpress CD4/8 coreceptor molecules.

phenotype, thus this method is a powerful tool for studying thymocyte lineage commitment *(12–15)*.

2. Materials

2.1. Cell Sorting

The staining antibody for cell sorting depends on your purpose of the experiment. Usually, total thymocytes are stained for CD4, CD8 and an additional surface antigen (e.g., CD5, CD69) to define the sorting population of interest.

1. Antibodies: FITC conjugated anti-CD8 (53.6.72), PE conjugated anti-CD4 (GK1.5), (Becton Dickinson, San Jose, CA or Pharmingen, San Diego, CA). Use 10–20µg of fluorescein conjugated antibodies for staining of 1×10^8 thymocytes.
2. Staining media: Hanks balanced salt solution (HBSS) (without phenol red) containing 0.1% bovine serum albumin and 0.1% NaN_3. Two percent fetal calf serum (FCS) may be used instead of 0.1% (BSA).

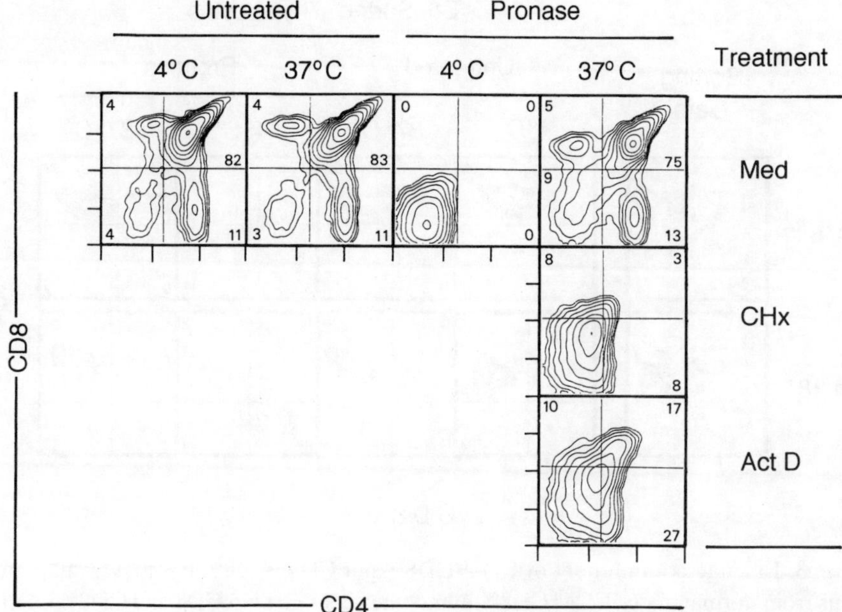

Fig. 2. Coreceptor reexpression requires active transcription and protein synthesis. Single cell suspensions of B6 thymocytes were preincubated with medium or 0.04% pronase to remove preexisting surface coreceptor molecules. Where indicated, some of the reexpression cultures contained 10µg/mL cycloheximide (Chx) or 3µg/mL actinomycin D (Act D).

3. Collection tube for sorting: RPMI-1640 media containing 25% FCS, 10µg/mL gentamycin. For this, put 1.5 mL of media into Falcon 2058 tube and freeze before use.

2.2. Pronase Digestion

1. PBS, pH 7.2
2. Pronase solution: Prepare 0.04% Pronase (Calbiochem, San Diego, CA) in PBS and filter for sterilization. Addition of 100µg/mL DNase I (Boehringer-Mannheim, Indianapolis, IN) greatly increases cell recovery by preventing cell aggregation.

3. Methods

3.1. Cell Sorting

1. Prepare single-cell suspension of thymocytes and stain them with appropriate antibodies (typically CD4 and CD8). 10µg of fluorescein-conjugated antibody is sufficient for 10^8 thymocytes.
2. Set desired gate (e.g., CD4^{hi} CD8^{lo} of CD4^{lo} CD8^{hi}) (*see* **Fig. 3**) and collect the cells using a cell sorter (FACStar, FACS Vanatage, Becton Dickinson). If the

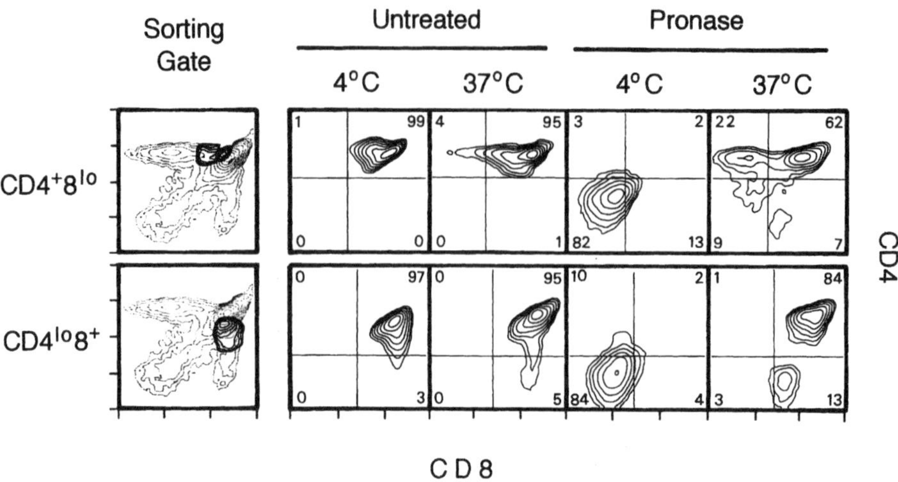

Fig. 3. Lineage commitment of CD4^{hi}CD8^{lo} and CD4^{lo}CD8^{hi} thymocyte subpopulations from normal mice. CD4^{hi}CD8^{lo} thymocytes contain both CD4 and CD8 committed cells, but CD4^{lo}CD8^{hi} thymocytes contain only CD8-committed cells. Purified populations of CD4^{hi}CD8^{lo} and CD4^{lo}CD8^{hi} thymocytes were obtained by electronically sorting B6 thymocytes according to the sorting gates superimposed on the original thymocyte population displayed (left). Sorted thymocyte populations were then assessed for lineage commitment by the coreceptor reexpression assay.

cell sorter does not have a cooling device for collection tubes, collecting cells into a tube containing frozen media will increase the viability of sorted cells. For detailed analysis, more than 2×10^6 sorted cells should be collected.

3. Spin collected cells at $500g$ for 30 min, and gather all of the sorted cells into one tube. Wash with 1mL of PBS twice and resuspend with 0.2–0.5mL of PBS for cell counting (*see* **Note 1**).

3.2. Pronase Treatment

1. Divide sorted cells into 2 groups (one for pronase treatment and the other for untreated controls) and spin again ($500g \times 10$min).
2. Resuspend the pellet with 0.5–1mL of pronase solution (0.04% pronase, 100µg/mL DNase I in PBS) and incubate for 10 min at 37°C with frequent shaking.
3. Spin down the cells ($500g \times 10$min), discard the supernatant and add 1mL of pronase solution to the pellet again (without washing). Mix well and treat for another 10 min at 37° C.
4. After incubation, add 1mL of FCS to quench pronase activity and wash the cells with 0.5mL of culture media ($500g \times 10$min). Divide pronase treated cells into 2 groups for incubation either at 4°C or 37°C for 12–16 h in a 24-well culture plate (*see* **Notes 2** and **3**).

5. After 16–24 h incubation, harvest cells and stain them for CD4 and CD8 for analysis of coreceptor reexpression. The same staining antibody used for sorting may be used at this stage.

4. Notes

1. Centrifugation: Since you have to handle small number of cells, be careful about spinning. Spinning for a longer time with decreased volume will increase the cell recovery. It is important that the initial spin after sorting is for 30 min at 500*g*, because sorted drops are electronically charged and cells tend to stick to the tube wall. A longer spin does not hurt the cells but avoid spinning at high speeds.
2. CD28, HSA as well as CD4 and CD8 are sensitive for pronase digestion. Surprisingly, a lot of surface molecules such as TCRβ, CD3ε, CD5, etc. are pronase resistant. Thus, TCR-dependent signals may be delivered even after pronase treatment *(11)*. The possibility exists that removal of surface proteins by pronase treatment delivers some type of signal into the cell, although no change in surface activation markers has been detected.
3. CD4/8 molecules occupied with staining antibody are relatively resistant to pronase digestion compared to molecules without bound antibody. Specifically, PE-conjugated antibodies interferes much more with pronase digestion than FITC-conjugated antibodies (**Fig. 3**). Treating the cells twice with pronase is helpful for this. Alternatively, cells may be washed thoughly with PBS before treatment to remove any proteins in solution.
4. Other types of protease may be used (e.g., trypsin) for digestion of surface CD4 and CD8, however, pronase was the least harsh of all proteases we tested for their effect on cell viability.

References

1. von Boehmer H., Swat, W., and Kisielow, P. (1993) Positive selection of immature alpha beta T cells. *Immunol. Rev.* **135,** 67–79.
2. Kisielow, P., Teh, H. S., Bluthmann, H., and von Boehmer, H. (1988) Positive selection of antigen-specific T cells in thymus by restricting MHC molecules. *Nature* **335,** 730–733.
3. Sha, W. C., Nelson, C. A., Newberry, R. D., Kranz, D. M., Russell, J. H., and Loh, D. Y. (1988) Positive and negative selection of an antigen receptor on T cells in transgenic mice. *Nature* **336,** 73–76.
4. Robey, E., Fowlkes, B. J., Gordon, J. W., et al. (1991) Thymic selection in CD8 transgenic mice supports an instructive model for commitment to a CD4 or CD8 lineage. *Cell* **64,** 99–107.
5. Davis, C. B., Kileen, N., Crooks, M. E. C., et al. (1993) Evidence for a stochastic mechanism in the differentiation of mature subsets of T lymphocytes. *Cell* **73,** 237–247.
6. Chan, H. S., Cosgrove, D., Waltzinger, C., Benoist, C., and Mathis, D. (1993) Another view of the selective model of thymocyte selection. *Cell* **73,** 225–236.

7. Suzuki, H., Punt, J. A., Granger, L. G., and Singer, A. (1995) Asymmetric signaling requirements for thymocyte commitment to the CD4+ versus CD8+ T cell lineage: a new perspective on lineage commitment and positive selection. *Immunity* **2,** 413–425.
8. Itano, A., Salmon, P., Kioussis, D., Tolaini, M., Corbella, P., and Robey, E. (1996) The cytoplasmic domain of CD4 promotes the development of CD4 lineage T cells. *J. Exp. Med.* **83,** 731–741.
9. Matechak, E. O., Killeen, N., Hedrick, S. M., and Fowlkes, B. J. (1996) MHC class II-specific T cells can develop in the CD8 lineage when CD4 is absent. *Immunity* **4,** 337–347.
10. Robey, E., Chang, D., Itano, A., Cado, D., Alexander, H., Lans, D., Weinmaster, G., and Salmon, P. (1996) An activated form of Notch influences the choice between CD4 and CD8 T cell lineages. *Cell* **87,** 483–492.
11. Kearse, K. P., Takahama, Y., Punt, J. A., Sharrow, S. O., and Singer, A. (1995) Early molecular events induced by T cell receptor (TCR) signaling in immature CD4$^+$CD8$^+$ thymocytes: Increased synthesis of TCR-α protein is an early response to TCR signaling that compensates for TCR-α instability, improves TCR assembly, and parallels other indicators of positive selection. *J. Exp. Med.* **181,** 193–202.
12. Punt, J. A., Suzuki, H., Granger, L. G., Sharrow, S. O., and Singer, A. (1996) Lineage commitment in the thymus: only the most differentiated (TCR^{hi}bcl-2^{hi}) subset of CD4$^+$CD8$^+$ thymocytes has selectively terminated CD4 or CD8 synthesis. *J. Exp. Med.* **184,** 2091–2099.
13. Lucas, B. and Germain, R. N. (1996) Unexpectedly complex regulation of CD4/CD8 coreceptor expression supports a revised model for CD4$^+$CD8$^+$ thymocyte differentiation. *Immunity* **5,** 461–477.
14. Ohoka, Y., Kuwata, T., Asada, A., Zhao, Y., Mukai, M., and Iwata M. (1997) Regulation of thymocyte lineage commitment by the level of classical protein kinase C activity. *J. Immunol.* **158,** 5707–5716.
15. Suzuki, H., Shinkai, Y., Granger, L. G., Alt, F. W., Love, P. E., and Singer, A. (1997) Commitment of immature CD4$^+$8$^+$ thymocytes to the CD4 lineage requires CD3 signaling but does not require expression of clonotypic T cell receptor (TCR) chains. *J. Exp. Med.* **86,** 17–23.

7

Intrathymic Delivery of MHC Genes Using Recombinant Adenoviruses

Ronald Rooke, Christophe Benoist, and Diane Mathis

1. Introduction

Advances in the study of thymic selection have relied heavily on animals that are genetically manipulated either by transgenesis and/or by knock out technology. Besides being costly and time consuming, these methods suffer inherent limitations (reviewed in **refs. *1–3***). In an effort to first, complement the existing panoply of methodologies used in the study of thymocyte selection and second, circumvent some of the problems inherent to these methods, we have developed an adenovirus-based vector system to deliver MHC class II genes to the thymic stroma. When injected into MHC class II-deficient animals (II°) *(4)*, these vectors punctually restore the expression of MHC class II molecules on the surface of transduced thymic stromal cells *(5)*. In turn, the block in T-cell development associated with the absence of MHC class II molecules in these thymi is relieved and significant numbers of mature CD4 single positive thymocytes appear *(5)*. Alternatively, this gene delivery system has also been used to look at positive selection of T cell receptor (TCR) transgenic thymocytes by a known peptide engineered in the invariant chain gene *(6)*. Although variability is seen in the reconstitution of injected animals, this method is a reliable delivery tool for punctual expression of genes in the thymic stroma. The experiments we have carried out indicate that the cortex of the thymus is the main target for MHC class II expression. Here, we will first describe the procedures to make, characterize, and produce high titer stocks of recombinant viruses, followed by the surgical procedure allowing intrathymic delivery of the virus.

From: *Methods in Molecular Biology, Vol. 134: T Cell Protocols: Development and Activation*
Edited by: K. P. Kearse © Humana Press Inc., Totowa, NJ

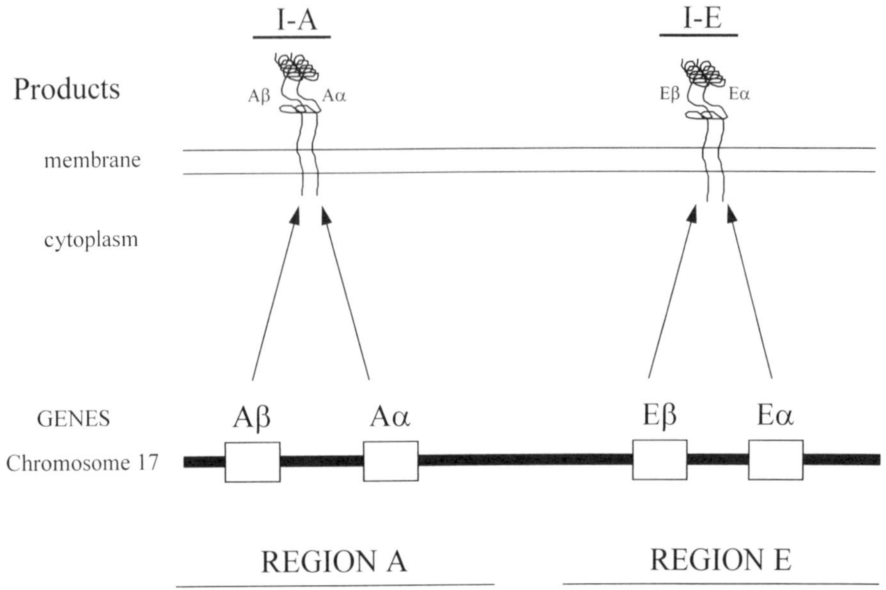

Fig. 1. Genomic organization and expression of MHC class II products. *See text* for details.

1.1. Murine MHC Class II Molecular Structure and Expression

The vast majority of MHC class II molecules that reach the cell surface are heterotrimers made up of one α chain, one β chain and a peptide of variable length (12–24 amino acids). The α and β chains are 33–35 and 26–28 kDa, respectively, whereas the peptide comes from a protein usually taken up from the extracellular milieu (reviewed in **ref. 7**). In the mouse, the H-2 complex, located on chromosome 17, contains two MHC class II regions (I-A and I-E). Each region is made up of two genes that encode polypeptides that associate to make αβ heterodimers (**Fig. 1**). The α chains pair noncovalently, in the endoplasmic reticulum, with the β counterpart of the same region. This complex can then associate with the proteins involved in further processing and transport to the cell surface (reviewed in **ref. 8**), thus generating the I-A and I-E MHC molecules. MHC class II deficient animals have been generated *(4)* by disrupting the β chain of the I-A locus in an embryonic cell line obtained from a mouse strain that is incapable of expressing the I-Eα chain, because of a naturally occurring mutation in its promoter *(9)*. The virtual absence of MHC class II expression in animals bearing both mutations is explained by the necessity of having the two chains of each region for proper processing and cell surface expression of MHC class II molecules, as well as by the absence of cross-pairing of the α and β chains from different regions *(10)*. In cells taken from mutated animals, the intracellular orphan chains (I-Aα and I-Eβ) are targeted for destruction. With this in mind, we have constructed adenovirus vectors that express a MHC class II cDNA that is complementary to either intracytoplasmic orphan chain, which rescues it from destruction and allows its expression on the cell surface *(5)*.

1.2. Adenoviruses Vectors

To target the thymic stroma, first-generation adenovirus vectors are ideal in that they infect numerous cell types of various animals, can transduce non-dividing cells, and may contain up to 7.5 kb of extraneous DNA. Another particularly interesting feature of adenovirus vectors, especially relative to the limited volume that can be injected in a mouse thymus (10 µL per lobe), is the extremely high titers that stock viruses can reach (10^{10} to 10^{12} plaque forming units [PFU]/mL) (reviewed in **ref. *11***).

The plasmid used to generate the vectors that express MHC class II is designed so that the MHC class II cDNA is introduced in a rabbit β-globin exon placed between the I-Eα promoter and the SV40 polyA sequences (**Fig. 2**) *(12)*. The entire cassette is 4.2 kb in size. We have streamlined the procedure to generate recombinant viruses so that batteries of vectors can be made and compared (*see* **Subheading 2.1.**). The ease with which recombinant viruses can be obtained makes this method highly versatile and numerous other applications can be envisaged.

2. Materials
2.1. Making Adenovirus Vectors

1. Transfer of plasmids: We have made the pNV4 transfer plasmid by modifying the pRSV-βgalpIX vector *(13)* so that a unique *Eco*RI site, within the exon, can be used to clone the cDNA to be expressed from the MHC class II promoter (**Fig. 2**).
2. Viral backbone: The replication-deficient first generation vector, Ad5dl324, contains one deletion in the E1 region (bp 456–3361 relative to wild-type Ad5 sequences) and a deletion in the E3 region (bp 28592–30470). This virus genome has a unique *Cla*I site at bp position 916 that allows removal of the packaging sequence contained in its 5' part.
3. The human embryonic kidney carcinoma cell line 293 (ATCC, cat no. CRL 1573) is used for transfections (generation of recombinant adenoviruses), and to propagate Ad5dl324 recombinant viruses. This cell line complements E1 deleted adenoviruses because it contains the 5' part of the adenovirus genome (bp 1–4344) *(14)*. The lowest possible passage number should be used for successful transfections (below passage 45). Higher passage numbers can be used for virus propagation and amplification (maximum passage 60) but higher yields are obtained at lower passage.
4. Minimal essential medium (MEM) supplemented with 10% fetal calf serum (FCS) for growth of adherent 293 cells. Joklik medium supplemented with 10%

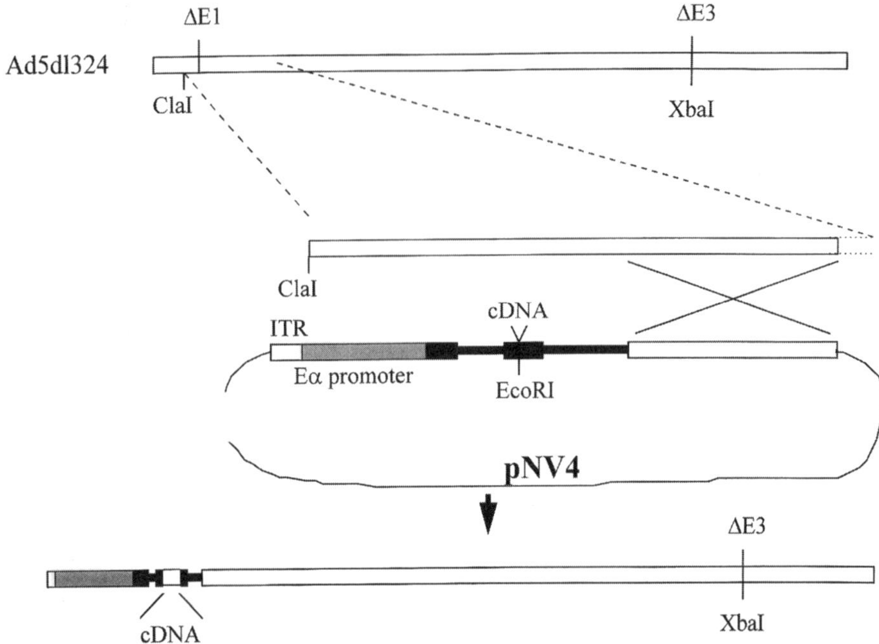

Fig. 2. Construction of adenovirus vectors using a MHC class II expression cassette. The homologous recombination event (shown by the cross) happens between the *ClaI*-digested genome and the linearized pNV4 plasmid. The pNV4 plasmid contains the MHC class II expression cassette taken from the pDOI-5 plasmid *(12)* (open bars: adenovirus sequences; hatched bars: Eα promoter/enhancer; solid bars: rabbit β-globin gene; solid line: plasmid backbone). ITR, inverted terminal repeat of the adenovirus genome essential in virus production.

FCS for growth of 293 cells in suspension. Adherent cells are put in suspension with 1 mM EDTA in PBS.
5. 2 M CaCl$_2$.
6. 100X PO$_4$$^{-3}$ solution: 25g/L Na$_2$HPO$_4$ 2H$_2$O.
7. 2X HEPES-buffered saline (HeBS), pH 7.08: 10 mM KCl, 0.275 M NaCl, 10 mM dextrose, 42 mM HEPES.
8. Sterile noble agar in H$_2$O (5%).
9. Sterile low melting point agar in H$_2$O (5%).
10. CsCl powder.
11. Sterile PBS.
12. Lysis buffer: 0.1% SDS, 10 mM Tris-HCl, pH 7.5, 1 mM EDTA.
13. Proteinase K: stock 20 mg/mL.
14. 2X Proteinase K buffer: 20 mM Tris-HCl, pH 7.8, 10 mM EDTA, 1% SDS.
15. Dialysis tubing.
16. Dialysis buffer: 500 mM NaCl, 20 mM Tris-HCl, pH 7.8.
17. Trichlorotrifluoromethane.

2.2. Intrathymic Injections

See **Notes 1** and **2**.

1. Hamilton syringe (50 µL).
2. No-dead-volume Hamilton needle (2 cm in length, beveled type end: SPE RN L20MM.31/.1694).
3. Surgical glue.
4. Heating lamp.

3. Methods

3.1. Making Recombinant Adenoviruses

Before starting this work, one should check with the legislation of one's country so that the rules and regulations relative to confinement for growth and manipulation of genetically modified organisms or their elimination are respected.

3.1.1. Transfection

1. Seed low-passage adherent 293 cells at 1×10^6 in 6-cm culture dishes 24 h prior to transfection. This allows the cells to be at optimal density for transfection (approx 80% confluent). Prepare two dishes per desired recombinant plus two for controls.
2. Prepare virus DNA (Ad5dl324) by digesting with *Cla*I (2 µg per transfection), and transfer plasmid (pNV4 with a transgene) by linearizing it with a restriction enzyme that does not cut in the adenovirus sequences nor in the transgene (total of 6 µg per desired recombinant virus). After digestion, the DNA is extracted once with phenol:chloroform and precipitated once in ethanol. No further purification steps are required.
3. Change medium 4 h before the addition of the DNA. For each recombinant to be obtained, mix 2 µg of *Cla*I-digested vector DNA (Ad5dl324) (*see below* for preparation) with 2 and 4 µg of linearized transfer plasmid in sterile H_2O so that the final volume reached is 437.5 µL. As controls, prepare one tube with 2 µg of *Cla*I digested vector alone and one with 2 µg of uncut vector. The former gives background transfection (presumably from uncut vector and/or homologous recombination between digested vector and the Ad5 sequences in the 293 cells), whereas the latter gives transfection efficiency. To each tube containing the DNA add 62.5 µL of 2 *M* $CaCl_2$. In a separate tube, mix 500 µL of 2X HeBS with 5 µL 100X PO_4^{-3}. Slowly add the DNA-$CaCl_2$ solution to the tube containing the HeBS-PO_4^{-3} while continuously vortexing or by blowing in air with a sterile pipet. Leave 30 min at room temperature, then add dropwise to the culture dish with gentle agitation. Incubate 24 h at 37°C in 5% CO_2.
4. Melt the 5% Noble agar and 5% LMP agarose stocks in the microwave and equilibrate at 65°C for 1 h. Equilibrate the Dulbecco medium containing 5% FCS at 37°C for 1 h. Prepare the agar mixture by mixing, per culture dish, 4 mL of medium and 0.5 mL of each type of agar. Prepare no more than 25 mL at once to

prevent the mixture from solidifying. Remove the medium and immediately but gently add 5 mL of the medium-agar mixture. Leave at room temperature for 1 h. Plaques appear about 5 d after the addition of agar in the control dish (uncut vector DNA) while an additional 2 d is required for recombinants.

3.1.2. Plaque Isolation and Purification

1. Ten days after transfection 12 viral plaques for each recombinant are picked by puncturing the agar layer with a sterile Pasteur pipet, gently aspirating the agar plug, and placing it in 200 µL of MEM containing 5% FCS by rinsing the pipet. Freeze and thaw the plug-containing medium once and place individually in a well confluent with 293 cells of a 24-well plate prepared 24 h before. To this end, aspirate the medium, add the 200 µL of supernatant, incubate 1 h at 37°C in 5% CO_2 and add 1 mL MEM with 5% FCS. When the cytopathic effect of each individual well reaches 100%, collect the cells and the supernatant and spin in a microfuge tube (2 min, 10,000g). Store the clarified supernatant at –80°C and extract the total DNA content of the corresponding cell pellet *(15)*. Alternatively, DNA can be extracted by the Hirt's method *(16)* which precipitates low molecular weight DNA (*see* **Note 3**). Precipitate and resuspend the DNA pellet in 50 µL Tris-EDTA (TE) (10 m*M* Tris-HCl, pH 8.0, 1 m*M* EDTA, pH 8.0). Digest 5 µL of DNA with relevant restriction enzymes and resolve on a 0.8–1% agarose gel. Direct identification of recombinants is possible by a judicious choice of enzyme. Alternatively, the DNA may be blotted and probed for the MHC II cDNA insert.
2. Select one or two of the supernatants corresponding to the viral DNA that contains the desired insert and genomic organization and prepare at least 3 mL of each of 10^{-3} to 10^{-6} dilutions in MEM supplemented with 5% FCS. Add 2.8 mL of each dilution to 48 wells (50 µL/well) of a 96-well plate, prepared 24 h before by plating 100 µL per well of a 293 cell suspension at 10^5 cells/mL. Seven days after infection, select 8–12 wells of the highest dilution showing cytopathic effect to infect individual wells of a 24-well plate confluent with 293 cells. Rescreen infected wells as described above (DNA extraction, restriction digest and southern blotting) and repeat the limiting dilution step twice. Finally, select only one clone per recombinant showing the proper genomic organization for amplification to high titers and reconstitution experiments.

3.1.3. Preparation of High Titer Virus Stock

1. In order to achieve the multiplicity of infection (MOI) necessary for optimal virus yield on infection of the 2 L suspension culture of 293 cells, amplify the selected clone by infecting one 75-cm² culture flask confluent with 293 cells with half of the supernantant (500 µL) obtained at the last step of purification. When the flask shows 100% lysis, collect cells and supernatant and submit to one freeze-thaw cycle and clarify by centrifuging at 1500g for 10 min at 4°C (total vol, approx 30 mL). Infect 6 × 125 cm² culture flasks confluent with 293 cells with 5 mL of the clarified supernatant for 1 h and complete to a final volume of 50 mL. When 100% cytopathic effect is seen, harvest the virus by pooling the infected cells from the

six flasks by centrifugation. Resuspend the cell pellet in approx 10 mL of medium and freeze-thaw twice. Rid the supernatant of cell debris by centrifugation (1800g, 10 min, 4°C) and store at –20°C until further use.

2. High titer virus stock is produced by infecting 2 L of 293 cells grown in suspension. To this end, adherent 293 cells grown in 175 cm^2 are seeded at a density of 1×10^5 cells/mL in 2 L of Joklik medium in a suspension culture vessel. Infect the suspension culture when it reaches a density of 5 to 7×10^5 cells/mL by centrifuging (800g, 15 min, 15°C) and resuspend in 200 mL of complete Joklik medium to which 10 mL of virus preparation is added. Under those conditions, the MOI is about 10. Cells are incubated in close proximity to virus particles for 1 h at 37°C with agitation. Dilute the culture in 4 L of complete Joklik medium and further incubate for 48 h at 37°C with agitation. At this point, close to 100% of the cells should be infected.

3. Harvest the virus by spinning the infected culture (1800g, 15 min, 15°C), remove the supernatant and wash the cell pellet once in 50 mL cold phosphate buffered saline (PBS). Resuspend the pellet in 10 mL of cold 20 mM Tris, pH 7.8, put on ice and subject to three rounds of sonication of 20 s each, with intervals of 30 s. Extract the cell lysate twice with an equal volume of trichlorotrifluoromethane. Weigh the aqueous phase, add one-half its weight of CsCl, transfer to ultracentrifuge tubes and spin in a Vti65.2 rotor (300,000g for 1 h at 10°C). Extract the lower virus band by puncturing the side of the centrifuge tube with an 18-gage needle fixed to a 5 mL syringe and gently aspirating it (puncturing a hole in the top of the tube allows air intake).

4. Transfer the concentrated virus stock to a dialysis bag and dialyse by gravity for 1 h at room temperature in 1 L of dialysis buffer (*see* **Subheading 2.1.16.**) followed by an overnight dialysis in 2 L of the same buffer at 4°C with agitation. Aliquot in small volumes and store at –80°C (*see* **Note 4**).

5. Stocks are ultimately verified for their molecular structure and their titer. For every virus preparation, thaw 1 aliquot and verify its genomic structure by extracting the DNA (*see below*) of 5 µL of the stock. Digest a small amount of DNA with relevant restriction enzymes, resolve the digestion on an 0.8–1% agarose gel that is blotted onto a membrane and probed with a ^{32}P-labeled fragment of DNA corresponding either to adenovirus sequences or to the total or part of the insert DNA. This procedure rules out the possibilities that the high-titer virus stocks are contaminated either by another recombinant and/or by parental strain and/or wild-type virus the (former two may originate from contamination while the latter was shown to occur from a recombination event with endogenous Ad5 sequences present in the 293 cell line) (Monika Lusky, Transgene, Strasbourg, France, personal communication). In parallel, titer the stock by doing serial dilutions (10^{-8}–10^{-12}) and by plating these dilutions in 96-well plates as described for the limiting dilution purification procedure (*see* **Subheading 3.1.2.2.**). The titer is determined by the following calculation; number of lysed wells at a particular dilution/dilution $\times$ 2.4 (or the total volume plated at that particular dilution), and is expressed as PFU/mL. Alternatively, the titer can be determined by doing a 20-

fold dilution of an aliquot of the virus stock in lysis buffer, incubating at 56°C for 10 min under agitation and reading the OD at 260 nm. The titer is determined by the following formula: $OD_{260} \times$ dilution factor (20 or more)$/9.09 \times 10^{-13}$. The first method determines the number of infectious/replication competent particles, and the latter estimates the total number of particles in the virus stock (*see* **Note 5**).

3.1.4. Preparation of Viral DNA

1. Take 200 µL of high titer-virus stock, dilute with an equal volume of 2X proteinase K buffer and add 50 µg/mL proteinase K. Incubate at 56°C for 1 h. Extract twice with phenol:chloroform and precipitate with ethanol. Resuspend in 100 µL TE buffer and estimate the DNA concentration by optical density (OD) at 260 nm. Verify DNA integrity by restriction enzyme digest and resolution on an agarose gel. For transfection, digest the viral genome with *Cla*I enzyme, extract once with phenol:chloroform and ethanol precipitate. Resuspend to get 0.5 µg/mL in TE and evaluate the amount of DNA either by OD_{260} or agarose gel quantitation.

3.2. Intrathymic Injection

1. Prepare virus for injection by diluting the least concentrated stock 1:3 in MEM without any additives. Plan 10 µL per thymic lobe (20 µL per mouse) of the diluted stock. Prepare other virus stocks (e.g., control virus) by estimating the number of particles contained in 10 µL of the diluted stock and adapt the volume so that the same number of particles are contained in the same volume for each virus stock. The diluted virus stocks are stable at room temperature for at least a few hours and we believe that they should not be put on ice before thymic injection.
2. We have essentially followed the protocol described by Scollay, R., et al. *(17)*. Anesthetize the mice by intraperitonial injection of a mixture of ketamine (2%), chlorobutanol (0.1%), and xylazine (0.2%). Inject no more than 10 µL per gram body weight of animal. Strap down the animals on a styrofoam board as shown in **Fig. 3A**, with two elastic bands holding each side of the animal and one across its chin (take care not to impair its breathing), so that the head is held back. Place the board so that the head of the animal is toward you. Charge the 50 µL Hamilton syringe with 20 µL of the virus stock to be injected. As quickly as possible, wet the entire neck area with ethanol, and using scissors make a longitudinal incision, in the middle of the animal, from the apex of the maxillary to the middle of the rib cage. In the middle of the opening, using forceps, pinch the skin on each side and stretch it outward (**Fig. 3A**). With forceps, pinch the apex of the submandibular muscles (the end pointing away from you) and gently pull it in your direction while cutting the connective tissue attaching it to the rib cage until the entire top of the rib cage is visible (*see* **Note 6**) (**Fig. 3B**). Hold the lower part of the mouse's rib cage between your thumb and index finger, and introduce blunt scissors into the small invagination located at the top center of the rib cage. Push the scissors down to the sternal angle while pointing the tip of the scissors away from the heart and lungs. With a brisk movement, cut the rib cage open with an upward movement. Use the tip of blunt, curved forceps to slit open the pleura from the rib

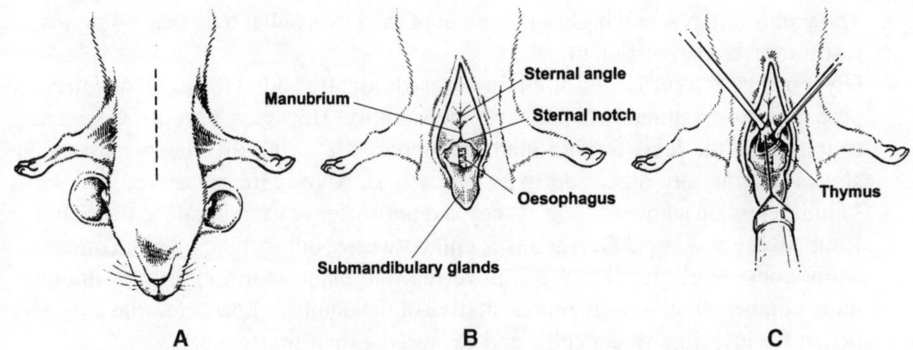

Fig. 3. Intrathymic injection procedure. *See text* for details.

cage towards the neck. Maintain the slit open by pushing it to the side with the same forceps. With the other hand, introduce the needle of the 50-µL Hamilton syringe 3–4 mm under the thymic capsule and inject 10 µL of the viral suspension (**Fig. 3C**). Allow the needle to remain in the lobe a few seconds after the injection so that the internal pressure decreases (this will prevent any backflow). Usually, a small white nodule, internal to the lobe (resulting from decreased blood flow associated with increased internal pressure) can be seen and is indicative of a successful injection. Repeat this procedure for the other lobe if needed. Push the submandibular muscles in place, thereby blocking the pleura and rib cage openings. Although not compulsory, a small drop of surgical glue can be used to attach these muscles to the rib cage. Close the opening of the skin with a few drops of surgical glue. Keep the animals under a heating lamp while still under anesthesia to prevent hypothermia.

4. Notes

1. This procedure is traditionally done in 4–6-wk-old-mice but younger and older animals have been used with success. Because of age-related thymus involution, it is very difficult to inject animals older than 9–10 wk for females and 8–9 wk for males. Also, we have empirically noticed that stress due to transport is a major problem in getting good reconstitution of the CD4 compartment. Best results (in levels of reconstitution attained and in consistency) were obtained with young animals bred in our facility. When mice had to be transported, an isolation period of at least 2 wk had to be observed prior to injection in order to see reconstitution. As a consequence, animals were often quite old and difficult to inject. We circumvent this problem by injecting animals on arrival (not respecting the usual 1 wk period to allow the animals to relax).

2. The dosing of anesthetics is crucial and should be evaluated relative to the weight, sex, and strain of mice as a function of the product used. The highly traumatic nature of the surgery requires profound anesthesia. We have found a mixture of Xylazine (Rompun), ketamine and chlorobutanol (Imalgene) to work best.

3. The yields of DNA and high salt content of the DNA pellet may make diagnostic restriction digest inefficient.
4. Glycerol, FCS, sucrose, or albumin are traditionally added to stored adenovirus preparations presumably to increase the stability. However, because we wanted to introduce the least foreign material as possible in the thymus, we froze our stocks without any other additives. Our stocks were regularly titered and were found to remain stable as long as they did not suffer any temperature fluctuation.
5. Routinely, a 1–2 log difference is found between both methods, the OD method being consistently higher. We believe that the plaque forming assay, although more cumbersome, is more representative of the number of particles that are competent for infecting target cells, and expressing their transgene.
6. Cutting too close to the blood vessels under the maxillary will cause bleeding that will blind the opening. In this situation, blood can be soaked up with a clean absorbent pad.

Acknowledgments

The authors would like to thank Benoit Heller for drawing **Fig. 3**.

References

1. Mittrücker, H. W., Pfeffer, K., Schmits, R., and Mak, T. W. (1995) T-lymphocyte development and function in gene-targeted mutant mice. *Immunol. Rev.* **148,** 115–150.
2. Banks, T. A. and Mucenski, M. L. (1994) Gene targeting of the immune system: the surprises continue. *Curr. Opin. Biotechnol.* **5,** 604–610.
3. von Boehmer, H. (1996) CD4/CD8 lineage commitment: back to instruction? *J. Exp. Med.* **183,** 713–715.
4. Corgrove, D., Gray, D., Dierich, A., Kaufman, J., Lemeur, M., Benoist, C., and Mathis, D. (1991) Mice lacking MHC class II molecules. *Cell* **66,** 1051–1066.
5. Rooke, R., Waltzinger, C., Benoist, C., and Mathis, D. (1997) Targeted complementation of MHC class II deficiency by intrathymic delivery of recombinant adenoviruses. *Immunity* **7,** 123–134.
6. Nakano, N., Rooke, R., Benoist, C., and Mathis, D. (1997) Positive selection of T cells induced by viral delivery of neopeptides to the thymus. *Science* **275,** 678–683.
7. Watts, C. (1997) Capture and processing of exogenous antigens for presentation on MHC molecules. *Annu. Rev. Immunol.* **15,** 821–850.
8. Harding, C. V. (1995) Intracellular organelles involved in antigen processing and the binding of peptides to class II MHC molecules. *Semin. Immunol.* **6,** 355–360.
9. Mathis, D. J., Benoist, C., Williams, V. E., Kanter, M., and McDevitt, H. O. (1983) Several mechanisms can account for defective Eα gene expression in different mouse haplotypes. *Proc. Natl. Acad. Sci. USA* **86,** 273–277.
10. Germain, R. N. and Malissen, B. (1986) Analysis of expression and function of class II major histocompatibility complex encoded molecules by DNA-mediated gene transfer. *Ann. Rev. Immunol.* **4,** 281–315.
11. Ali, M., Lemoine, N. R., and Ring, C. J. A. (1994) The use of DNA viruses as vectors for gene therapy. *Gene Ther.* **1,** 367–384.

12. Kouskoff, V., Fehling, H. J., Lemeur, M., Benoist, C., Mathis, D. (1993) A vector driving the expression of foreign cDNAs in the MHC class II-positive cells of transgenic mice. *J. Immunol. Methods* **166,** 287–291.
13. Stratford-Perricaudet, L. D., Levrero, M., Chasse, J. F., Perricaudet, M., and Briand, P. (1990) Evaluation of the transfer and expression in mice of an enzyme-encoding gene using a human adenovirus vector. *Human Gene Ther.* **1,** 241–256.
14. Louis, N., Evelegh, C., and Graham, F. L. (1997) Cloning and sequencing of the cellular-viral junctions from the human adenovirus type 5 transformed 293 cell line. *Virology* **233**, 423–429.
15. Sambrook, J., Fritsch, E. F., and Maniatis, T., eds. (1989) *Molecular Cloning,* Cold Spring Harbor Laboratory Press, Cold Spring Harbor, NY.
16. Hirt, B. (1967) Selective extraction of polyoma DNA from infected mouse cell cultures. *J. Mol. Biol.* **26,** 365–369.
17. Scollay, R., Butcher, E., and Weissman, I. (1980) Thymus cell migration: quantitative studies on the rate of migration of cells from the thymus to the periphery in mice. *Eur. J. Immunol.* **10,** 210–217.

8

Quantitative Analysis of the Usage of Human T-Cell Receptor α and β Chain Variable Regions by Reverse Dot-Blot Hybridization

Takaji Matsutani, Takeshi Yoshioka, Yuji Tsuruta,
Shoji Iwagami, Tomoko Toyosaki-Maeda, and Ryuji Suzuki

1. Introduction

Mature T lymphocytes specifically recognize antigens through interaction between MHC/peptide complex and αβ or γδ TCR. Variable region genes created by recombination of variable (V), diversity (D), and joining (J) locus contribute to shaping T cell receptor (TCR) repertoires *(1,2)*. Thus, TCRαV and TCRβV repertoires have been studied for characterizing of T cells that may play major role in peripheral blood or pathological lesions of patients with autoimmune diseases *(3–6)*.

Quantitative polymerase chain reaction (PCR) method with many sets of primers specific for variable regions has been used *(7)*. However, different amplification efficiencies among individual primers or cross-reactivity between subfamilies hampered the accurate estimation of the frequency of individual families *(8)*. Moreover, previously described V segment-specific primers cannot amplify all the TCR segments. Anchored PCR and inverse PCR have also been developed *(9–11)*, however homopolymeric tailing is somewhat tricky and the tailing reaction needs to be titrated. Furthermore, inverse PCR is less efficient in the ligation reaction. On the contrary, adaptor ligation-mediated PCR method developed by us is more efficient than other PCR-based methods, and less skewing through PCR cycles between TCR V segments occurs, because common primers are used for amplification *(12,13)*.

In this chapter, we describe our quantitative methods for analyzing TCR repertoires. Our method consists of an adaptor ligation-mediated PCR and various solid support, e.g., nylon membrane (RDB method) or microplate wells

From: *Methods in Molecular Biology, Vol. 134: T Cell Protocols: Development and Activation*
Edited by: K. P. Kearse © Humana Press Inc., Totowa, NJ

(MHA method) *(14–16)*. Another advantage of our method is reverse-phase hybridization. Standard hybridization methods that utilize a large number of probes take plenty of time and labor. However, our method does not require many sets of PCR tubes, but only requires a single tube for determining the frequencies of almost all TCR V families. In the RDB method, 44 and 39 sequence-specific oligonucleotide probes (SSCPs) for TCRαV and TCRβV, respectively, are tailed with T nucleotides at the 3' end by terminal deoxynucleotidyl transferase in order to facilitate binding of probes onto nylon membrane. Biotinylated 21-dUTP is internally incorporated into amplified PCR products. PCR products are specifically captured, and then detected by chemiluminescent enzyme immunoassay.

We have recently developed a simpler MHA method. In this technique, 5' biotinylated primer is used for labeling PCR products instead of incorporation of biotinylated dUTP. Oligonucleotide probes are covalently immobilized onto 96-well microplate wells, and automated colorimetric reading is performed after the reaction. This procedure is simpler and the results are more reproducible.

Accurate estimation of TCR repertoires using our simple methods will provide deep insight into the role of T cells in immunological reactions.

2. Materials

2.1. Isolation of Total RNA from Peripheral Blood Mononuclear Cells (PBMCs) or Tissue Samples

1. Trizol reagent and Trizol LS reagent (Gibco-BRL, Bethesda, MD).
2. 10 mg/mL yeast transfer RNA (tRNA), extracted once with Trizol reagent and then adjusted to 10 mg/mL.
3. Phenol/chloroform/isoamyl alcohol (25:24:1).
4. Chloroform (not containing isoamyl alcohol).
5. Isopropanol.
6. Ribonuclease (RNase)-free distilled water (DEPC-treated).
7. 80% Ethanol.

2.2. Synthesis of Single- and Double-Stranded cDNA from mRNA

1. 200 μM BSL-18 primer (*see* **Table 1**).
2. 5X first strand synthesis buffer: 250 mM Tris-HCl, pH 8.3, 375 mM KCl, 15 mM MgCl$_2$ (Gibco-BRL).
3. 0.1 M Dithiothreitol (DTT) (Gibco-BRL).
4. 10 mM dNTPs solution: 10 mM aqueous solutions of each of dATP, dCTP, dGTP, and dGTP (Pharmacia, Uppsala, Sweden).
5. RNase H-reverse transcriptase (Superscript II), 200 U/μL, Gibco-BRL. Store at –20°C.
6. RNasin (10,000 U/mL) (Promega, Madison, WI).
7. 5X second-strand synthesis buffer: 100 mM Tris-HCl, pH 6.9, 450 mM KCl, 23 mM MgCl$_2$, 0.75 mM β-NAD⁺, 50 mM (NH$_4$)$_2$SO$_4$ (Gibco-BRL).

Table 1
Oligonucleotide Primers

Oligonucleotide primers	Sequence
BSL-18	5'-GACTAGTCAAAGCGGCCGCGAGCTCTTTTTTTTTTTTTTTTTTTT
P10EA	5'-GGGAATTCGG-3'
P20EA	5'-TAATACGACTCCGAATTCCC-3'
CA1	5'-TGTTGAAGGCGTTTGCACATGCA-3'
CA2	5'-GTGCATAGACCTCATGTCTAGCA-3'
CA3	5'-ACTTTGTGACACATTTGTTTGAG-3'
CB1	5'-GAACTGGACTTGACAGCGGAACT-3'
CB2	5'-AGGCAGTATCTGGAGTCATTGAG-3'
CB3	5'-ACTGTGCACCTCCTTCCCATTCA-5'
CA4BIO	5'-Bio-ATAGGCAGACAGACTTGTCACTG-3'
CB4BIO	5'-Bio-ACACCAGTGTGGCCTTTTGGGTG-3'

8. *Escherichia coli* DNA polymerase I, 10 U/μL (Gibco-BRL). Store at –20°C.
9. RNase H, 2 U/μL, Gibco-BRL. Store at –20°C.
10. *E. coli* DNA ligase, 10 U/μL (Gibco-BRL). Store at –20°C.
11. T4 DNA polymerase, 1 U/μL (Gibco-BRL). Store at –20°C.
12 Phenol/chloroform/isoamyl alcohol.
13. Chloroform.
14. Poly (A), 1 mg/mL (Pharmacia).
15. 20% Polyethylene glycol 6000 (PEG), 2.5 M NaCl solution, filtrated with 0.22 nm membrane filter.
16. TE buffer: 10 mM Tris-HCl, pH 8.0, 1 mM EDTA, autoclaved.
17. Ethanol.
18. RNase-free distilled water, DEPC-treated.
19. 5X T4 ligase buffer: 250 mM Tris-HCl, pH 7.6, 50 mM MgCl$_2$, 5 mM ATP, 5 mM DTT, 25% (w/v) PEG8000 (Gibco-BRL).
20. T4 ligase, 1 U/μL, (Gibco-BRL). Store at –20°C.
21. 50 μM P20EA/P10EA primer adaptor (*see* **Table 1**): Dissolve primer adaptor in distilled water incubate at 95°C for 5 min, and slowly cool down to room temperature. Store at –20°C.
22. *Not*I, 50 U/μL (TaKaRa-Syuzo, Kyoto, Japan).

2.3. PCR

1. 10X PCR buffer, 100 mM Tris-HCl, pH 9.0, 500 mM KCl, 1% Triton X-100 (Promega, Madison, WI).
2. 25 mM Mg^{2+} solution (Promega).
3. 10 mM dNTPs solution (Pharmacia).
4. *Taq* Polymerase, 5 U/μL (Promega).
5. Oligonucleotide primers: P20EA, CA, and CB primers (*see* **Table 1**).

6. 5' Biotinylated oligonucleotide primers (for MHA): CA4BIO, CB4BIO.
7. 10 m*M* d(AGC)TP mix (for RDB): contain 10 m*M* dATP, dGTP and dCTP (Pharmacia).
8. 0.5 m*M* dTTP, Pharmacia (for RDB).
9. 0.5 m*M* BIOTIN-21-dUTP (for RDB) (Clonetech, Palo Alto, CA).
10. Distilled water.
11. Mineral oil (Sigma, St. Louis, MO).

2.4. Quantitative Analysis of TCRαV and TCRβV Repertoires

2.4.1. Reverse Dot-Blot Method (RDB Method)

2.4.1.1. IMMOBILIZATION ONTO NYLON MEMBRANE

1. 5X 3' tailing buffer: 400 m*M* potassium cacodylate, pH 7.2, 10 m*M* CoCl$_2$, 1 m*M* dithiothreitol (Gibco-BRL).
2. Terminal deoxynucleotidyl transferase (TdT), 3.25 U/µL (Toyobo, Tokyo, Japan).
3. 100 µ*M* sequence-specific oligonucleotide probe (SSOP) (*see* **Table 2**).
4. 20 m*M* dTTP solution.
5. 20X SSC: 3.0 *M* NaCl, 0.3 *M* sodium citrate.
6. Hybond-Nfp (Amersham, Buckinghamshire, UK).
7. 48-well slot type filtration manifold system (Gibco-BRL).
8. Strata linker 2400 (Stratagene, La Jolla, CA).
9. 0.5 *M* EDTA, pH 8.0.

2.4.1.2. DETECTION BY CHEMILUMINESCENT ENZYME IMMUNOASSAY

1. GMC buffer: 0.5 *M* Na$_2$HPO$_4$, pH 7.0, 7% SDS, 1% BSA, 10 m*M* EDTA. Store at room temperature.
2. 2X SSC, 0.1% SDS.
3. 0.2X SSC, 0.1% SDS.
4. T-TBS buffer: 10 m*M* Tris-HCl, pH 7.4, 0.5 *M* NaCl, 0.5% Tween 20.
5. TB-TBS buffer: 10 m*M* Tris-HCl, pH 7.4, 0.5 *M* NaCl, 0.5% Tween 20, 0.5% blocking reagent. Blocking reagent is purchased from Boehringer Mannheim Biochemica (Mannheim, Germany).
6. Alkaline phosphatase working buffer: 10 m*M* Tris-HCl, pH 9.6, 10 m*M* NaCl, 1 m*M* MgCl$_2$.
7. AMPPD working buffer: 10 m*M* Tris-HCl, pH 9.6, 10 m*M* NaCl, 1 m*M* MgCl$_2$, 1.13 m*M* cetyltrimethylammonium bromide (CTAB), 0.75 *M* 2-amino-2-methyl-1-propanol.
8. Alkaline-phosphatase conjugated streptavidin (Gibco-BRL). Store at 4°C; do not freeze.
9. AMPPD (Tropix system, Bedford, MD).
10. X-ray film (Eastman Kodak, Rochester, NY).

2.4.2. Microplate Hybridization Assay (MHA Method)

2.4.2.1. IMMOBILIZATION ONTO MICROPLATE WELLS

1. Carboxylate-modified ELISA plate (Sumitomo Bakelite Co., Ltd., Tokyo, Japan).
2. 10 µ*M* 5' amino-modified SSOP (*see* **Table 3**).

3. 10 m*M* 2(*N*-morpholine)ethansulfonic acid (MES); adjust with 0.4 *N* NaOH to pH 5.4. Reagent from Sigma.
4. 0.2 *M* 1-ethyl-3-(3-dimethylaminopropyl) carbodiimide HCl (EDC) in 10 m*M* MES buffer, pH 5.4, freshly prepared. Reagent from Pierce (Rockford, IL).
5. 4 m*M* *N*-Hydroxysulfosuccinimide (Sulfo-NHS) in 10 m*M* MES buffer, pH 5.4, freshly prepared. Reagent from Pierce.
6. 1X PBS, phosphate-buffered saline tablets (Sigma).
7. 0.4 *N* NaOH.

2.4.2.2. DETECTION BY ENZYME-LINKED IMMUNOSORBENT ASSAY

1. GMC buffer (*see* **Subheading 2.4.1.2., item 1**).
2. 2X SSC, 0.1% SDS.
3. 0.4X SSC, 0.1% SDS (VA high stringency washing buffer).
4. 0.6X SSC, 0.1% SDS (VB high stringency washing buffer).
5. T-TBS buffer (*see* **Subheading 2.4.1.2., item 4**).
6. TB-TBS buffer (*see* **Subheading 2.4.1.2., item 5**)
7. Alkaline-phosphatase conjugated streptavidin.
8. 20% Diethanolamine (DEA) buffer, 1 m*M* MgCl$_2$, pH 9.8; adjust with 0.4 *N* NaOH.
9. 4 mg/mL p-nitrophenyl phosphate (pNPP) in 20% DEA buffer, 1 m*M* MgCl$_2$, pH 9.8. Reagent from Sigma.
10. Stop solution: 0.2 *M* EDTA, pH 8.0.

3. Methods (Fig. 1)

3.1. Isolation of Total RNA from PBMCs and Tissue Samples (see Note 1)

1. Suspend cell pellet in 1 mL of Trizol reagent.
2. Add 1 µL of 10 mg/mL yeast tRNA as carrier, shake the resulting preparation vigorously, and keep at room temperature for 5 min.
3. Add 200 µL (0.2 vol) of chloroform (not containing isoamylalcohol) to the cell lysate, shake vigorously, and leave at room temperature for 5 min. Centrifuge at 10,000*g* for 10 min at 4°C.
4. Transfer the aqueous phase to the new tube.
5. Mix the RNA present in the aqueous phase, with an equal volume of isopropanol and leave for 10 min at room temperature.
6. Centrifuge at 10,000*g* for 20 min. Dissolve the pellet in 1 mL of Trizol reagent (*see* **Note 2**).
7. Repeat the extraction procedure as in **steps 3–5**. Rinse RNA with 80% ethanol, vacuum-dry, and dissolve in 10 µL of distilled water.

3.2. Adaptor-Ligation Mediated PCR Method (see Note 3)

3.2.1. Synthesis of Single-Stranded cDNA

1. Anneal approx 1–10 µg of total RNA with >50 pmol of BSL-18 primer containing *Not*I cutting site at 70°C for 8 min.

Table 2
Specific Probes Used in Reverse Dot-Blot Hybridization

TCRαV	Sequence (5'-3')	Target segment	TCRβV	Sequence (5'-3')	Target segment
Vα1-1	ATCAAGGGCTTTGAGGCTGAA	αV1S1	Vβ1-1	ACAACAGTTCCCTGACTTGCA	βV1S1, 1S2
Vα1-2	ATCAACGGTTTTGAGGCTGAAT	αV1S2, 1S3, 1S5	Vβ2-1	TCATCAACCATGCAAGCCTGA	βV2S1, 2S2, 2S3
Vα1-3	GCATTAAAGGCTTTGAGGCTG	αV1S4	Vβ2-2	CCATCAACCATCCAAACCTGA	βV2S4
Vα1-4	CATCACGGTTTTGAGGCTGAA	αV1S6	Vβ3-1	GTCTCTAGAGAGAAGAAGGAG	βV3S1, 3S2
Vα2-1	ACAGCTCAATAAAGCCAGCCA	αV2S1	Vβ4-1	TTGACAAGTTTCCCATCAGCC	βV4S1, 4S2, 4S3
Vα2-2	CACAGGTCGATAAATCCAGCA	αV2S2	Vβ5-1	CTTCAGTGAGACACAGAGAAA	βV5S1
Vα2-3	AGAGCCAGCCAGTATATTTCC	αV2S3	Vβ5-2	ATTATGAGGAGGAAGAGAGACA	βV5S2
Vα3-1	GTGGAAGATTAAGAGTCACGC	αV3S1	Vβ5-3	TATTATGAGAAAGAAGAGAGAGG	βV5S3
Vα4-1	AACAACAGAATGGCCTCTCTG	αV4S1	Vβ5-4	TGACGAGGGTGAAGAGAGAAA	βV5S8
Vα4-2	CCTCTCTGATCATCACAGAAG	αV4S2, 4S3	Vβ5-5	ATTATAGGGAGGAAGAGAATGG	βV5S6
Vα5-1	CTGAAGGTCACCTTTGATACC	αV5S1	Vβ6-1	ACGATCGGTTCTTTGCAGTCA	βV6S1
Vα6-1	TGACACCAGTGATCCAAGTTAT	αV6S1, DV4	Vβ6-2	TCAACTAGACAAATCGGGGCT	βV6S3
Vα7-1	ATTCCTTAGTCGCTCTGATAGT	αV7S1, 7S3	Vβ6-3	CCAACAAGACAAATCAGGGCT	βV6S4
Vα7-2	TTCCTTAGTCGGTCTAAAGGG	αV7S2	Vβ6-4	AAGGCTGCTCAGTGATCGGT	βV6S5
Vα8-1	TGGGCGAAAAGAAAGACCAAC	αV8S1	Vβ6-5	TCGCTTCTCTGCAGAGAGGA	βV6S7
Vα8-2	GGCCAAAGAGTCACCGTTTTA	αV8S2	Vβ6-6	AACTGGAAAAATCAGGGCTGC	—
Vα9-1	CATCAAAGGCTTCACTGCTGA	αV9S1	Vβ7-1	CTGAATGCCCCAACAGCTCT	βV7S1,7S2,7S3
Vα10-1	GTGGAGAAGTGAAGAAGCTGA	αV10S1	Vβ8-1	TTTACTTTAACAACAACGTTCCG	βV8S1, 8S2
Vα11-1	AGGGACGATACAACATGACCT	αV11S1	Vβ8-2	AAGGACTGGAGTTGCTGGCT	βV8S3
Vα12-1	GTCGGTATTCTTGGAACTTCC	αV12S1	Vβ9-1	AAACAGTTCCAAATCGCTTCTC	βV9S1,9S2
Vα13-1	AAGATTAAGCGCCACGACTGT	αV13S1	Vβ10-1	CCAAAAACTCATCCTGTACCTT	βV10S1
Vα14-1	CGTTTCTCTGTGAACTTCCAG	αV14S1	Vβ11-1	TCAACAGTCTCCAGAATAAGGA	βV11S1
Vα15-1	GACCAAAGACTCACTGTTCTAT	αV15S1	Vβ12-1	CAAAGGAGAAGTCTCAGATGG	βV12S2, 12S3
Vα16-1	CAGCTATGGCTTTGAAGCTGA	αV16S1, 16S2	Vβ13-1	CAATGGCTACAATGTCTCCAG	βV13S1, 13S3
Vα17-1	GAAGGAAGATTCACAATCTCCT	αV17S1	Vβ13-2	GGTCCCTGATGGCTACAATG	βV13S2
Vα18-1	GGACGATATAGTGCCACTCTT	αV18S1	Vβ13-3	TGATGGTTATAGTGTCTCCAG	βV13S5
Vα19-1	GCATGGAAGATTAATTGCCACA	αV19S1	Vβ13-4	CCGAATGGCTACAACGTCTC	βV13S6
Vα20-1	GACTATACTAACAGCATGTTTGA	αV20S1	Vβ14-1	GTCTCTCGAAAAGAGAAGAGG	βV14S1

Vα21-1	AACAAAAGTGCCAAGCACCTC	αV21S1, DV5	Vβ15-1	AGTGTCTCTCGACAGGCACA	βV15S1
Vα22-1	TGACAAGGGAAGCAACAAAGG	αV22S1, 22S2	Vβ16-1	GTGAAAGAGTCTAAACAGGAT	βV16S1
Vα23-1	AAGTGGAAGACTTAATGCCCC	αV23S1	Vβ17-1	CACAGATAGTAAATGACTTTCAG	βV17S1
Vα24-1	CAACTCTGGATGCAGACACAA	αV24S1	Vβ18-1	GATGAGTCAGGAATGCCAAAG	βV18S1
Vα25-1	AAGACTGACTGCTCAGTTTGG	αV25S1	Vβ19-1	CTCAATGCCCCAAGAACGCA	βV19S1
Vα26-1	AGATAACTGCCAAGTTGGATGA	αV26S1	Vβ20-1	TCTGAGGTGCCCCAGAATCT	βV20S1
Vα27-1	GGACGATTAATGGCCTCACTT	αV27S1	Vβ21-1	TCTGCAGAGAGGCTCAAAGG	βV21S1,21S3, 21S4
Vα28-1	GTCAGGAAGACTAAGTAGCATA	αV28S1	Vβ22-1	TTCAGTGACTATCATTCTGAACT	βV23S1
Vα29-1	GGAGAACAGATGCGTCGTGA	αV29S1	Vβ23-1	AATCTTGGGGCAGAAAGTCGA	βV22S1
Vα29-2	TGGAGAACAGAAGGGTCATGA	αV29S2	Vβ24-1	CCAGGAGGCCGAACACTTC	βV24S1
Vα30-1	TGAAGAAGCAGAAAAGACTGAC	αV30S1	Vβ25-1	AACAGGTATGCCCAAGGAAAG	βV25S1
Vα31-1	CTGTATTCAGCTGGGGAAGAA	αV31S1	CβI	CACCCGAGGTCGCTGTGTT	TCRBC
Vα32-1	TCAGAGAGAGACAATGGAAAAC	αV32S1	CβII	GCTGTGTTTGAGCCATCAGAA	TCRBC
VD1	GAAACAAGTTGGTGGTCATATTA	DV1			
VD2	AAAGGAGAAGCGATCGGTAAC	DV2			
VD3	GACACTGTATATTCAAATCCAGA	DV3			
CAI	TATCCAGAACCCTGACCCTG	TCRAC			

Table 3
Specific Probes Used in Microplate Hybridization Assay

TCRαV	Sequence (5'-3')	Target segment	TCRβV	Sequence (5'-3')	Target segment
Vα1-1	CTTTTCAGGGGATCCACTGG	αV1S1	Vβ1-1	ACAACAGTTCCCTGACTTGCA	βV1S1
Vα1-2	GTACACATCAGCGGCCACC	αV1S2, 1S5	Vβ2-1	TCATCAACCATGCAAGCCTGA	βV2S1
Vα1-3	GACACTCTGGTTCAAGGCAT	αV1S4	Vβ2-2	CCATCAACCATCCAAACCTGA	—
Vα1-4	TTTATCAGGATCCACCCTGGT	αV1S3, 1S6	Vβ3-1	GTCTCTAGAGAGAAGAAGGAG	βV3S1
Vα2-1	TATTCTGGGAAAAGCCCTGAG	αV2S1	Vβ4-1	TTGACAAGTTTCCCATCAGCC	βV4S1, BV4S2
Vα2-2	CACAGGTCGATAAATCCAGCA	αV2S2	Vβ5-1	ACTTCAGTGAGACACAGAGAAA	βV5S1
Vα2-3	CAGGATTGCAGGAAAGAACCT	αV2S3	Vβ5-2	ATTATGAGGAGGAAGAGAGACA	βV5S2
Vα3-1	AGCAGTTCCTTGTTGATCACG	αV3S1	Vβ5-3	TATTATGAGAAAGAAGAGAGAGG	βV5S3, BV5S7
Vα4-1	AACAACAGAATGGCCTCTCTG	αV4S1	Vβ5-4	TGACGAGGGTGAAGAGAGAAA	βV5S8
Vα4-2	CACCTTGATCCTGCCCCAC	αV4S2, 4S3	Vβ5-5	ATTATAGGGAGGAAGAGAATGG	βV5S6
Vα5-1	GGTCACCTTTGATACCACCC	αV5S1	Vβ6-1	ACGGGTGCGGCAGATGACT	βV6S1
Vα6-1	TCCAGAAGGCAAGAAAATCCG	αV6S1, DV4	Vβ6-2	TCAACTAGACAAATCGGGGCT	βV6S3
Vα7-1	TCGCTCTGATAGTTATGGTTACC	αV7S1, 7S3	Vβ6-3	CCAACAAGACAAATCAGGGCT	βV6S4
Vα7-2	TTCCTTAGTCGGTCTAAAGGG	αV7S2	Vβ6-4	AAGGCTGCTCAGTGATCGGT	βV6S5
Vα8-1	TGGGCGAAAAGAAAGACCAAC	αV8S1	Vβ6-5	TCCAAGGCAACAGTGCACCA	βV6S7
Vα8-2	GGCCAAAGAGTCACCGTTTTA	αV8S2	Vβ6-6	AACTGGAAAAATCAGGGCTGC	—
Vα9-1	GCGAGACATCTTTCCACCTG	αV9S1	Vβ7-1	CTGAATGCCCCAACAGCTCT	βV7S1, 7S2, 7S3
Vα10-1	TGGTGATGCAAGAAAGGACAG	αV10S1	Vβ8-1	TTTACTTTAACAACAACGTTCCG	βV8S1, 8S2
Vα11-1	AGGGACGATACAACATGACCT	αV11S1	Vβ8-2	AAGGACTGGAGTTGCTGGCT	βV8S3
Vα12-1	CGTCGGAACTCTTTTGATGAG	αV12S1	Vβ9-1	AAACAGTTCCAAATCGCTTCTC	βV9S1, 9S2
Vα13-1	CTTGGGGACGCTCATCAAC	αV13S1	Vβ10-1	CCAAAAACTCATCCTGTACCTT	βV10S1
Vα14-1	TGTGAACTTCCAGAAAGCAGC	αV14S1	Vβ11-1	ATAAGGACGGAGCATTTTCCC	βV11S1
Vα15-1	TGGACATGAAACAAGACCAAAG	αV15S1	Vβ12-1	CAAAGGAGAAGTCTCAGATGG	βV12S2, 12S3
Vα16-1	ACCTGGTTAAAGGCAGCTATG	αV16S1, 16S2	Vβ13-1	AGTTGGTGCTGGTATCACTGA	βV13S1, 13S6
Vα17-1	TGATAGCCATACGTCCAGATG	αV17S1	Vβ13-2	GAATTTCCTGCTGGGGTTGG	βV13S2
Vα18-1	GGACGAATAAGTGCCACTCTT	αV18S1	Vβ13-3	ACAAACGGGAGTTCTCGCTC	βV13S3
Vα19-1	GCATGGAAGATTAATTGCCACA	αV19S1	Vβ13-4	TGATGGTTATAGTGTCTCCAGA	βV13S5
Vα20-1	CCTGTTTATCCCTGCCGACA	αV20S1	Vβ14-1	GTCTCTCGAAAAGAGAAGAGG	βV14S1

Vα21-1	TGCTGAAGGTCCTACATTCCT	αV21S1, DV5	Vβ15-1	AGTGTCTCTCGACAGGCACA	βV15S1, 15S2
Vα22-1	GACAAGGGAAGCAACAAAGGT	αV22S1	Vβ16-1	TTGTGAAAGAGTCTAAACAGGAT	βV16S1
Vα23-1	CGCTGGATAAATCATCAGGAC	αV23S1	Vβ17-1	CACAGATAGTAAATGACTTTCAG	βV17S1
Vα24-1	CAACTCTGGATGCAGACACAA	αV24S1	Vβ18-1	GATGAGTCAGGAATGCCAAAG	βV18S1
Vα25-1	TTGACCTCAAATGGAAGACTGA	αV25S1	Vβ19-1	CTTCAAGAAACGGAGATGCAC	βV19S1
Vα26-1	AGATAACTGCCAAGTTGGATGA	αV26S1	Vβ20-1	TCTCAGCCTCCAGACCCCA	βV20S1
Vα27-1	GGACGATTAATGGCCTCACTT	αV27S1	Vβ21-1	TCTGCAGAGAGGCTCAAAGG	βV21S1,21S3, 21S4
Vα28-1	GTGGAATTGAAAAGAAGTCAGG	αV28S1	Vβ22-1	TGCAGAGCGATAAAGGAAGCA	βV23S1
Vα29-1	CACCCGTCTTCCTGATGATAT	αV29S1	Vβ23-1	AATCTTGGGGCAGAAAGTCGA	βV22S1
Vα30-1	TGACATTTCAGTTTGGAGAAGC	αV30S1	Vβ24-1	GCCCCAAAGCTGCTGTTCC	βV24S1
Vα31-1	CTGTATTCAGCTGGGGAAGAA	αV31S1	Vβ25-1	AACAGGTATGCCCAAGGAAAG	βV25S1
Vα32-1	GAGAGACAATGGAAAACAGCAA	αV32S1	CBI	CACCCGAGGTCGCTGTGTT	TCRBC
VD1	CCTTATTCGCCAGGGTTCTG	DV1	CBII	GCTGTGTTTGAGCCATCAGAA	TCRBC
VD2	AAAGGAGAAGCGATCGGTAAC	DV2			
VD3	CTCAAGGACGGTTTTCTGTGA	DV3			
CAI	TATCCAGAACCCTGACCCTG	TCRAC			
CAII	CTGCCGTGTACCAGCTGAG	TCRAC			

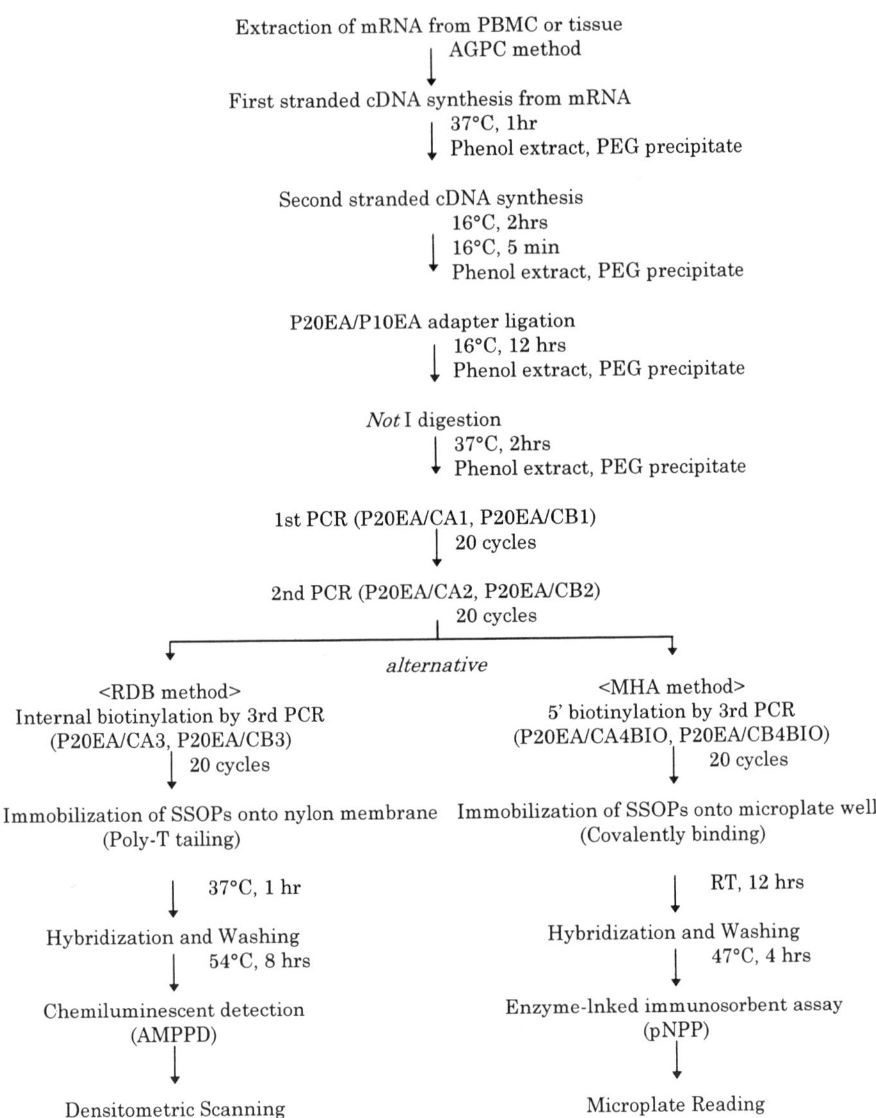

Fig. 1. Flow chart of quantitative analysis of TCR repertoires.

2. Convert the RNA to cDNA using the SuperScript II reverse transcriptase in 10 µL of reaction mixture (*see* **Table 4**).

3.2.2. Synthesis of Double-Stranded DNA

1. Add directly 9 µL of the cDNA to second-stranded synthesis buffer containing *E. coli* DNA polymerase, RNase H, and *E. coli* DNA ligase, and incubate at 16°C for 2 h (*see* **Table 5**).

Table 4
First-Strand Synthesis

Reagent	Volume (μL)	Final concentration/condition
RNA solution (1–10 μg)	3.25	
200 μM BSL-18	1.25	25 μM
	Total 4.5	Annealed at 70°C for 8 min
5X first-strand buffer	2	50 mM Tris-HCl, pH 8.3, 75 mM KCl, 3 mM MgCl$_2$
0.1 M DTT	1	10 mM DTT
10 mM dNTPs	0.5	0.5 mM dNTP
Distilled water	0.5	
RNasin, 40 U/μL	0.5	2 U/μL
Superscript II, 200 U/μL	1	20 U/μL
	Total 10	Incubate at 37°C for 1 h

Table 5
Second-Strand Synthesis

Reagent	Volume (μL)	Final concentration/condition
First strand mixture	9	
DEPC-treated water	46.5	
5X second-strand buffer	15	25 mM Tris-HCl, pH 7.5, 100 mM KCl, 5 mM MgCl$_2$, 10 mM (NH$_4$)SO$_4$, 0.15 mM β-NAD$^+$, 1.2 mM DTT
10 mM dNTPs	1.5	0.2 mM
E. coli DNA ligase, 10 U/μL	0.5	0.067 U/μL
E. coli DNA polymerase,	2	0.27 U/μL
10 U/μL; RNase H,	0.5	0.013 U/μL
2 U/μL	Total 75	Incubate at 16°C for 2 h
T4 DNA polymerase, 5 U/μL	1	0.067 U/μL
		Incubate at 16°C for 5 min

2. Add 1 μL of T4 DNA polymerase to second-stranded synthesis mixture and incubate at 16°C for 5 min.
3. Stop the reaction by adding of 5 μL of 0.5 M EDTA.
4. Extract the reaction mixture with the equivalent volume of phenol/chloroform/isoamyl alcohol. Then, extract reversely with 25 μL of TE solution.
5. Extract once with 500 μL of ether for removal of phenol.
6. Add 2 μL of 1 mg/mL of Poly (A) solution as carrier and PEG solution at a final concentration of 6.5%. Store on ice for 1 h.

7. Centrifuge at 10,000*g* for 20 min.
8. Dissolve the pellet with 27 μL of TE solution and then precipitate with 13 μL of 20% PEG solution for removal of excess linkers and small cDNA fragments. Store on ice for 1 h (*see* **Note 4**).
9. Centrifuge at 10,000*g* for 10 min.
10. Rinse the pellet with 80% ethanol and dry in a vacuum desiccator.

3.2.3. Ligation of Primer Adaptor to ds cDNA (Note 5)

1. Dissolve the ds cDNA pellet in 12.5 μL of distilled water.
2. Add P20EA/P10EA primer adaptor and buffer as shown in **Table 6**.
3. Add 2.5 U of T4 DNA ligase and incubate the tube at 16°C overnight.
4. Extract the reaction mixture with the equivalent volume of phenol/chloroform/isoamyl alcohol. Then, extract reversely with 25 μL of TE solution.
5. Extract once with 300 μL of ether for removal of phenol.
6. Add 2 μL of 1 mg/mL Poly (A) solution as carrier and then add 25 μL of 20% PEG solution (final concentration is 6.5%). Store on ice for 1 h.
7. Centrifuge at 10,000*g* for 20 min.
8. Rinse the pellet with 80% ethanol and dry in vacuum desiccator.
9. Dissolve DNA pellet in 34 μL of distilled water.

3.2.4. Digestion of Adaptor-Ligated ds cDNA with Not*I* (Note 6)

1. Cut an adapter present at the 3' end of the ds cDNA with *Not* I restriction enzyme (*see* **Table 7**). Incubate at 37°C for 2 h.
2. Extract with an equivalent volume of phenol/chloroform/isoamyl alcohol. Extract reversely with 50 μL of TE solution.
3. Add 2 μL of 1 mg/mL Poly (A) solution as carrier and 49 μL of 20% PEG solution (final concentration is 6.5%). Store on ice for 1 h.
4. Recover the ds cDNA by centrifugation at 10,000*g* for 20 min.
5. Rinse the pellet with 80% ethanol and then dry in a vacuum desiccator.
6. Dissolve the pellet with 40 μL of distilled water and store at –20°C.

3.3. PCR (see Note 7)

1. Add buffers, reagents, and primer solutions (CA1/P20EA, CB1/P20EA) to the first PCR tube on ice as shown in **Table 8**.
2. Add 2 μL of the ds cDNA solution.
3. Add 20 μL of mineral oil and spin down once at 10,000*g*.
4. Perform PCR reaction for 20 cycles.
5. Add buffers, reagents, and primer solutions (CA2/P20EA, CB2/P20EA) to the second PCR tube.
6. Add 10 μL of the first PCR mixture. Perform PCR reaction for 20 cycles.
7. Electrophorese the aliquots of the second PCR mixture on a 1% agarose gel.

Table 6
Ligation of P20EA/10EA Primer Adapter

Reagent	Volume (μL)	Final concentration/condition
ds DNA solution	12.5	
T4 ligase buffer	5	50 mM Tris-HCl, pH 7.6, 10 mM MgCl$_2$, 1 mM ATP, 5% PEG5000, 1 mM DTT
50 μM P20EA/10EA adapter	5	10 μM
T4 DNA ligase, 1 U/μL	2.5	0.1 U/μL
	Total 25	Incubate at 16°C for over 12 h

Table 7
***Not*I Digestion of dsDNA**

Reagent	Volume (μL)	Final concentration/condition
ds DNA solution	34	
H buffer	5	50 mM Tris-HCl, pH 7.5, 10 mM MgCl$_2$, 1 mM DTT, 100 mM NaCl
0.1% BSA	5	0.01%
0.1% Triton X-100	5	0.01%
*Not*I, 50 U/μL	1	1 U/μL
	Total 50	Incubate at 37°C for over 2 h

Table 8
PCR

Reagent	Volume (μL)	Final concentration/condition
10X PCR buffer	10	10 mM Tris-HCl, pH 9.0, 50 mM KCl, 0.1% Triton X-100
25 mM MgCl$_2$	6	1.5 mM
10 mM dNTP	2	0.2 mM
10 μM P20EA	1 (1st PCR), 10 (2nd)	0.1 μM (1st), 1 μM (2nd)
10 μM C-specific-primer	1 (1st), 10 (2nd)	0.1 μM (1st), 1 μM (2nd)
Distilled water	77.5 (1st), 51.5 (2nd)	
Taq Polymerase, 5 U/μL	0.5	0.025 U/μL
Template DNA	2 (1st), 10 (2nd)	1/50 vol (1st), 1/10 vol (2nd) 94°C: 1 min, 55°C: 1.5 min, 72°C: 2 min
	Total 100	
		20 cycles

3.4. Quantitative Analysis of TCRαV and TCRβV Repertoire

3.4.1. RDB Method

3.4.1.1. BIOTINYLATION OF PCR PRODUCTS

1. Add reagents and primer solution (CA3, CB3) into the PCR tube (*see* **Table 9**).
2. Add 1 µL of the second PCR solution to the mixture.
3. Add 20 µL mineral oil and spin down at 10,000*g*.
4. Perform PCR reaction for 20 cycles.

3.4.1.2. POLY T-TAILING OF SSOPS

1. To perform the poly T-tailing, add reagents to 1.5 mL tube (as shown in **Table 10**).
2. Incubate the tube at 37°C for 1 h.
3. Stop the reaction by boiling.

3.4.1.3. IMMOBILIZATION OF TCRαV AND TCRβV-SPECIFIC PRIMERS ONTO MEMBRANE FILTER

1. Cut the Hybond-Nfp membrane to the appropriate size (80 × 115 mm).
2. Soak the Hybond-Nfp membrane with distilled water and absorb excess water of the membrane into paper towels.
3. Soak the membrane in 20X SSC and absorb excess 20X SSC of the membrane into paper towels.
4. Put the membrane on the 48-well slot type filtration manifold system.
5. Add 1 mL of 20X SSC containing 2.5 µL of SSOPs (5 pmol) into wells on the filtration manifold system (**Note 8**).
6. Aspirate the solution using a water aspirator.
7. Add 1 mL of 20X SSC into each well for complete blotting.
8. Aspirate the solution using a water aspirator.
9. Rinse the membrane once with 20X SSC.
10. Leave the membrane on the 3 MM chromatography paper soaked with 20X SSC.
11. Illuminate UV to the membrane with Strata linker 2400 (UV autocrosslink mode) (*see* **Note 9**).

3.4.1.4. DETECTION BY CHEMILUMINESCENT ENZYME IMMUNOASSAY

1. Prehybridize SSOP-immobilized membrane filter with 10 mL of GMC buffer per sheet at 54°C for 2 h in sealed film.
2. Denature 100 µL of biotinylated PCR mix with equivalent volume of 0.4 *N* NaOH/10 m*M* EDTA for 5 min at room temperature.
3. Mix 10 mL of preheated GMC buffer with the denatured solution. Hybridize at 54°C for 8 h in sealed film.
4. After hybridization, wash the filter three times with washing buffer (2X SSC, 0.1% SDS) at 35°C. Then, wash twice with 0.2X SSC, 0.1% SDS at 35°C.
5. Incubate the filter in TB-TBS buffer for 30 min at room temperature in order to block nonspecific binding.

Table 9
Biotinylation of PCR Products

Reagent	Volume (µL)	Final concentration/condition
10X PCR buffer	10	10 m*M* Tris-HCl, pH 9.0, 50 m*M* KCl, 0.1% Triton X-100
25 m*M* MgCl$_2$	6	1.5 m*M*
10 m*M* d(AGC)TP mix	2	200 µ*M*
0.5 m*M* dTTP	36	180 m*M*
0.5 m*M* BIOTIN-21-dUTP	4	20 µ*M*
Distilled water	40.5	
Taq Polymerase, 5 U/µL	0.5	0.025 U/µL
Template DNA	1	1/100 vol
		94°C: 1 min, 55°C: 1.5 min, 72°C: 2 min
	Total 100	
		20 cycles

Table 10
Poly T-Tailing of SSOPs

Reagent	Volume (µL)	Final concentration/condition
5X 5' tailing buffer	20	40 m*M* potassium cacodylate, pH 7.2, 1 m*M* CoCl$_2$, 0.2 m*M* dithiothreitol
100 µ*M* SSOP	2	2 µ*M*
20 m*M* dTTP	6	1.2 m*M*
Distilled water	68	
Terminal deoxynucleotidyl Transferase (3.25 U/µL)	4	0.13 U/µL
	Total 100	37°C for 1h

6. Incubate the filter for 30–45 min at room temperature in TB-TBS containing a 1/1000 dilution of alkaline-phosphatase-conjugated streptavidine.
7. Wash six times with T-TBS at room temperature.
8. Soak the filter with coloring buffer to replace buffer.
9. Absorb excess coloring buffer of the membrane into the 3 MM chromatography paper.
10. Soak the filter in AMPPD buffer contain 1/1000 vol of AMPPD for 30 min in a darkroom.
11. Get rid of excess AMPPD buffer on the 3 MM chromatography paper.
12. Expose to a X-ray film for 15–30 min (**Fig. 2**).

3.4.1.5. ESTIMATION OF THE FREQUENCIES OF TCRαV AND TCRβV REPERTOIRES (*SEE* **NOTE 10**)

1. Measure the visualized films by an image scanner GT-9000 (Epson, Tokyo, Japan).

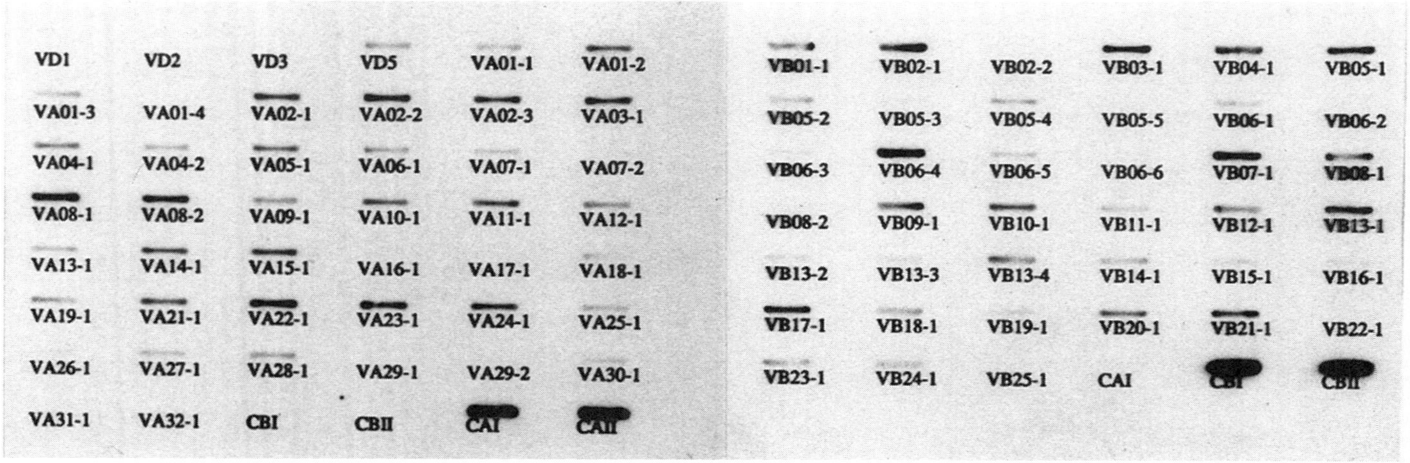

Fig. 2. Representative result of human TCRαV and TCRβV repertoire analysis using reverse dot-blot analysis.

96

2. Estimate the signals by the Quantity One Image Analysis software (pdi Huntington Station, NY).
3. Compensate the difference of hybridization intensities among these TCR SSOPs using V/C value (*see* **Table 2**).
4. Calculate the relative frequency (%) of each TCRAV or TCRBV usage according to this formula:

$$\text{relative frequency (\%)} = \frac{(\text{corrected absorbance with TCRV-specific probe} \times 100)}{(\text{sum of corrected absorbances with TCRV-specific probes})} \tag{1}$$

3.4.2. MHA Method

3.4.2.1. BIOTINYLATION OF PCR PRODUCTS

1. Add each reagent and 5' biotinylate primer solution (CA4BIO, CB4BIO) to the PCR tube.
2. Mix 1 µL of the second PCR solution to the tube.
3. Add 20 µL of mineral oil and spin down at 10,000g.
4. Perform PCR reaction for 20 cycles.
5. Electrophorese the aliquots of the PCR mixture on 1% agarose gel.

3.4.2.2. IMMOBILIZATION OF TCRαV AND TCRβV SPECIFIC PRIMERS ONTO MICROPLATE (*SEE* NOTE 11)

1. Add 25 µL of 10 pmol amino-modified oligonucleotides into each well of carboxylate-modified ELISA plate, C type, Sumitomo Bakelite.
2. After adding 50 µL of 0.2 M EDC and 25 µL of 4 mM Sulfo-NHS in MES buffer (pH 5.4) to each well, incubate overnight at room temperature in a container.
3. Wash plate wells twice with phosphate-buffered saline (PBS).
4. Add 200 µL of 0.4 N NaOH to wells and incubate for 2 h at 47°C to remove noncovalently bound oligonucleotides.
5. Wash the plate wells with PBS.
6. Dry up oligonucleotide-immobilized plates in vacuum desiccator and store at 4°C in sealed film (*see* **Note 12**).

3.4.2.3. ENZYME-LINKED IMMUNOSORBENT ASSAY (*SEE* NOTE 13)

1. Prehybridize oligonucleotide-immobilized plates with 200 µL per well of GMC buffer at 47°C for 30 min in a humidified incubator.
2. Denature 60 µL aliquots of 5'-biotinylated PCR mix with equivalent volume of 0.4 N NaOH/10 mM EDTA for 5 min at room temperature.
3. Add the denatured mixture to 6 mL of GMC buffer. Add 100 µL of hybridization solution (1/100 dilution in GMC buffer) to each well of the micro-titer plate. Hybridize at 47°C for 4 h.
4. After the hybridization, wash the wells six times with washing buffer (2X SSC, 0.1% SDS) at room temperature.
5. Prewash the wells twice with VA (0.4X SSC, 0.1% SDS) or VB (0.6X SSC, 0.1% SDS) high stringency washing buffer. Add 200 µL each of stringency

washing buffer to each well and incubate for 10 min at 37°C. Finally, wash two times with each high stringency washing buffer.

6. Add 200 µL of TB-TBS buffer to wells and sit at room temperature for 10 min in order to block nonspecific binding.
7. To detect hybridized 5'-biotinylated PCR products, Add 100 µL of a 1/1000 dilution of alkaline-phosphatase-conjugated streptavidine in TB-TBS per well and incubate at 37°C for 30 min.
8. Wash the wells six times in T-TBS.
9. Add 100 µL of substrate solution containing 4 mg/mL *p*-nitrophenylphosphate in 20% diethanolamine, pH 9.8, to wells.
10. After color development, measure absorbance at 405 nm by using an immunoreader (**Fig. 3,** *see* **Note 14**).

3.4.2.4. ESTIMATION OF FREQUENCIES OF TCRAV AND TCRBV REPERTOIRES

1. Measure the absorbance units of each well.
2. Divide absorbance of TCRV segments by each V/C value for normalization of different hybridization intensities between probes (**Table 3**).
3. Calculate the relative frequency (%) of each TCRAV or TCRBV probe according to the formula described in (**Subheading 3.4.1.5., step 4**).

4. Notes

1. Although we use commercially available Trizol reagent kit, the procedure can be substituted by the acid-guanidinium phenol chloroform (AGPC) method described by Chomzensky et al. *(17)*. One million cells can be generally obtained from 1 mL of whole peripheral blood. PBMCs are isolated by Ficoll-Paque (Pharmacia Biotech, Uppsala, Sweden) gradient centrifugation, cells are washed once with RPMI-1640 medium, and collected by centrifugation. At least 1 mL of Trizol reagent should be added to ~1 × 10⁷ cells for extraction of total RNA. Total RNA extracted from 1–5 mL of whole blood is sufficient for precise analysis of TCR repertoires. However, it is difficult to analyse TCR repertoires of T cells in tissues, such as skin or mucosal lesion, because a limited number of T cells are present in the pathogenic lesions even when inflammatory reactions occur. When tissue samples are used as a mRNA source, the samples should be fresh and contain a large number of T cells. Two milliliters of Trizol LS reagent is added to samples (3–5 mm³) in a glass homogenizer instead of Trizol reagent because the Trizol LS reagent is composed of high concentration of guanidinium salt, which can inhibit RNase activity. After the samples are completely homogenized, 530 µL of chloroform is added to the mixture.
2. A second extraction step with Trizol reagent may be required for the purification of RNA from tissue samples, or the extensive removal of a large amount of cell debris. It is difficult to directly dissolve the RNA pellet recovered by isopropanol precipitation in Trizol reagent. Thus, the pellet should be first dissolved in a small volume of DEPC-treated water.

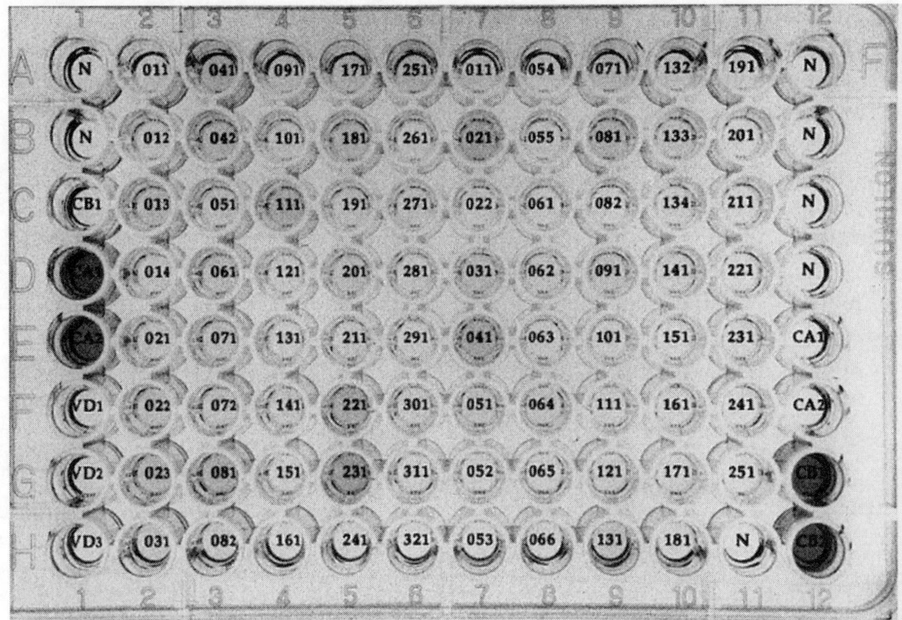

Fig. 3. Representative result of human TCRαV and TCRβV repertoire analysis using microplate hybridization assay. Columns 1–6 indicate plate format for TCRαV repertoire analysis, columns 7–12 for TCRβV. N indicates wells containing no oligonucleotide. CA1, CA2 (column 1) and CB1, CB2 (column 12) were positive controls. CB1 (column 1) and CA1, CA2 (column 12) were negative controls.

3. The procedure follows the instruction manual for Trizol reagent from Gibco-BRL. This procedure is previously described by Okayama et al. *(18)* and Gubler et al. *(19)*. If necessary, you can use the second-strand synthesis kit (Superscript plasmid system) supplied by Gibco-BRL.

4. Throughout this protocol, PEG precipitation is used for recovery of DNA instead of ethanol precipitation, which is sufficient for removal of residual primers or small fragments of DNA from ds cDNA. Further precipitation with PEG is effective for complete purification of DNA.

5. Primer adapters should not be phosphorylated at the 5' end to prevent the ligation of the adapter to the 5'-end of the antisense strand. The adapter may be ligated to the 5'-end of antisense strand, however, if the nucleotide at this end is removed by the 5'→3' exonuclease activity of *E. coli* DNA polymerase I.

6. The adapter is completely removed from 3' end of ds cDNA by digestion with *Not*I. When mRNA from T cells is abundant, TCR gene segments may be efficiently amplified without *Not*I digestion.

7. To specifically amplify TCR gene segments, the first PCR reaction is performed using a relatively lower concentration of primers (final concentration: 0.1 μ*M*).

8. Addition of a small amount of bromophenol blue dye to the 20X SSC solution can visualize SSOPs blotted onto membranes.

9. The nylon membrane with bound SSOPs can be stored at room temperature in sealed film, and is stable for at least 3 mo.

10. The corrected absorbance should be used for determination of TCR repertoires because potential of hybridization with target V segment is different among SSOPs. It is important that signals obtained with individual probes is normalized with respect to relative hybridization potential (V/C value). Thus, ratio of hybridization intensity of each TCRV-specific probe to that of TCRC-specific probe (V/C value) should be precisely determined by using TCR cDNA clones bearing both the V segment and the universal C segment. The V/C values should preferrably be determined in each laboratory, because this may be influenced by synthesized probes, experimental devices, or other factors. These V/C values can dramatically alter the frequency of TCR repertoires.

11. Plate format is shown in **Fig. 3**. As a positive control, specific probes (CβI and CβII) for the TCRβC segment are used for TCRβV repertoire assays, whereas specific probes for TCRαC (Cα and Cα2) are used as a negative control. On the same way, CA probes are used as a positive control, CB probe as a negative control in TCRαV repertoire assays.

12. The microplate with covalently bound SSOPs is stable at 4°C for at least 3 mo.

13. Use of GMC buffer effectively decreases the levels of background signal on hybridization. The high stringency washing buffer should be prepared exactly according to the format because some biotinylated PCR products may be washed out at low salt concentration.

14. The measurement should be done before absorbance units reach plateau, which is approximately over 1.5.

References

1. Davis, M. M. and Bjorkman, P. K. (1988) T-cell antigen receptor genes and T-cell recognition. *Nature* **334,** 395–402.

2. Wilson, R. K., Lai, E., Concannon, P., Barth, R. K., and Hood, L. E. (1988) Structure, organization and polymorphism of murine and human T-cell receptor α and β chain gene family. *Immunol. Rev.* **101,** 149–172.

3. Jenkins, R. N., Nikaein, A., Zimmermann, A., Meek, K., and Lipsky, P. E. (1993) T cell receptor Vβ gene bias in rheumatoid synovial fluid T lymphocytes. *Clin. Exp. Immunol.* **92,** 2688–2701.

4. Plushke, G., Ricken, G., Taube, S., Kroninger, S., Melchers, I., Peter, H., Eickmann, K., and Krawinkel, U. (1991) Biased T cell receptor V region repertoire in the synovial fluid of rheumatoid arthritis patients. *Eur. J. Immunol.* **21,** 2749–2754.

5. Ben-nun, A., Liblau, R. S., Cohen, L., Lehmann, D., Tournier-Lasserve, A., Rosenzweig, A., Zhang, J., Raus, J. C. M., and Bath, M.-A. (1991) Restricted T-cell receptor Vβ gene usage by myelin basic protein-specific T-cell clones in multiple sclerosis: predominant genes vary in individuals. *Proc. Natl. Acad. Sci. USA* **88,** 2466–2470.

6. O'Hanlon, T. P, Dalakas, M. C., Plotz, P. H., and Miller, F. W. (1994) Predominant TCR-αβ variable and joining gene expression by muscle-infiltrating lymphocytes in idiopathic inflammatory myopathies. *J. Immunol.* **152,** 2569–2576.

7. Choi, Y., Kotzin, B., Herron, L., Callahan, P., Marrack, P., and Kapper, J. (1989) Interaction of Staphylococcus aureus toxin "superantigen" with human T-cells. *Proc. Natl. Acad. Sci. USA* **86,** 8941–8945.

8. Diu, A., Romagne, F., Genevee, C., Rocher, C., Bruneau, J. M., David, A., Praz, F., and Hercend, T. (1993) Fine specificity of monoclonal antibodies directed at human T cell receptor variable regions: comparison with oligonucleotide-deriven amplification for evaluation of Vβ expression. *Eur. J. Immunol.* **23,** 1422–1429.

9. Loh, E. Y., Elliot, J. F., Cwirla, S., Lanier, L. L., and Davis, M. M. (1989) Polymerase chain reaction with single-sided specificity: analysis of T cell receptor γ chain. *Science* **243,** 217–220.

10. Roman-Roman, S., Ferradini, L., Azocar, J., Genevee, C., Hercevd, T., and Triebel, F. (1991) Studies on the human T cell receptor α/β variable region genes. I. Identification of 7 additional Vα subfamilies and 14 Jα gene segments. *Eur. J Immunol.* **21,** 927–933.

11. Uematsu, Y., Wege, H., Straus, A., Ott, M., Bannwarth, W., Lanchbury, J., Panayi, G., and Steinmetz, M. (1991) The T-cell receptor repertoire in the synovial fluid of a patient with rheumatoid arthritis is polyclonal. *Proc. Natl. Acad. Sci. USA* **88,** 8534–8538.

12. Tsuruta, Y., Iwagami, S., Furue, S., Teraoka, H., Yoshida, T., Sakata, T., and Suzuki, R. (1993) Detection of human T cell receptor cDNA (α, β, γ, and δ) by ligation of a universal adaptor to variable region. *J. Immunol. Methods* **161,** 7–21.

13. Tsuruta, Y., Yoshioka, T., Suzuki, R., and Sakata, T. (1994) Analysis of the population of human T cell receptor γ and δ chain variable region subfamilies by reverse dot blot hybridization. *J. Immunol. Methods* **169,** 17–23.

14. Matsutani, T., Oishi, C., Kaneshige, T., Igimi, H., Uchida, K., Tsuruta, Y., Yoshioka, T., Suzuki, R., and Sakata, T. (1994) Molecular analysis of T-cell receptor Vβ chain to detect leukemia cell clonality in patients by adaptor ligation-mediated polymerase chain reaction. *J. Immunol. Methods* **177,** 9–15.

15. Yoshioka, T., Matsutani, T., Iwagami, S., Tsuruta, Y., Kaneshige, T., Toyosaki, T., and Suzuki, R. (1997) Quantitative analysis of the usage of human T cell receptor α and β chain variable regions by reverse dot blot hybridization. *J. Immunol. Methods* **201,** 145–155.

16. Matsutani, T., Yoshioka, T., Tsuruta, Y., Iwagami, S., and Suzuki, R. (1997) Analysis of TCRαV and TCRβV repertoires in healthy individuals by microplate hybridization assay. *Human Immunol.* **56,** 57–69.

17. Chomczynski, P. and Sacchi, N. (1987) Single-step method of RNA isolated by acid guanidium-thiocyanate-phenol-chloroform extraction. *Anal. Biochem.* **162,** 156–159.

18. Okayama, H. and Berg, P. (1982) High-efficiency cloning of full length cDNA. *Mol. Cell. Biol.* **2,** 161–170.

19. Gubler, U. and Hoffman, B. J. (1983) A simple and very effective method for generating cDNA libraries. *Gene* **25,** 263–269.

9

Flow Cytometric Detection of Cytoplasmic and Surface CD3-ε Expression in Developing T Cells

Karl J. Franek and Robert Chervenak

1. Introduction

The pathway of T-cell development follows a series of highly regulated steps beginning with the differentiation of bone marrow-resident pluripotent hemato-poietic stem cells (HSCs) into T-cell progenitors that migrate to the thymus. Upon colonizing the thymic microenvironment, T-cell progenitors further differentiate into mature immunocompetent T lymphocytes through a series of stages that are characterized by the regulated expression of the coreceptor molecules CD4 and CD8. However, the acquisition of a functional T-cell antigen receptor (TCR)/CD3 complex is perhaps the most significant of the events that take place during early thymocyte development. This multisubunit complex consists of two disulfide-linked variant TCRα/β (or TCRγ/δ) chains, which are responsible for recognition of MHC-restricted antigenic peptides. Noncovalently associated with the TCR heterodimer is a signal transducing complex, which is comprised of the invariant chains CD3γ, δ, ε, and ζ. The expression of the components of the TCR/CD3 complex is developmentally regulated, and evidence in recent years has suggested that immature signaling receptor complexes composed of CD3 chains may, in part, direct very early intrathymic development. Prior to their assembly and transport to the cell surface, however, CD3 subunits accumulate in the intracellular compartment of immature thymocytes. The current chapter describes a flow cytometric technique that enables the study of CD3 expression both on the surface and in the cytoplasm of developing thymocytes.

1.1. Intrathymic T-Cell Development

Intrathymic differentiation can be divided into major developmental stages based on the expression of CD4, CD8, and the TCR/CD3 subunits (reviewed in

From: *Methods in Molecular Biology, Vol. 134: T Cell Protocols: Development and Activation*
Edited by: K. P. Kearse © Humana Press Inc., Totowa, NJ

refs. *1–4*). Early thymocytes lack expression of cell surface TCR/CD3 and the coreceptors CD4 and CD8, and are referred to as triple negative (TN; CD3⁻ CD4⁻ CD8⁻) *(1–4)*. The earliest (thymic seeding) cells, however, have been identified as a population that expresses low levels of CD4 (i.e., CD3⁻ CD4^{Lo} CD8⁻) *(5)*. The CD3⁻ CD4^{Lo} CD8⁻ population lacks surface CD3 expression and contains TCRα, β, γ, and δ genes in germline configuration *(5)*. The rearrangement and expression of TCRβ genes occurs at the TN stage, and the TCRβ chain initially is expressed on the cell surface as a heterodimer with the pre-Tα chain *(6,7)* within the context of a pre-T-cell receptor *(6–8)*. Signaling through the pre-TCR leads to β-selection (allelic exclusion), the upregulation of CD4 and CD8, and promotes the differentiation of thymocytes to the CD4⁺ CD8⁺ double positive (DP) stage *(4)*. During the DP stage, TCRα genes are rearranged and expressed in association with the TCRβ and CD3 chains in complete TCR complexes that are expressed on the cell surface *(9)*. T cells are finally selected on the basis of the specificities of their T-cell receptors to advance to the CD4⁺ CD8⁻ or CD4⁻ CD8⁺ single positive (SP) stage *(9,10)*.

1.2. CD3 Expression During T-Cell Development

The expression, assembly, and transport of TCR/CD3 complexes differs significantly in mature T cells and immature thymocytes. In mature T cells, only complete receptor complexes consisting of TCRα/β and the CD3γ, δ, ε, and ζ chains are transported from the endoplasmic reticulum (ER), where they are synthesized, to the Golgi, and finally to the cell surface (for reviews *see* **refs.** *11,12*). Each component must be available in stoichiometric amounts before assembly and transport of the receptor complex can occur *(11,12)*. Incomplete TCR/CD3 complexes are retained in the ER and subsequently degraded *(13)*. In immature thymocytes, however, rare partial TCR complexes consisting of CD3γ, δ, and ε subunits that are competent for signal transduction, may be present on the surface of DN thymocytes.

Expression of CD3 genes is evident very early in the developmental pathway, before the onset of TCRβ gene rearrangement. The earliest thymus seeding (CD4^{Lo}) cells express transcripts from the CD3γ, δ, ε, and ζ genes *(14)*. Several studies have provided evidence of incomplete T-cell receptor complexes consisting of CD3 subunits that are associated with a TCRβ chain *(15–17)* or of CD3 chains alone *(18–21)*. CD3 receptor complexes consisting of CD3γε and CD3δε dimers *(23)* are present on the cell surface prior to the expression of TCRβ chains in normal immature thymocytes, and are thought to be involved in very early signaling events that promote DN thymocytes to differentiate to the DP stage *(20–22)*.

Because signaling via cell surface CD3 complexes appears to be important in the early stages of intrathymic differentiation, the status of CD3 gene and protein expression may be indicative of developmental progression. In particular, the intracellular accumulation of free CD3 chains and partially assembled subcomplexes, prior to the appearance of cell surface-associated receptors, may be exploited to characterize phenotypic changes during very early T-cell development (i.e., TN thymocytes). This chapter describes a method by which the expression of cytoplasmic CD3ε (and likely other intracellular targets) may be monitored by flow cytometry during intrathymic development. This technique complements very well other cellular, biochemical, and molecular methods of analysis of TCR/CD3 expression during T-cell development.

2. Materials

2.1. Staining of Cytoplasmic CD3ε, Surface CD3ε, and Multiple Surface Markers

1. Phosphate-buffered saline (PBS): 1.5 mM KH$_2$PO$_4$, 2.7 mM KCl, 13.7 mM NaCl, 8 mM Na$_2$HPO$_4$, pH 7.4 (Dulbecco PBS; Sigma, St. Louis, MO), sterilized by passage through a 0.2-μm filter. Store at 4°C.
2. Staining buffer (SB): PBS with 2% fetal bovine serum, 0.1% NaN$_3$ (all purchased from Sigma). Sodium azide is a hazardous material and must be handled with caution (*see* **Note 1**). Store at 4°C.
3. Paraformaldehyde: Paraformaldehyde is extremely toxic! Consult MSDS for safe handling procedures. Wear proper protective clothing (latex gloves, lab coat, goggles, and so forth) and handle under a ventilated fume-hood (*see* **Note 1**). Paraformaldehyde (Sigma) is prepared as a 4% (w/v) stock solution in PBS, pH 7.3. Paraformaldehyde dissolves very slowly and may require stirring overnight at room temperature under a fume-hood. Alternatively, one can raise the pH using 1 N NaOH until the paraformaldehyde completely dissolves (~ pH 10.0). Then, lower the pH to 7.3 with HCl. Filter and store at 4°C in a lightproof bottle for up to 2 wk. Dilute to 2% with sterile PBS just prior to use.
4. Saponin: Saponin (Sigma) is prepared as a 10% (w/v) stock solution in PBS. Store at room temperature.
5. Digitonin: Digitonin (Sigma) is prepared as a stock solution of 0.25% (w/v) in PBS. The mixture is boiled for 10 min to dissolve digitonin. Store at room temperature.
6. Bovine serum albumin (BSA): A stock solution of 10% (w/v) BSA (Sigma) is prepared in PBS. Store at 4°C.
7. Antibody reagents: Prepare fluorochrome-conjugated antibodies for the staining of surface molecules in SB. Anti-CD3ε-PE, anti-CD3ε-FITC (YCD3, clone 29B), and anti-CD4-RED613 (clone H129.19) were purchased from Gibco-BRL (Gaithersburg, MD). Anti-CD8α-APC (clone 53-6.7) was purchased from PharMingen (San Diego, CA). Unlabeled YCD3 used in blocking surface CD3 was purified from hybridoma supernatants in our laboratory. Purified antibody was diluted in SB containing 2% BSA (*see* **Note 2**).
8. Digitonin/BSA/saponin (DBS) detergent solution: Prepare a mixture of 0.025% digitonin, 2% BSA, and 0.5% saponin in PBS. This solution is used to

permeabilize cells during the staining of cytoplasmic CD3ε and as a post-stain wash to remove nonspecifically bound anti-CD3ε.

9. Cytoplasmic staining reagents: Fluorochrome-conjugated anti-CD3ε (YCD3-FITC or YCD3-PE) is diluted in DBS (DBS-CD3ε-FITC).

10. An isotypic control, matched to the monoclonal antibody used to stain cytoplasmic CD3ε (i.e., rat IgG2b-FITC; PharMingen) is diluted in DBS.

3. Methods

3.1. Simultaneous Staining of Surface and Cytoplasmic CD3ε

The procedure described below is a modification of the methods previously described by Franek et al. *(24)*.

1. Prepare single-cell suspensions of freshly isolated lymphoid tissue or cultured cells. Thymocytes and splenocytes are obtained by macerating whole thymus or spleen through a fine wire mesh, or by crushing the organ between the frosted ends of two microscope slides and washing with ice-cold Hanks balanced salt solution (HBSS; Sigma). Single-cell suspensions of thymocytes or splenocytes are obtained by passing the crude tissue homogenate through a syringe fitted with a 26-gage needle. Adherent cells grown in culture should be removed from the plastic surfaces by treatment with EDTA or Versene; enzymatic treatments (i.e., trypsinization) should be avoided to preserve cell surface molecules. Centrifuge fresh or cultured cells at 200g at 4°C for 10 min, resuspend the cells in cold SB, and keep on ice.

2. The following staining procedure (**steps 2–9**) is depicted as a flow diagram in **Fig. 1**. Place 1×10^6 cells in the wells of a 96-well round bottom microtiter plate, centrifuge at 200g for 3 min at 4°C. Remove the supernatant and resuspend each cell pellet in 50 μL of unlabeled anti-Fc receptor (anti-FcR; clone 2.4G2) to block cell surface Fc receptors. Incubate the cells on ice for 15 min.

3. Wash the cells by adding 150 μL of SB, centrifuging at 200g for 3 min at 4°C, and removing the supernatant.

4. Fix the cells by resuspending the cell pellet in 50 μL of 2% paraformaldehyde. Incubate the cells at room temperature for 15 min, and wash as in **step 3**.

5. Resuspend the cell pellet in 50 μL of anti-CD3ε-PE and incubate as described above (**step 2**) to stain surface CD3ε (*see* **Note 2**). Keep the cells protected from light in this and in subsequent steps to avoid degradation of fluorochromes. Wash the cells free of the antibody as described in **step 3**.

6. Block any unstained surface CD3ε by incubating the cells with excess unconjugated anti-CD3ε on ice for 15 min (*see* **Note 3**). Wash the cells as in **step 3**.

7. Resuspend the stained cells in 0.5% saponin and incubate at 4°C for 10 min. Wash the cells in SB to permeabilize the cells. Resuspend the cells in DBS-anti-CD3ε-FITC and incubate at 4°C for 15 min to stain intracellular CD3ε. Wash the cells as in **step 3**.

8. Incubate the cells in DBS (without antibody) to remove nonspecifically bound antibody by incubation at 4°C for 15 min. Wash the cells twice in SB as in **step 3**.

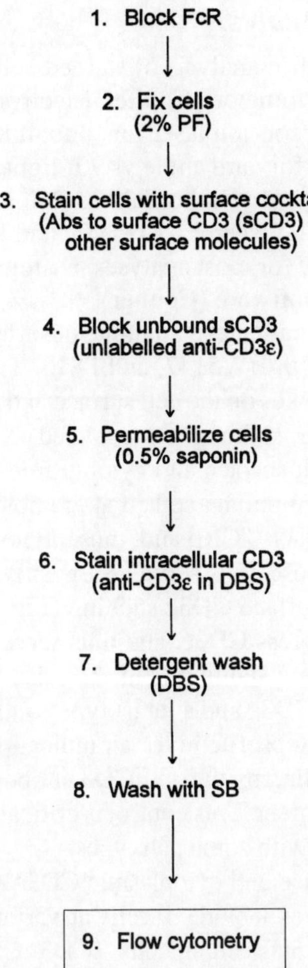

Fig. 1. Procedure for the simultaneous staining of surface and cytoplasmic CD3ε: The flow diagram outlines the protocol for the detection of surface molecules (such as CD3ε) and cytoplasmic CD3ε on freshly isolated and cultured cells by flow cytometry. Procedures are as outlined in the text. Cells are fixed with paraformaldehyde to preserve structural integrity (**step 2**). Surface targets, such CD3ε, CD4, and CD8, are then stained (**step 3**). In preparation for staining of cytoplasmic CD3ε, any remaining unstained surface CD3 molecules are then blocked with unconjugated anti-CD3 (using the same monoclonal antibody idiotype; **step 4**). Cells are then permeablized with saponin and cytoplasmic CD3ε is stained (**steps 5,6**). Sustained cells are then washed in detergent (**step 7**) and finally washed in SB (**step 8**). PF, Paraformaldehyde; DBS, Digitonin:BSA:Saponin solution; SB, staining buffer; SA, streptavidin-fluorochrome conjugate.

9. Finally, resuspend the stained cells in SB at a concentration of 1×10^6 cells/mL for analysis by flow cytometry.

3.2. Flow Cytometric Analysis

Two-color flow cytometric analysis of stained cells was performed using a EPICS Profile II flow cytometer (Coulter Electronics, Inc., Hialeah, FL), equipped with a 15 mW argon-ion laser tuned to 488 nm. The cell population of interest was gated using forward angle vs 90° light scatter. Electronic gating was set to omit dead cells and cellular debris. Color compensation was set to minimize spectral overlap between FL1 (FITC) and FL2 (PE). A minimum of 10,000 events was collected for most analyses. Histograms were analyzed using EPICS Elite Workstation software (Coulter).

Figure 2 illustrates the simultaneous staining of surface and cytoplasmic CD3ε using the cell lines DO11.10, BW5147, and P815. The DO11.10 cells express complete TCR/CD3 complexes on the cell surface and serve as a positive control for surface and cytoplasmic staining. As depicted in **Fig. 2**, a majority of the DO11.10 cells express both surface and cytoplasmic CD3ε. The BW5147 cell line represents murine T lymphoma cells that are able to synthesize the TCRα and CD3 components, but lack TCRβ and, thus, do not express complete receptors on the cell surface. These cells serve as a positive control for cytoplasmic CD3 but are negative for surface CD3ε staining (**Fig. 2**). The murine mastocytoma P815 cells do not express CD3ε, and thus serve as a negative control for both surface and cytoplasmic staining (**Fig. 2**). Also shown in **Fig. 2** are cells stained with anti- (surface)CD3ε and a rat isotype control (i.e., rat IgG2b-FITC). The isotype control staining profile gives an indication of the level of nonspecific (isotype-specific) binding by the anti-CD3 antibody, and antibody trapping in the intracellular compartment. This control is critical because levels of trapped antibody can be quite high with some cell types.

Figure 3 illustrates surface and cytoplasmic CD3ε expression by thymocytes and spleen cells. Thymocytes include T cells at various stages of development ranging from immature thymic seeding cells (sCD3⁻ CD4^Lo CD8⁻) that lack surface TCR complexes, to mature CD4⁺ CD8⁻ and CD4⁻ CD8⁺ single positive (SP) T cells that express high levels of the TCR complex (CD3^Hi). A vast majority (97.7%) of thymocytes expresses cytoplasmic CD3ε (quadrants 2 and 4), whereas 17% of the cells express both high level surface and cytoplasmic CD3ε, presumably CD4⁺ CD8⁺ and SP T cells. The spleen contains similar levels of mature T cells that express both surface and cytoplasmic CD3ε, approx 17%.

3.3. Staining of Cytoplasmic CD3
and Multiple Surface Targets—Intrathymic T-Cell Development

The procedure for staining multiple surface markers is similar to that used in staining cytoplasmic and surface CD3ε only (**Subheading 3.1.**), the major dif-

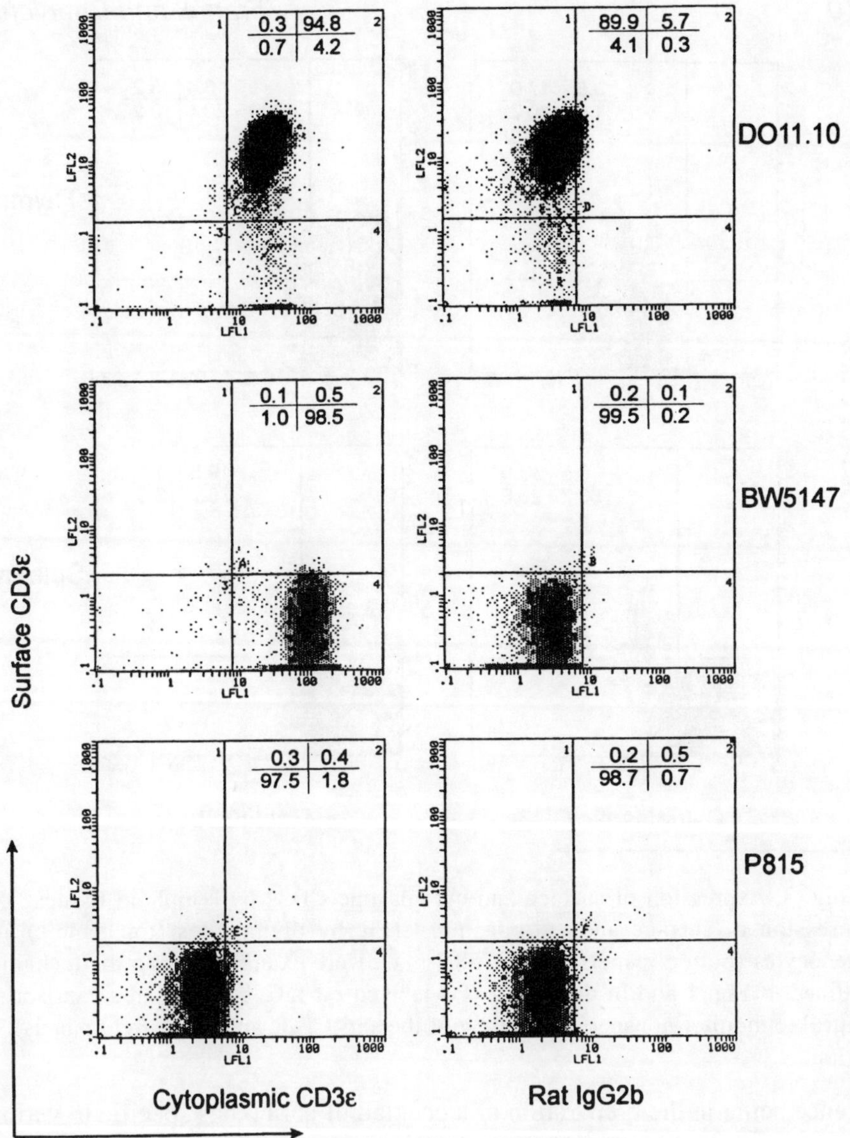

Fig. 2. Expression of surface and cytoplasmic CD3ε by cell lines: Various cell lines may be used as controls in optimizing a protocol for the staining of surface and cytoplasmic CD3ε (outlined in **Fig. 1** and in the text). DO11.10 cells are positive controls for both surface and cytoplasmic CD3ε expression (top panels). The BW5147 thymoma cells are positive controls for cytoplasmic CD3ε expression and negative controls for surface CD3ε expression (middle panels). P815 mastocytoma cells are negative controls for both surface and cytoplasmic CD3ε expression (bottom panels). Staining with an isotype control matched to the anti-CD3ε monoclonal antibody used to stain cytoplasmic CD3ε (e.g., rat IgG2b) is depicted in the right panels.

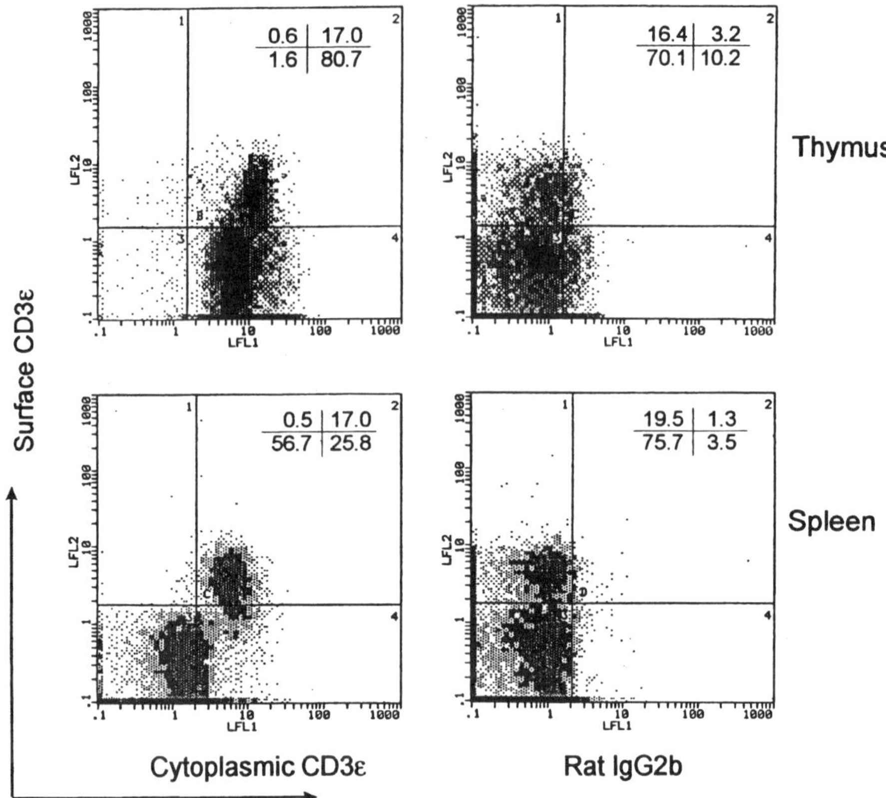

Fig. 3. Expression of surface and cytoplasmic CD3ε by lymphoid tissues: The expression of surface and cytoplasmic CD3ε by thymocytes (top panels) and splenocytes (bottom panels) from C58/J mice were examined using the technique outlined in **Fig. 1** and in the text. FITC-labeled rat IgG2b was used as an isotype control to monitor nonspecific binding of the anti-CD3ε antibody (right panels).

ference being in the preparation of a cocktail of antibodies specific to various surface markers (*see also* **Fig. 1.**). In this section we describe the staining of thymocytes from C58/J mice with antibodies to surface CD4, CD8, and CD3ε, as well as cytoplasmic CD3ε. Control staining reactions are summarized in **Table 1**. The same general scheme should be applicable to a wide range of cell surface markers expressed by thymocytes or other cell types.

1. Harvest thymocytes as described in **Subheading 3.1., step 1**.
2. Block Fc receptors with anti-FcR (unconjugated 2.4G2): Incubate on ice for 15 min. Wash the cells in SB.
3. Fix thymocytes in 2% paraformaldehyde at room temperature for 15 min. Wash the cells in SB.

Table 1
Control Staining Reactions[a]

Intact cells	Staining step		
Well	1	2	3
1.	—[b]		
2.	αCD3-FITC[c]		
3.	αCD3-PE		
4.	αCD4-RED613		
5.	αCD8-APC		
6.	αCD3-PE, αCD4-RED613, αCD8-APC		
7.	αCD3-PE	αCD3-Un	αCD3-FITC

Fixed cells	Staining step					
Well	1	2	3	4	5	6	7
8.	PF	—	—	Sap	DBS	DBS	SB wash
9.	PF	αsCD3-PE, αCD4-R613, αCD8-APC	αsCD3-Un	Sap	αcCD3-FITC-DBS	DBS	SB wash
10.	PF	αsCD3-PE, aCD4-R613, αCD8-APC	αsCD3-Un	Sap	rt IgG2b-FITC-DBS	DBS	SB wash

[a]Before staining, all cells are incubated with anti-FcR (2.4G2) to block surface Fc receptors.

[b]Well 1 contains unstained control cells. Wells 2–5 represent single-color stained cells used to set instrument color compensation. The cells in well 6 are used to inspect the populations of interest. Well 7 represents a control which monitors the efficiency of blocking of surface CD3ε by unconjugated anti-CD3ε. Well 8 contains fixed and permeabilized unstained cells used to assess changes in forward angle and 90° light scatter. Well 9 contains cells with stained surface markers and cytoplasmic CD3ε. Well 10 contains cells stained with antibodies to surface markers and with the appropriate rat isotype control (i.e., rat IgG2b-FITC)

[c]αsCD3 = anti-surface CD3ε; αcCD3 = anti-cytoplasmic CD3ε; αsCD3-Un = unlabeled anti-surface CD3ε; αCD4 = anti-CD4; αCD8 = anti-CD8; rt IgG2b = isotype control; PF = 2% paraformaldehyde; Sap = 0.5% saponin; DBS = digitonin:BSA:saponin solution

4. Stain thymocytes with a cocktail of anti-CD4-RED613, anti-CD8α-APC, and anti-CD3ε-PE. Incubate the cells on ice for 15 min in the dark. Wash the cells as described in (**Subheading 3.1., step 3**). Be sure to keep the stained cells protected from light in all subsequent steps to prevent degradation of fluorochromes.
5. Block remaining unbound surface CD3ε with unconjugated anti-CD3ε. Wash the cells in SB.
6. Permeabilize the cells with 0.5% saponin. Wash the cells in SB.
7. Stain cytoplasmic CD3ε and wash the cells in SB.
8. Incubate the cells with despeciated bovine serum (DBS) for 15 min at 4°C, followed by two washes in SB.
9. Resuspend stained thymocytes in SB at $0.5–1.0 \times 10^6$ cells/mL and analyze by flow cytometry.

3.4. Flow Cytometry

Stained thymocytes were analyzed using a FACS Vantage flow cytometer (Becton Dickinson, San Jose, CA) made available through the Core Facility for Flow Cytometry at LSUMC (Shreveport). The instrument is equipped with a 35 mW helium-neon laser (Spectra-Physics, Mountain View, CA) tuned to 633 nm and an Enterprise (Coherent, Santa Clara, CA) argon-ion laser producing 125 mW of 488 nm light. The thymocyte population of interest was gated using forward angle versus 90° light scatter. Electronic gating was set to omit dead cells and cellular debris. Spectral overlap between FL1 (FITC), FL2 (PE), and FL3 (RED613) was compensated using single-color controls (*see* **Table 1**). A minimum of 50,000 events was collected for most analyses. Histograms were analyzed using CELLQuest software (Becton Dickinson).

The representative experiment described here (**Fig. 4**) involves the phenotypic analysis of the expression of CD4, CD8, and surface and cytoplasmic CD3ε by thymocytes. The principal stages in intrathymic T-cell development are represented in **Fig. 4A** beginning with the CD4^{Lo} CD8$^-$ thymic immigrant cells (R2), followed by the CD4$^-$ CD8$^-$ (R3), CD4$^+$ CD8$^+$ thymocytes (R4), and finally the CD4$^+$ CD8$^-$ and CD4$^-$ CD8$^+$ single positive mature thymocytes (R5 and R6, respectively). **Fig. 4B** depicts the expression of surface and cytoplasmic CD3ε by each of these thymic subpopulations. A majority of the proposed earliest thymic immigrant CD4^{Lo} CD8$^-$ cells (~83%) expresses cytoplasmic CD3ε; about half of these cells also express CD3ε on the surface. A large portion (~ 73%) of the DN thymocytes (R3) express only cytoplasmic CD3ε, and many of these thymocytes express high levels of the protein. This may be indicative of the accumulation of CD3ε polypeptides in intracellular compartments (e.g., ER, Golgi), perhaps as free subunits or in partial complexes with CD3 and TCR chains awaiting assembly and/or transport to the cell surface.

The DP thymocyte population (R4) includes a large proportion of thymocytes that express cytoplasmic CD3ε, but do not yet express CD3e on the

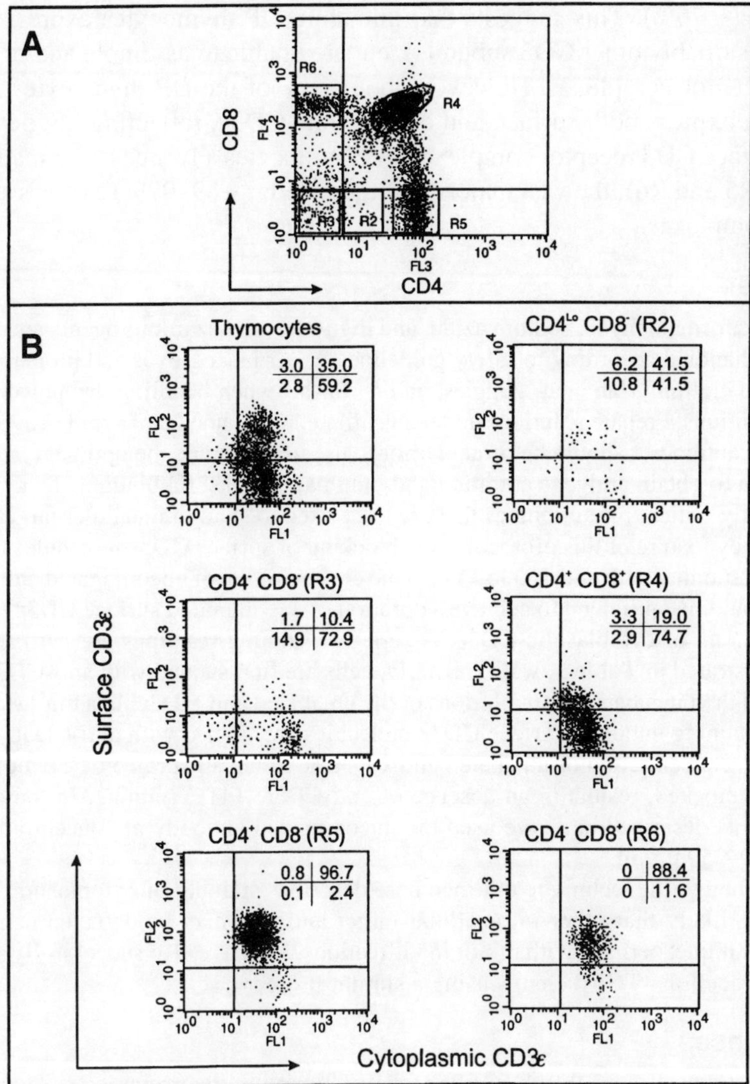

Fig. 4. Expression of surface and cytoplasmic CD3ε during stages of intrathymic development: C58/J thymocytes were stained with anti-CD4-RED613 and anti-CD8α-APC. Surface CD3ε was stained with anti-CD3ε-PE and cytoplasmic CD3ε was stained with anti-CD3ε-FITC according to the protocol outlined in **Fig. 1** and in the text. (**A**) expression of CD4 and CD8 by thymocytes. The major stages of intrathymic development are delineated by gated regions in order of increasing maturity: CD4^Lo CD8^- (R2), CD4^- CD8^- (R3), CD4^+ CD8^+ (R4), CD4^+ CD8^- (R5), and CD4^- CD8^+ (R6). (**B**) Expression of surface and cytoplasmic CD3ε by each population.

surface (~ 75%). This suggests that immature DP thymocytes express CD3ε and presumably other CD3 subunits), but are unable to assemble and/or transport receptor complexes. However, about 20% of the DP thymocytes in this fraction express both surface and cytoplasmic CD3ε, reflecting low levels of cell surface CD3 receptor complexes. As thymocytes advance to the mature SP stage (R5 and R6), the vast majority of these cells (~ 89–97%) express surface CD3 complexes.

4. Notes

1. Paraformaldehyde, sodium azide, and digitonin are hazardous agents and should be handled according to safety guidelines. Wear latex gloves and proper protective clothing (lab coat, goggles, and so forth.) when handling dry powders and solutions. Prepare solutions under a ventilated fume hood and avoid skin contact.
2. All antibodies should be titrated prior to use to determine the optimal concentration to obtain antigen saturation and minimal nonspecific binding. This is especially critical for antibodies that are to be used to stain intracellular targets.
3. A key feature of this protocol is the blocking of surface CD3ε molecules following staining with anti-CD3ε-FITC. The concentration of unconjugated anti-CD3ε should be optimized to achieve saturation of any unbound surface CD3ε prior to staining of cytoplasmic CD3ε. A series of staining reactions are performed as illustrated in **Table 1**, well 7. Briefly, cells are first stained with anti-CD3ε -PE, and then incubated with dilutions of the unlabeled anti-CD3ε. In a third step, any remaining unbound surface CD3ε molecules are stained with anti-CD3ε -FITC. The concentration of unlabeled anti-CD3ε at which all surface CD3ε molecules are blocked, results in an absence of anti-CD3ε -FITC staining. In the experiments described here, we used the unconjugated antibody at concentrations of 140–250 µg/mL.
4. Although the technique outlined here describes staining of cytoplasmic CD3ε, it is likely that other intracellular target antigens may be detected using this technique, perhaps with minor modifications. We have also successfully stained intracellular TCRβ chains using a similar protocol.

References

1. Shortman, K. and Wu, L. (1996) Early T lymphocyte progenitors. *Annu. Rev. Immunol.* **14,** 29–47.
2. Zúñiga-Pflücker, J. C. and Lenardo, M. J. (1996) Regulation of thymocyte development from immature progenitors. *Curr. Opin. Immunol.* **8,** 215–224.
3. Anderson, G., Moore, N. C., Owen, J. T., and Jenkinson, E. J. (1996) Cellular interactions in thymocyte development. *Annu. Rev. Immunol.* **14,** 73–99.
4. Fehling, H. J. and von Boehmer, H. (1997) Early αβ T cell development in the thymus of normal and genetically altered mice. *Curr. Opin. Immunol.* **9,** 263–275.
5. Wu, L., Scollay, R., Egerton, M., Pearse, M., Spangrude, G. J., and Shortman, K. (1991) CD4 expressed on earliest T-lineage precursor cells in the adult murine thymus. *Nature* **349,** 71–74.

6. Groettrup, M., Ungewiss, K., Palacios, R., Owen, M. J., Hayday, A. C., and von Boehmer, H. (1993) A novel disulfide-linked heterodimer on pre-T cells consists of the T cell receptor β-chain and a 33kDa glycoprotein. *Cell* **75**, 283–294.
7. Saint-Ruf, C., Ungewiss, K., Groettrup, M., Bruno, L., Fehling, H. J., and von Boehmer, H. (1994) Analysis and expression of a cloned pre-T cell receptor gene. *Science* **266**, 1208–1212.
8. Malissen, B. and Malissen, M. (1996) Functions of TCR and pre-TCR subunits: lessons from gene ablation. *Curr. Opin. Immunol.* **8**, 383–393.
9. Robey, E and Fowlkes, B. J. (1994) Selective events in T cell development. *Annu. Rev. Immunol.* **12**, 675–705.
10. Blackman, M. J., Kappler, J., and Marrack, P. (1990) The role of the T cell receptor in positive and negative selection of developing T cells. *Science* **248**, 1335–1341.
11. Klausner, R. D., Lippincott-Schwartz, J., and Bonifacino, J. S. (1990) The T cell antigen receptor: insights into organelle biology. *Annu. Rev. Cell Biol.* **6**, 403–431.
12. Bonifacino, J. S., Lippincott-Schwartz, J., and Klausner, R. D. (1991) The T cell antigen receptor: assembly and expression of a multisubunit complex, in *Intracellular Trafficking of Proteins,* (Steer, C. J. and Hanover, J. A., eds.), Cambridge University Press, Cambridge, UK, pp. 549–574.
13. Lippincott-Schwartz, J., Bonifacino, J. S., Yuan, L., and Klausner, R. D. (1989) Degradation from the endoplasmic reticulum: disposing of newly synthesized proteins. *Cell* **54**, 209–220.
14. Wilson, A. and MacDonald, H. R. (1995) Expression of genes encoding the pre-TCR and CD3 complex during thymus development. *Intl. Immunol.* **7**, 1659–1664.
15. Punt, J., Kubo, R. T., Saito, T., Finkel, T. H., Kathiresan, S., Blank, K. J., and Hashimoto, Y. (1991) Surface expression of a T cell receptor β (TCR-β) chain in the absence of TCR-α, -δ, -γ proteins. *J. Exp. Med.* **174**, 775–783.
16. Groettrup, M., Baron, A., Griffiths, G., Palacios, R., and von Boehmer, H. (1992) T cell receptor (TCR) β chain homodimers on the surface of immature but not mature α–, γ–, δ– chain deficient T cell lines. *EMBO J.* **11**, 2735–2745.
17. Levelt, C. N., Carsetti, R., and Eichmann, K. (1993) Regulation of thymocyte development through CD3. II. Expression of T cell receptor β CD3ε and maturation to the CD4⁺8⁺ stage are highly correlated in individual thymocytes. *J. Exp. Med.* **178**, 1867–1875.
18. Ley, S. C., Tan, K.-N., Kubo, R., Sy, M.-S., and Terhorst, C. (1989) Surface expression of CD3 in the absence of T cell receptor (TcR): evidence for sorting of partial TcR/CD3 complexes in a post-endoplasmic reticulum compartment. *Eur. J. Immunol.* **19**, 2309–2317.
19. Carrel, S., Mack, J. P., Miescher, G., Salvi, G., Giuffre, L., Schreier, M., and Isler, P. (1987) Phorbol 12-myristate 13-acetate induces surface expression of T3 on human immature T cell lines with and without concomitant expression of the T cell antigen receptor complex. *Eur. J. Immunol.* **17**, 1079–1087.
20. Levelt, C. N., Mombaerts, P., Iglesias, A., Tonegawa, S., and Eichmann, K. (1993) Restoration of early thymocyte differentiation in T-cell receptor β-chain-deficient

mutant mice by transmembrane signaling through CD3ε. *Proc. Natl. Acad. Sci. USA* **90,** 11,401–11,405.
21. Levelt, C. N., Ehrfeld, A., and Eichmann, K. (1993) Regulation of thymocyte development through CD3. I. Timepoint of ligation of CD3ε determines clonal deletion of induction of developmental program. *J. Exp. Med.* **177,** 707–716.
22. Jacobs, H., Vandeputte, D., Tolkamp, L., deVries, E., Borst, J., and Berns, A. (1994) CD3 components at the surface of pro-T cells can mediate pre-T cell development in vivo. *Eur. J. Immunol.* **24,** 934–939.
23. Wiest, D. L., Kearse, K., Shores, E. W., and Singer, A. (1994) Developmentally regulated expression of CD3 components independent of clonotypic T cell antigen receptor complexes on immature thymocytes. *J. Exp. Med.* **180,** 1375–1382.
24. Franek, K. J., Wolcott, R. M., and Chervenak, R. (1994) Reliable method for the simultaneous staining of surface CD3ε expression by murine lymphoid cells. *Cytometry* **17,** 224–236.

10

Assessing Apoptosis of Developing T Cells by Flow Cytometry

Caroline D. V. A. Bishop, Amy Jost, Elizabeth Crane, and Jennifer A. Punt

1. Introduction

Apoptosis is a highly regulated process by which eukaryotic cells undergo cell death *(1–4)*. Often synonymous with "cell suicide" and "programmed cell death," apoptosis is distinguishable from another major form of cell death, necrosis, by a number of key morphological and biochemical features *(3–6)*. First and arguably most importantly, plasma membrane integrity is maintained throughout apoptosis. On the other hand, membrane damage is a key characteristic of necrosis, which often occurs as a result of gross tissue and cellular injury. The containment of cytosolic material during apoptosis likely abrogates inflammatory reactions which could be detrimental to normal biological events. Second, apoptosis is an active process and requires cellular energy to systematically activate both signaling and catabolic enzymes. Necrosis, on the other hand, occurs as a result of a loss in a cell's ability to maintain energy levels and does not involve the regulated activation of signaling or enzyme cascades.

Apoptosis is the dominant form of physiological cell death and is integral to the development of organisms and their response to environmental input and insult *(1–8)*. Furthermore, a variety of diseases, including cancer, autoimmunity, and neurodegeneration, are in large part a consequence of dysregulation in apoptosis *(3,7)*.

A wide variety of natural stimuli can trigger apoptosis in cells, including receptor/ligand interactions *(9)*, growth factor withdrawal *(10)*, DNA damage *(11)*, and hypoxia *(12)*. Although initiating signals may differ, the "execution" events of apoptotic processes share multiple intracellular features, effectors, and regulators:

From: *Methods in Molecular Biology, Vol. 134: T Cell Protocols: Development and Activation*
Edited by: K. P. Kearse © Humana Press Inc., Totowa, NJ

1. Caspases, a family of cysteine proteases which cleave after aspartate residues, are key activators of apoptosis *(13–15)*.
2. Mitochondria appear to play a central role in apoptosis and are responsible for the release of factors which propel the apoptotic process, including cytochrome c *(16–18)*.
3. A component of the phospholipid bilayer, phosphatidyl serine (PS), is externalized relatively early in most apoptotic processes *(19)*.
4. DNA is digested by endonucleases into approx 200 base-pair fragments (DNA fragmentation) relatively late in the apoptotic process *(20)*. It is important to note, however, that this is not as universal an event as was once supposed *(21)*.
5. Members of the bcl-2 family appear to be universal regulators of eukaryotic cell apoptosis *(22,23)*.

Investigators have taken advantage of some of these characteristic molecular changes to establish assays to evaluate apoptosis. Some of the most useful assays allow one to examine apoptosis at the single cell level using flow cytometry. These assays have been invaluable tools in immunological research, particularly in the evaluation of cell death in distinct subpopulations of developing lymphocytes. Developing T cells, particularly CD4$^+$CD8$^+$ thymocytes, can be induced to undergo apoptosis via a number of stimuli, including fas/fasL and TNF/TNF-R interactions, irradiation, glucocorticoid exposure, and T-cell receptor (TCR) interactions *(8,13,24–26)*. Described here are three methods that have been shown to be useful for identifying apoptotic thymocytes on a single cell level by flow cytometry:

1. Annexin V staining for externalized phosphatidyl serine residues on the cell membrane;
2. Terminal deoxynucleotidyl transferase-mediated dUTP-biotin nick-end labeling (TUNEL) staining for DNA fragmentation; and
3. Ethidium bromide (EtBr) exclusion staining.

We will discuss the strategy, advantages, and disadvantages of each of these methods. Although each technique is amenable to the evaluation of apoptosis in a wide variety of cell types, the protocols described are optimized for murine thymocytes.

1.1. Introduction to Annexin V Staining

Annexin V staining, first described for use with the flow cytometer by Koopman et al. in 1994 *(27)* and further modified by Reutelingsperger et al. in 1995 *(28)*, is a relatively new method to assess apoptosis that is gaining popularity. This assay takes advantage of a phenomenon whereby PS, normally confined to the inside of the membrane lipid bilayer, is redistributed to the outside in response to apoptotic stimuli *(19)*. (For a recent review, *see* **ref. 29**) It has been speculated that this early PS "flip" is a feature of most if not all apoptotic processes *(19)* and that externalized phosphatidylserine residues can be recognized and subsequently eliminated by neighboring phagocytic cells *(30)*. Annexin V, a member of a family of proteins that bind to aminophospholipids, will specifically bind externalized PS in a Ca^{2+}-dependent manner *(31–33)*. Fluorescent conjugates of Annexin V (usually available as a human recombinant protein) will bind apoptotic murine thymocytes and allow them to be identified by flow cytometry.

1.1.1. Advantages

This is one of the simplest and quickest staining procedures which assesses a well-defined molecular event specific for apoptosis. The technique also permits multiparameter analysis by flow cytometry. Because it does not involve cell permeabilization and is apparently not detrimental to cells, Annexin V staining is one of the only techniques that allows sorting of live cells by flow cytometry. In addition, PS externalization is thought to occur relatively early in the apoptotic process (e.g., prior to the activation endonuclease activity) *(19)*. However, it is of interest to note that we have consistently found no striking differences in the kinetics of Annexin V vs TUNEL vs EtBr staining in thymocytes (**Fig. 1**).

1.1.2. Disadvantages

Annexin V conjugates tend to be rather expensive ($200/100 tests is a typical price, regardless of the company source), although we have found that Annexin V conjugates can be used very successfully at lower than recommended concentrations. In addition, we and others have found that cells that are not undergoing apoptosis by other criteria (e.g., freshly isolated cells) tend to stain broadly with Annexin V conjugates, regardless of technique or source of Annexin V (**Figs. 1,3**, and **4** in **ref. *34***). We do not yet understand the significance (if any) of this broad staining and it can confound interpretations of multiparameter staining.

1.2. Introduction to TUNEL Staining

Terminal deoxynucleotide transferase (TdT)-mediated dUTP nick end labeling or TUNEL is an assay established by Gavrieli et al. in 1992 to identify cells undergoing DNA fragmentation *in situ* *(35)*. It is based on the ability of terminal deoxynucleotide transferase (TdT) to add nucleotides to double-stranded DNA breaks which are a feature of many, though not all apoptotic processes *(20,21)*. The TUNEL technique has been adapted by multiple groups for use with the flow cytometer *(36)* and numerous kits based on this method are available from multiple companies. We prefer the *in situ* Cell Death Detection Kit sold by Boehringer Manheim (#1684795), but find that the protocol

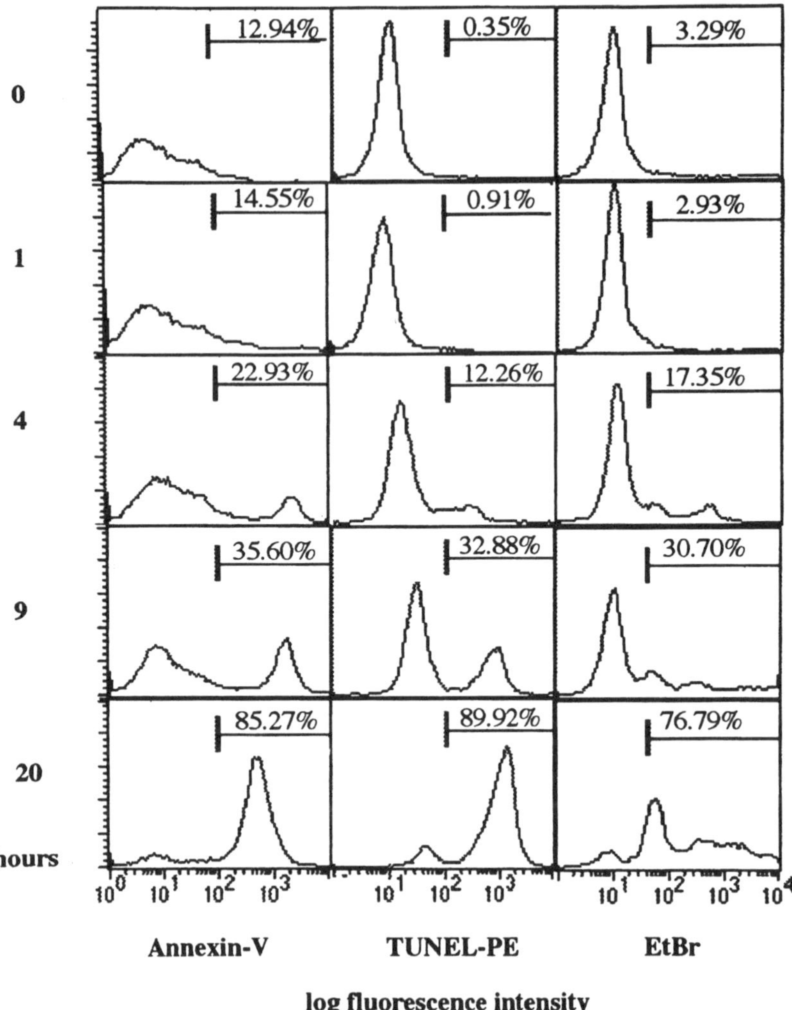

Fig. 1. Comparison of kinetics of Annexin-V, TUNEL, and EtBr staining. Histograms compare the results of Annexin-V, TUNEL, and EtBr staining techniques on freshly isolated whole thymocytes cultured in parallel for 0, 1, 4, 9, and 20 h in the presence of a stimulator of apoptosis, dexamethasone ($10^{-8}M$). The percentage of cells staining above background is indicated. Although Annexin V has been speculated to provide an earlier measure of apoptosis, each of the three measures of apoptosis display similar kinetics. Apoptotic cells are clearly evident at 4 h in all three assays and increase steadily over time. Annexin-V staining of freshly isolated (nonapoptotic) cells is consistently broader than TUNEL or EtBr staining.

can be performed as easily and less expensively "from scratch." One of the best protocols was originally described by Kishimoto et al. *(36)* and an adaptation of this method is outlined in **Subheading 3.2.**

1.2.1. Advantages

The TUNEL assay is sensitive and specific for a well-characterized molecular event associated with apoptosis in thymocytes. Multiparameter analysis can also be performed with this method (*see* **Note 11** and **ref.** *37* for suggestions).

1.2.2. Disadvantages

The TUNEL assay is relatively expensive and more labor intensive than alternative methods described in this chapter. It also requires cell fixation and permeabilization so cannot be performed on live cells. It is important to note that although DNA fragmentation is a common feature of thymocyte apoptosis, it is not a universal consequence of apoptosis.

1.3. Introduction to EtBr Staining

Ethidium bromide (EtBr) has been used as a measure of cell apoptosis in a number of systems *(25,38,39)*. The EtBr molecule, very similar in structure to propidium iodide (PI), is considered a more sensitive indicator of cell death *(38)*. It appears as if EtBr will cross the plasma membrane of cells undergoing apoptosis. Given that the cell membrane is known to retain its gross integrity during apoptosis, the biochemical basis for cell uptake of EtBr is not fully understood, but may be related to membrane changes that occur early in the apoptotic process *(38)*. After entry into the cell, EtBr will intercalate between nucleic acid bases and will stain DNA much more intensely than RNA.

1.3.1. Advantages

This is a very inexpensive and simple method for analyzing cell death on a single-cell level. No cell permeabilization is required. Two-color stains with a FITC conjugated antibody or reagent are straightforward. Three-color analyses can be done with a two laser flow cytometer.

1.3.2. Disadvantages

The biological basis for the entry of EtBr into apoptotic cells is not well understood and the specificity of this method for apoptotic versus necrotic cells has been called into question. In addition, three-color stains are difficult to perform on single laser machines because EtBr fluoresces in both the FL2 and FL3 channels. This technique works best with primary cells (thymocytes or splenocytes); it does not work well with many cell lines or tumor lines, presumably because their membranes are not as permeable to EtBr during apoptosis.

2. Materials

2.1. Annexin V Staining

1. Binding buffer: 2.5 mM CaCl$_2$, 25 mM HEPES, 150 mM NaCl. Store at 4°C.
2. Annexin V-FITC solution: Human recombinant Annexin V-FITC (Caltag AnnexinV01) 200 μg/mL. Make a 1:200 dilution (1 μg/mL) in binding buffer. This can be stored at 4°C in the dark for 1 mo or more.
3. Staining buffer: 0.1% BSA (1 g/1000 mL), 0.1% NaN$_3$ (1 g/1000 mL) in Hanks buffered saline solution (HBSS) without phenol red and with Ca^{2+} and Mg^{2+} (Gibco-BRL #14025-076 Bethesda, MD). Can store at room temperature for several weeks. Storage at 4°C probably increases shelf life.
4. 96-well round bottom plates (e.g., Nunc #163320, Costar #3596).

2.2. TUNEL Staining

1. Paraformaldehyde (PFA) 1%: To make 100 mL of 1% paraformaldehyde (PFA) add 1 g PFA to 10 mL of H$_2$O in a 100 mL glass bottle and bring to a near boil in microwave (watching carefully so solution does not bubble over). PFA fumes are toxic, so it is important to cap bottle and to work in fume-hood as soon as possible. Add 1 drop of 10 M NaOH in fume-hood. Solution should clarify. Add 90 mL of HBSS (or PBS) and neutralize by adding 1 drop of 12 M HCl in fume-hood. pH should be approx 7.0. This solution is best used fresh although it can also be aliquotted and stored at 4°C in the dark for up to one month.
2. TdT buffer: 100 mM cacodylic acid, 0.2 mM cobalt chloride, 0.1 mM dithiothreitol, 100 μg/mL BSA. Adjust pH to 6.8. Just before using, supplement needed volume with 5 μM biotin-21-dUTP (CLONTECH #5021-1) and 0.1 U/μL TdT (Promega #M1871 or M1875) for labeling reaction (*see* **Note 16**). Supplement with biotin-21-dUTP alone when using as negative control for labeling. Store buffer in 1–10 mL aliquots at –20°C or –80°C. Buffer should be stable for several months (without TdT or biotin-21-dUTP added).
3. Staining buffer: 0.1% BSA (1.0 g in 1000 mL), 0.1% NaN$_3$ (1.0 g in 1000 mL) in HBSS. Store at room temperature for several weeks. Storage at 4°C will increase shelf life.
4. Streptavidin conjugates (1 μg/mL): Dilute Phycoerythrin-streptavidin (PE-SA) or RED-670-streptavidin (Gibco-BRL #19539-014 and #19543-024, respectively) by adding 4 μL of stock (250 μg/mL) to 1 mL of staining buffer. This dilution can be stored in the dark at 4°C for at least 1 mo.

2.3. Ethidium Bromide Staining

1. Buffer A: 133 mM NaCl (2.66 mL of 5 M NaCl in 100 mL), 4.5 mM KCl (0.45 mL of 1 M KCl in 100 mL), 10 mM HEPES, pH 7.4 (1 mL of 1 M HEPES, pH 7.4, in 100 mL).
2. EtBr stock solution (100 μg/mL): Add 10 μL of a 10 mg/mL solution of EtBr to 990 μL of Buffer A. Store at 4°C in the dark for up to 1 yr.
3. EtBr working solution (1 μg/mL): Add 10 μL of EtBr stock solution to 990 μL of Buffer A. Store at 4°C in the dark for up to 1–2 wk.

4. Staining buffer: 0.1% BSA (1.0 g in 1000 mL), 0.1% NaN_3 (1.0 g in 1000 mL) in HBSS, (Gibco-BRL #24020-109). Store at room temperature for several weeks or 4°C for longer.

3. Methods

3.1. Annexin V Staining

1. Distribute positive controls, negative controls and experimental cells (*see* **Note 1**) in 96-well round bottom plate.
2. Pellet by spinning at 800*g* for 1.5 min. (This is equivalent to 2000 rpm on a Forma table top centrifuge [Model #5682].)
3. Flick out supernatant and wipe any excess liquid from the plate top on a paper towel.
4. Vortex plate (by placing one finger on each of two opposite corners of a covered 96-well plate and pressing lightly on Vortex set at 3–4) to resuspend cells in residual liquid.
5. Add 50 µL Annexin V-FITC solution to each well. Nonapoptotic cells are an excellent negative control for staining.
6. Vortex again to mix.
7. Wrap plate in foil.
8. Incubate at 4°C (refrigerator or on ice) for 10 min.
9. Wash wells by adding 150 µL staining buffer to each well and pelleting as above (wash #1). (Do not vortex wells with more than 100 mL vol.)
10. Flick out supernatant, resuspend cells by vortexing briefly, and wash again by adding 150 µL staining buffer (wash #2).
11. Flick out supernatant, add another 150 µL staining buffer, and transfer cells (mixing well before transferring) into 12 × 75 mm plastic tubes (VWR #60818-408) containing 250 µL staining buffer.
12. Assay by flow cytometry.

3.2. TUNEL Staining

1. Distribute $5 \times 10^5 - 1 \times 10^6$ cells into 12 × 75 mm tubes (VWR #60818-408 or Falcon #2052). *See* **Note 10** in **Subheading 4.2.** for suggestions for positive and negative controls.
2. Pellet cells at 300*g* for 5 min (this is equivalent to 1200 rpm on a Forma table top centrifuge [Model #5682]) and flick out supernatant so you have minimal residual volume.
3. Fix by adding 0.5 mL 70% ice-cold ethanol drop-wise (with a pipetman or pipetaid) while vortexing cell pellet continuously in the residual volume. Place tubes on ice for 15 min. Cells can be stored overnight at this point (*see* **Note 12**).
4. Pellet cells at 800*g* for 1.5 min (2000 rpm on Forma Table top centrifuge). Flick out supernatant.
5. Add 500 µL 1% paraformaldehyde (mix well) and incubate on ice for 15 min.
6. Pellet cells again at 800*g* for 1.5 min and flick out supernatant.

7. Add 150 μL PBS to pellet and transfer all cells to 96-well round-bottom plate. Cells can be stored overnight at this time.

8. Pellet cells in plate at 800*g* for 1.5 min (2000 rpm on a Forma Table Top Centrifuge). Flick out supernatant and vortex gently but thoroughly to resuspend in residual liquid.

9. Wash two more times in 150 μL TdT buffer (by repeating **steps 7** and **8**) and resuspend cells by vortexing them in residual liquid.

10. Add 50 μL TdT buffer containing 0.1 U/μL TdT and 5 μ*M* biotin-21-dUTP to experimental samples and 50 μL TdT buffer containing only 5 μ*M* biotin-21-dUTP to negative control samples. Vortex cells to mix.

11. Incubate for 30 min at 37°C (A tissue culture incubator works well).

12. Wash cells three times in 150 μL staining buffer and resuspend cells as above.

13. Add 30 μL per well of a fluoresceinated streptavidin (SA) conjugate (phycoerythrin-SA [PE-SA] or RED670-SA [Gibco-BRL #19539-014 and #19543-024, respectively].)

14. Incubate at 4°C for 15 min.

15. Wash three times in 150 μL staining buffer. Resuspend in 150 μL staining buffer.

16. Transfer cells to 12 × 75 mm plastic tubes containing 450 μL staining buffer for analysis by flow cytometry.

3.3. EtBr Staining

1. Distribute 5×10^5 cells per well in a 96-well round bottom plate. *See* **Note 1** for suggestions for positive and negative controls. *See* **Subheading 3.1.** for more detailed descriptions of washing and resuspending cells in 96-well plates.

2. Pellet cells at 800*g* for 1.5 min and flick out supernatant.

3. Vortex gently to resuspend cells in residual volume.

4. Add 30 μL of the EtBr working solution to each well. Vortex to mix.

5. Incubate for 20–30 min at 4°C.

6. Wash two times with 150 μL of staining buffer. (*See* **Subheading 3.1.**) for a more detailed description of the washing techniques.

7. Transfer cells to 12 × 75 mm plastic tubes containing 250 μL staining buffer.

8. Analyze by flow cytometry.

4. Notes

1. Positive/negative controls: For positive controls (cells undergoing apoptosis), treat thymocytes for 6–24 h with 10^{-8}M dexamethasone. (Distribute $1–2 \times 10^6$ cells in 500 μL in a well of a 24-well plate [Costar #3524] and incubate with dexamethasone. Culture 4–24 h at 37°C in a tissue culture incubator containing 5–7% CO_2). Culturing overnight without dexamethasone will also result in the apoptosis of a significant percentage of thymocytes (12–40% depending on the gentleness of the cell preparation). For negative controls (cells not undergoing apoptosis), use freshly isolated thymocytes or thymocytes stored in medium at 4°C (as long as overnight). These cells will not show any signs of apoptosis by the methods described in this chapter.

2. All of the assays described in this chapter can be streamlined considerably using a multichannel pipetor for the washes. Cells are distributed in every other well of a 96-well plate to avoid spillover contamination (during vortexing) and pipet tips are placed on every other prong of the multipipetor. A trough (the top of a pipet tip box) is filled with staining medium and, after the cells are vortexed to resuspend in residual volume, 150 µL of staining medium is added to six wells at a time. No additional mixing is required as long as the cells are resuspended by vortexing in residual volumes after flicking out supernatants and before adding staining medium. (Vortexing is not recommended if there is more than 100 µL in the well and is most efficient when there is less <50 µL in each well.)

3. Cells can also be easily redistributed from 96-well plates into 12×75-mm tubes for flow cytometry using the multipipetman. Cell samples (six at a time from a single row of the 96-well plate) are resuspended simultaneously with a multipipetman and distributed simultaneously to *(6)* 12×75-mm tubes (filled with 250 µL staining buffer) that are arranged in a rack where the spacing between the tubes is the same as the spacing between the wells. We find that Nalgene racks for 13-mm tubes work perfectly for this purpose.

4. Many laboratories continue to use 12×75-mm tubes for their staining protocols because of a concern that one cannot get adequate washing or mixing in the 96-well plate. (One cannot use the large volumes to wash the cells in plates versus tubes.) We have found that this is rarely a problem if the protocols are followed carefully (as described). Internal staining can pose more of a problem, which is why we recommend additional wash steps in the protocol. We feel that the efficiency of the 96-well staining technique outweighs any theoretical disadvantage.

5. Forward light scatter (FSC) generated by apoptotic cells can be a very revealing parameter. A reduction in FSC intensity correlates well with EtBr uptake, TUNEL staining, and Annexin V staining (**Fig. 2**) and can, in fact, be one of the earliest indicators of apoptosis (data not shown). Cells undergoing apoptosis do not scatter as much light because they shrink quite soon after the apoptotic process is initiated. We generally adjust FSC and side scatter (SSC) settings so that our cell populations are roughly in the center of the plot. Care must be taken not to set any live gates or thresholds that will exclude cells with reduced FSC intensity from the analysis. (Reminder: any staining protocol that requires fixation [especially with ethanol] will reduce the size of all cells, so FSC assessments must also be readjusted.)

6. Thymocytes are often thought of as cells that are extraordinarily susceptible to apoptotic stimuli. However, we have found that they are relatively hardy cells if handled gently from the beginning of isolation. We have reduced our background deaths after overnight culture to 12–15% (by all three assays described) by following some simple rules:

   a. Tease cells from the thymus after dissection by gently pulling the capsule apart with tweezers. Never grind the cells with tweezers or slides.

   b. Separate thymocytes from the fibrous capsule tissue by filtering over nylon membrane.

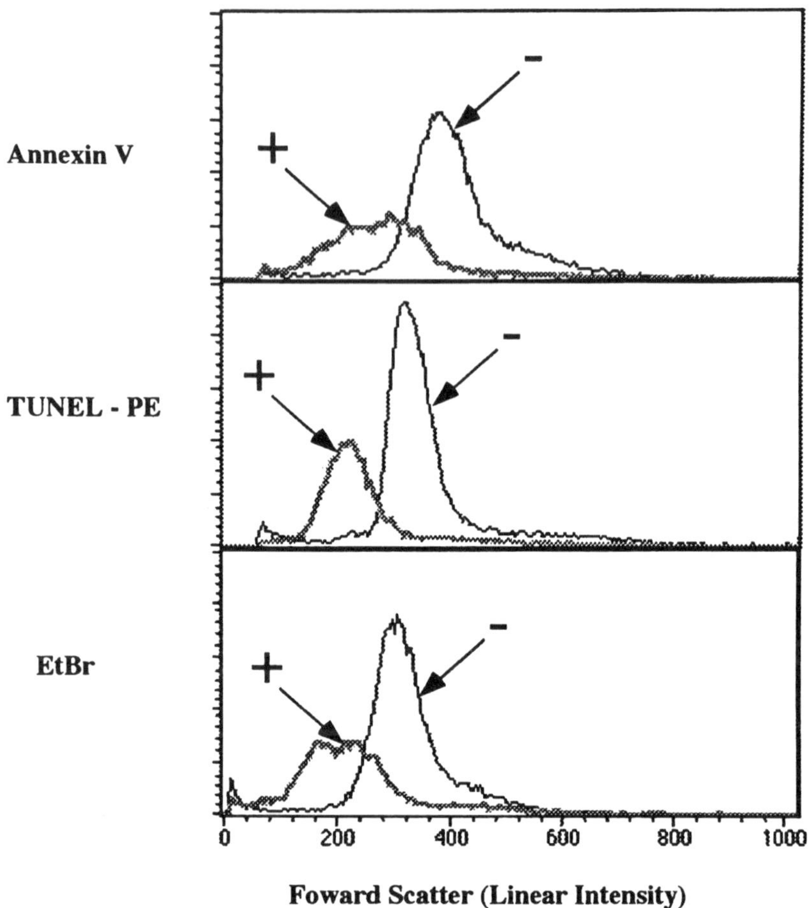

Foward Scatter (Linear Intensity)

Fig. 2. Forward scatter intensity is reduced among apoptotic thymocytes. Histograms compare the forward scatter profiles of apoptotic and nonapoptotic whole thymocytes treated for 9 h with 10^{-8} M dexamethasone. The ($^+$) arrow represents cells stained for apoptosis (via Annexin V, TUNEL, or EtBr) and the ($^-$) arrow represents cells that that did not fluoresce with the apoptotic staining procedure. Low forward scatter, an indicator of cell size reduction, is a feature of fluorescent (apoptotic) cells in all three cases. Forward scatter profile represents an additional although arguably less sensitive method by which apoptosis can be evaluated. It is a useful confirmation of the efficacy of the apoptotic stimuli and fluorescent staining method.

   c. Avoid spinning thymocytes in a centrifuge. (Suspend cells in a small enough volume so that you don't have to concentrate the cells.)

   d. Culture cells at low density (we typically culture 1×10^6 thymocytes in 24-well plates in a 0.5-mL volume [2×10^6 cells/mL].

e. Culture cells in medium that has been freshly supplemented with 1 mM L-glutamine (the most unstable of all of the amino acids).

f. Test your fetal calf serum (FCS) lots for their ability to support thymocyte viability. We have been very happy with Summit Biotechnology and Hyclone as FCS sources, but have found significant variation among lots.

g. Do not add HEPES to the culture medium; we have found, inexplicably, that it reduces cell viability. Our culture medium contains the following: RPMI (Gibco-BRL), 10% FCS (Hyclone or Summit Biotechnology), 1 mM L-glutamine, $5 \times 10^{-5}\,M$ 2-ME, sodium pyruvate, nonessential amino acids, and penicillin-streptomycin (optional).

h. Finally, if you are evaluating apoptosis of CD4$^+$CD8$^+$ thymocytes specifically it is clearly best to separate DP from SP cells. (Panning is a very gentle procedure that can enrich DP populations from 80% to >95%.) The presence of SP cells in the DP mix can influence their response to a number of stimuli, including TCR engagement (data not shown and **ref. 40**).

4.1. Annexin V Staining

1. Many companies sell kits that include both Annexin V-FITC and PI and suggest that cells be stained for both. Annexin V$^+$ PI$^-$ cells are considered early apoptotic cells and Annexin V$^+$ PI$^+$ cells are considered late apoptotic cells. (Annexin V$^+$ PI$^-$ cells were once described as apoptotic and the PI$^+$/Annexin V$^+$ cells as necrotic cells. This is no longer considered fully accurate, for PI$^+$ cells are clearly apoptotic in many cases.) Though useful in many experimental contexts, concomitant staining with PI reduces your ability to assess other cell features on a single laser flow cytometer.

2. CalTag is one of the few companies that identifies the concentration (rather than test-equivalents) of its Annexin V conjugates. It also sells a variety of fluorescent conjugates, allowing one more flexibility in performing multiparameter staining of cells.

3. The most important thing to remember with this staining technique is the Ca^{2+} dependence of the Annexin V/PS interaction. Many laboratories use staining buffers with PBS or HBSS that are Ca^{2+} and Mg^{2+}- free. These buffers will not, of course, permit the binding of Annexin V to PS.

4.2. TUNEL Staining

1. **Steps 1–6** can also be performed in 96-well round bottom plates but constant agitation (on a shaker in a cold room) is recommended so that cells do not aggregate with the fixation procedures.

2. If opting to perform multicolor staining in addition to the TUNEL assay, cells should be stained prior to ethanol fixation in **step 3**. Ethanol (EtOH) fixation can change protein epitopes and surface molecules can become unrecognizable to antibodies. (CD8 is a good example of a protein vulnerable to alteration by EtOH and paraformaldehyde fixation [data not shown].)

3. Cells can be stored for days and even months in EtOH following **step 3**. However, it is generally recommended to use them as soon as possible. Cells can also be stored overnight following **step 7**.

4. FITC-conjugated dUTP can also be used successfully in this assay. The biotinylated conjugate in combination with Phycoerythrin-streptavidin conjugate often gives us more intense staining on the FACSCalibur (Becton Dickinson), but other groups have reported the opposite *(37)*.

5. Higher centrifuge speeds must be used in protocol **step 4** and for the remainder of the procedure because cells are smaller and less dense after ethanol fixation. The cell pellet will not be as "tight" as it was before ethanol treatment; rather, it is often visible as a diffuse ring at the bottom of the tube.

6. Nonspecific 'background' staining is the most problematic feature of this methodology and thorough washing, particularly at **steps 12** and **15**, will help to wash excess fluorescence from the interior of the cells for the best signal-to-noise ratio. Although some suggest that tubes are better for internal staining because they permit higher wash volumes, we have not found plates to be problematic. It is, however, critical that the cell pellets are resuspended adequately (by gentle vortexing) before adding wash buffer. Wells can be mixed individually after the addition of TdT enzyme, but this is usually not necessary if the cells are resuspended as suggested.

7. 0.5–1.0 μ*M* concentrations of biotin-21-dUTP may be adequate and could even reduce background *(6,37)*. We have not yet optimized the procedure with these concentrations, but this modification would certainly reduce cost.

8. During flow cytometric analysis it may be necessary to raise the amplitude of FSC signals to adjust for the cell shrinkage caused by ethanol treatment.

4.3. EtBr Staining

1. Three fluorescent peaks are generally seen after EtBr staining of apoptotic thymocytes. Cells that stain with lowest intensity (EtBr⁻) represent live cells by all criteria available, while cells that stain with intermediate and high intensity (EtBr⁺) represent cells in the early and end process of dying by apoptosis, respectively *(25)*. Intermediate and high intensity EtBr⁺ cells, but not EtBr⁻ cells, have been shown to be undergoing DNA fragmentation *(25)*.

2. Two-color analysis can be performed easily with this technique. Because the buffers for stains differ, we generally stain sequentially with a fluorescein conjugated antibody to a surface marker, then with EtBr. However, there is no *a priori* reason that antibody and EtBr cannot be added simultaneously. We have, in fact, prepared EtBr in staining buffer and stained successfully for apoptosis. Although the total percentage of apoptotic (EtBr⁺) cells does not differ whether EtBr is prepared in staining solution versus Buffer A, we have noticed that the three peaks of EtBr cells are not as apparent when EtBr is added in staining solution. We do not know the reason for this difference.

3. EtBr will fluoresce predominantly in the FL2 channel. Unfortunately, EtBr fluorescence can be detected in both the FL2 and FL3 channels, so Tricolor (Pharmingen) or RED-670 (Gibco-BRL) conjugates are not useful when using EtBr as a measure of death.

References

1. Kerr, J. F. R., Wyllie, A. H., and Currie, A. R. (1972) Apoptosis: A basic biological phenomenon with wide ranging implications in tissue kinetics. *Br. J. Cancer* **26,** 239–257.
2. White, E. (1996) Life, death, and the pursuit of apoptosis. *Genes Devel.* **10,** 1–15.
3. Hetts, S. (1998) To die or not to die: an overview of apoptosis and its role in disease. *JAMA* **279,** 300–307.
4. Hale, A. J., Smith, C. A., Sutherland, L. C., Stoneman, V. E. A., Longthorne, V. L., Culhane, A. C., and Williams, G. T. (1996) Apoptosis: molecular regulation of cell death. *Eur. J. Biochem.* **236,** 1–26.
5. Thompson, B. E. (1998) Special topic: apoptosis. *Annu. Rev. Physiol.* **60,** 525–532.
6. Allen, R. T., Hunter, W. J., and Agrawal, D. K. (1997). Morphological and biochemical characterization and analysis of apoptosis. *J. Pharmacol. Toxicol. Methods.* **37,** 215–228.
7. Rudin, C. M. and Thompson, C. B. (1997) Apoptosis and disease: Regulation and clinical relevance of programmed cell death. *Annu. Rev. Med.* **48,** 267–281.
8. Osborne, B. (1996) Apoptosis and the maintenance of homeostasis in the immune system. *Curr. Opin. Immunol.* **8,** 245–254.
9. Nagata, S. (1997) Apoptosis by death factor. *Cell* **88,** 355–365.
10. Abbas, A. K. (1996) Die and let live: eliminating dangerous lymphocytes. *Cell* **84,** 655–657.
11. Elledge, R. M. and Lee, W. H. (1995) Life and death by p53. *Bioessays* **17,** 923–930.
12. Yun, J. K., McCormick, T. S., Judware, R., and Lapetina, E. G. (1997) Cellular adaptive responses to low oxygen tension: apoptosis and resistance. *Neurochem. Res.* **4,** 517–521.
13. Henkart, P. A. (1996) ICE family proteases: mediators of all apoptotic cell death? *Immunity* **4,** 195–201.
14. Cohen, G. M. (1997) Caspases: the executioners of apoptosis. *Biochem. J.* **326,** 1–16.
15. Patel, T., Gores, G. J., and Kaufmann, S. (1996) The role of proteases during apoptosis. *FASEB* **10,** 587–597.
16. Mignotte, B. and Vayssiere, J. L. (1998) Mitochondria and apoptosis. *Eur. J. Biochem.* **1,** 1–15.
17. Yang J., Liu, X., Bhalla, K., Kim, C. N., Ibrado, A. M., Cai, J., Peng, T. I., Jones, D. P., and Wang, X. (1997) Prevention of apoptosis by bcl-2: release of cytochrome c from mitochondria blocked. *Science* **275,** 1129–1132.
18. Kluck R. M., Bossy-Wetzel, E., Green, D. R., and Newmeyer, D. D. (1997) The release of cytochrome c from mtochondria: a primary site for bcl-2 regulation of apoptosis. *Science* **275,** 1132–1136.
19. Martin, S. J., Reutelingsperger, C. P. M., McGahon, A. J., Rader, J. A., van Schie, R. C. A. A., La Face, D. M., and Green, D. R. (1995) Early redistribution of plasma membrane phosphatidylserine is a general feature of apoptosis

regardless of the initiating stimulus: Inhibition by overexpression of Bcl-2 and Abl. *J. Exp. Med.* **182,** 1545–1556.

20. Arends, M. J., Morris, R. G., and Wyllie, A. H. (1990) Apoptosis: the role of endonuclease. *Am. J. Pathol.* **136,** 593–608.

21. Cohen, G. M., Sun, X. M, Snowden, T., Dinsdale, D., and Skilleter, D. N. (1992) Key morphological features of apoptosis may occur in the absense of internucleosomal DNA fragmentation. *Biochem J.* **286,** 331–334.

22. Chao, D. T. and Korsmeyer, S. J. (1998) BCL-2 family: regulators of cell death. *Annu. Rev. Immunol.* **16,** 395–419.

23. Golstein, P. (1997) Controlling cell death. *Science* **275,** 1081,1082.

24. Conroy, L. A. and Alexander, D. R. (1996) The role of intracellular signalling pathways regulating thymocyte and leukemic T cell apoptosis. *Leukemia* **9,** 1422–1435

25. Punt, J. A. and Osborne, B., Takahama, Y., Sharrow, S., and Singer, A. (1994) Negative selection of CD4$^+$ CD8$^+$ thymocytes by T cell receptor-induced apoptosis requires a costimulatory signal that can be provided by CD28. *J. Exp. Med.* **179,** 709–713.

26. Page, D. M., Kane, L. P., Allison, J. P., and Hedrick, S. M. (1993) Two signals are required for negative selection of CD4$^+$CD8$^+$ thymocytes. *J. Immunol.* **151,** 1868–1880.

27. Koopman, G., Reutelingsperger, C. P., Kuijten, G. A., Keehnen, R. M., Pals, S. T., and avan Oers, M. H. (1994) Annexin V for flow cytometric detection of phosphatidyl-serine expression on B cells undergoing apoptosis. *Blood* **84,** 1415–1420.

28. Vermes, I., Haanen, C., Steffens-Nakken, H., and Reuteingsperger, C. P. M. (1995) A novel assay for apoptosis: flow cytometric detection of phosphatidylserine expression on early apoptotic cells using fluorescein labelled annexin V. *J. Immunol. Methods* **184,** 39–51.

29. Van Engleand, M., Nieland, L. J. W., Ramaekers, F. C. S., Schutte, B., and Reutelingsperger, C.P.M. (1998) Annexin V-affinity assay: a review on an apoptosis detection system based on phosphatidylserine exposure. *Cytometry* **31,** 1–9.

30. Fadok, V. A., Voelker, D. R., Campbell, P. A., Cohen, J. J., Bratton, D. L., and Henson, P. M. (1992) Exposure of phosphatidylserine on the surface of apoptotic lymphocytes triggers specific recognition and removal by macrophages. *J. Immunol.* **148,** 2207–2216.

31. Thiagarajan, P. and Tait, J. F. (1990) Binding of annexin V/ placental anticoagu-lant protein 1 to platelets. Evidence for phosphatidylserine exposure in the procoagulant response of activated platelets. *J. Biol. Chem.* **265,** 17,420–17,423.

32. Andree, H. A., Reutelingsperger, C. P., Hauptmann, R., Hemker, H. C., Hermens, W. T., and Willems, G. M. (1990) Binding of vascular anticoagulant alpha (VAC alpha) to planar phospholipid bilayers. *J. Biol. Chem.* **265,** 4923–4928.

33. Tait, J. F., Gibson, D., and Fujikawa, K. (1989) Phospholipid binding properties of human placental anticoagulant protein-I, a member of the lipocortin family. *J. Biol. Chem.* **264,** 7944–7949.

34. Colby, S., Dohner, K., Gunn, D., Mayo, K., Tanner, K., Trelogan, S., and Zahl, N., eds. (1996) ApoAlert Annexin V apoptosis kit: fast, easy, early detection of apoptosis. *CLONTECHniques* **IX,** 9–11.
35. Gavrieli, Y., Sherman, Y., and Ben-Sasson, S. A. (1992) Identification of programmed cell death in situ via specific labeling of nuclear DNA fragmentation. *J. Cell. Biol.* **119,** 493–501.
36. Kishimoto, H., Surh, C. D., and Sprent, J. (1995) Upregulation of surface markers on dying thymocytes. *J. Exp. Med.* **181,** 649–655.
37. Coico, R., ed. (1998) Morphological, biochemical and flow cytometric assays of apoptosis. In <u>Current Protocols in Immunology, Vol. 1</u> , Section 3.17.
38. Lyons, A. B., Samuel, K., Sanderson, A., and Maddy, A. H. (1992) Simultaneous analysis of immunophenotype and apoptosis of murine thymocytes by single laser flow cytometry. *Cytometry* **13,** 809.
39. Swat, W., Ignatowiez, L. and Kisielow, P. (1991) Detection of apoptosis of immature CD4$^+$8$^+$ thymocytes by flow cytometry. *J. Immunol Methods* **137,** 79–87.
40. Punt, J. A., Havran, W., Abe, R., Sarin, A., and Singer, A. (1997) T cell receptor (TCR)-induced death of immature CD4+CD8+ thymocytes by two distinct mechanisms differing in their requirement for CD28 costimulation: Implications for negative selection in the thymus. *J. Exp. Med.* **186,** 1911–1922.

11

Isolation of T-Cell Subsets
by Magnetic Cell Sorting (MACS)

Luminita A. Stanciu and Ratko Djukanović

1. Introduction

T cells are defined by the expression of CD3 molecules on the cell surface in association with the T-cell receptor (TCR) to form the TCR/CD3 complex. Within the $CD3^+$ cell population there are two main subsets identified by the expression of CD4 ($CD4^+$ T cells) and CD8 ($CD8^+$ T cells) cell surface molecules. In addition, there is a small percentage of $CD3^+$ T cells which are either negative for both CD4 and CD8 ($CD4^-CD8^-$) or are double positive ($CD4^+CD8^+$).

In this chapter a separation method is described which enables purification of $CD4^+$ and $CD8^+$ T cells by negative selection. Positive selection using antibodies specific for the T-cell subsets is not recommended as ligation of CD4 or CD8 molecules can affect cell functions, such as cytokine generation *(1,2)*, and cell activation induced either by antigen *(3)*, anti-TCR antibodies *(4)*, or anti-CD3 antibodies *(5)*. In addition, anti-CD4 antibodies modulate responses in mixed leukocyte cultures *(6)*. A number of mechanisms for this effect have been proposed, including inhibition of the binding activity of nuclear factors NF-AT, NF-kB and AP-1 *(7)*.

Highly purified populations of both $CD4^+$ and $CD8^+$ T-cell subsets can be negatively selected with good cell viability and recovery using a number of methods, the most recent being the Magnetic Activated Cell Sorter (MACS) system *(8)*. Negative selection of cells by MACS involves:

1. Incubation of cells that one wishes to deplete with a cocktail of primary hapten-conjugated monoclonal antibodies (MAb) against the specific surface markers of all the cells that have to be removed.

From: *Methods in Molecular Biology, Vol. 134: T Cell Protocols: Development and Activation*
Edited by: K. P. Kearse © Humana Press Inc., Totowa, NJ

2. A second incubation with a secondary antihapten MAb conjugated to paramagnetic colloidal MicroBeads.
3. Passing the cells over a ferromagnetic column in a strong magnetic field where the cells with magnetic MicroBeads on their surface are retained and thus separated from the unbound cells that pass through the column (**Figs. 1** and **2**).

For CD4$^+$ T cells the purity is between 92 and 96% and the recovery between 83 and 96%. For CD8$^+$ T cells, the purity is generally lower, but can be as high as 98% using a modification of the protocol recommended by the manufacturers (*see* **Notes**).

2. Materials

1. Ficoll-Isopaque (Lymphoprep) (Nycomed Pharma, Oslo, Norway).
2. Phosphate buffered saline (PBS) without calcium and magnesium, pH 7.2, (Gibco-BRL, Uxbridge, UK), containing 2% fetal calf serum (FCS) (Gibco-BRL).
3. Washing buffer: PBS, pH 7.2, without calcium and magnesium, supplemented with 2 m*M* EDTA (Sigma, Poole, UK) and 0.5% bovine serum albumin (BSA) (Sigma). The washing buffer should be kept on ice.
4. CD4$^+$ and CD8$^+$ T-cell isolation kits (Miltenyi Biotec, Bergisch Gladbach, Germany), containing two reagents:
   a. A cocktail of primary hapten-conjugated MAb against CD4 or CD8 molecules, for selective depletion of CD4$^+$ and CD8$^+$ T cells, respectively, and against CD11b, CD16, CD19, CD36, and CD56 molecules in order to remove dendritic cells, monocytes, granulocytes, B cells, platelets, early erythroid precursors cells and NK cells, respectively; and
   b. MACS paramagnetic MicroBeads coated with secondary antihapten MAb (*see* **Note 4**).
5. There is a choice of 4 MACS magnetic separators (Miltenyi Biotec) that are used in conjunction with different types of single-use separation columns depending on the numbers of cells to be processed (**Table 1**):
   a. SuperMACS (used with columns types AS, BS, CS, and D.
   b. VarioMACS (used with columns AS, BS, and CS).
   c. MidiMACS (used with columns LS$^+$).
   d. MiniMACS (used with MS$^+$ columns).
   The method described below is applicable to the depletion columns AS, BS, CS, and D, which are used in conjunction with VarioMACS and SuperMACS magnetic separators.
6. MACS metallic stands that hold the magnets (Miltenyi Biotec).
7. Polystyrene 15 mL and 50 mL Falcon tubes (Becton Dickinson, Cowley Oxford, UK).
8. Preseparation 30-μm filters (Miltenyi Biotec).
9. Three way stop-cocks for the preparation of the columns (Miltenyi Biotec).
10. Disposable plastic syringes (20 mL).
11. Disposable needles (20G, 21G, 22G, and 24G).
12. CD3-PerCP, CD4-FITC and CD8-PE specific MAb and isotype control MAb for all three colors (Becton Dickinson).

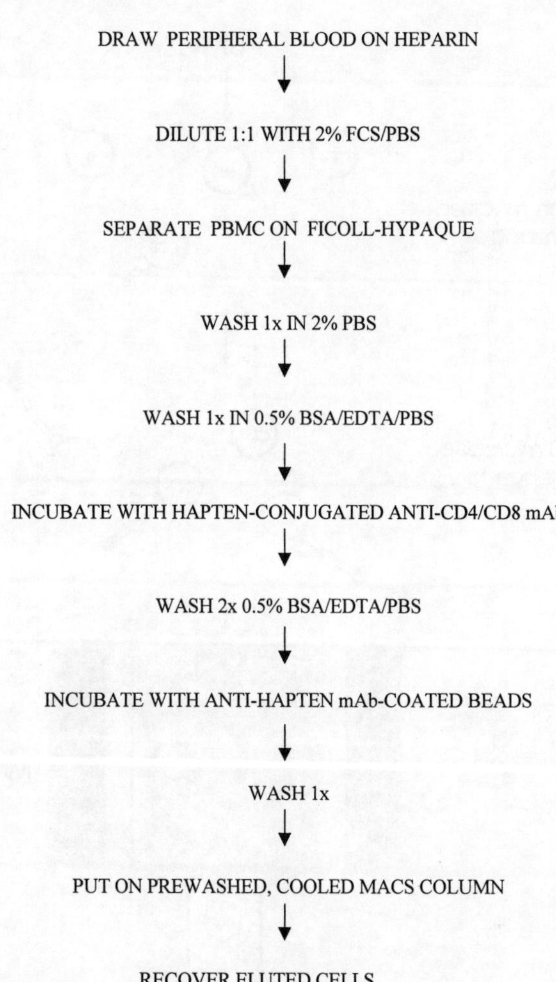

Fig. 1. The principles of negative separation of T-cell subsets (in this case CD4[+] cells) by magnetic cell sorting. PBMC are obtained by density gradient centrifugation. Cells are incubated with a cocktail of hapten-conjugated primary antibodies against cells that need to be removed, and subsequently with secondary antihapten antibody that are conjugated to paramagnetic microbeads. The bound cells are retained in the column and the desired cells are eluted.

3. Methods

3.1. Isolation of Peripheral Blood Mononuclear Cells (PBMC)

1. PBMC are obtained by density gradient centrifugation on Lymphoprep according to Boyum et al. *(9)*.

                                          Stanciu and Djukanović

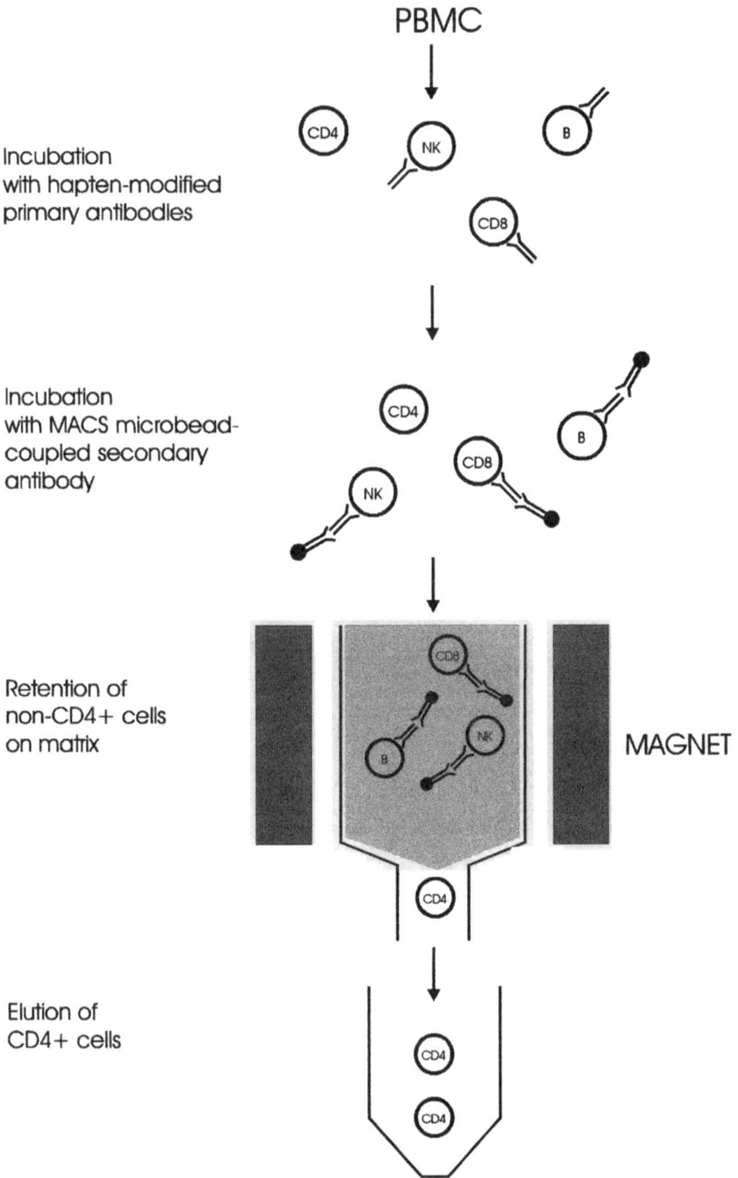

Fig. 2. Magnetic cells sorting procedure.

2. Draw peripheral blood into heparinized tubes, dilute 1:1 with PBS containing 2% FCS (at room temperature), and layer on Lymphoprep in a ratio 2.5:1 in 15 mL polystyrene Falcon tubes. Centrifuge without brake and acceleration for 25 min

**Table 1
Characteristics of Depletion Columns**

Columns	MS$^+$	LS$^+$	AS	BS	CS	D
MACS separator	Mini MACS	Midi MACS	VarioMACS or SuperMACS	Vario MACS Or SuperMACS	VarioMACS or SuperMACS	SuperMACS
Retained cells	10^7	10^8	3×10^7	10^8	2×10^8	10^9
Needle^a			24G	22G	22G	20G
Matrix Volume	60 µL	0.45 mL	1.0 mL	3.4 mL	6.3 mL	43 mL
Reservoir volume	2 mL	6 mL	1.3 mL	3 mL	6.5 mL	20 mL

^{a}MiniMACS and MidiMACS systems do not need needles to slow down the flow.

at 500*g* at room temperature. Aspirate PBMC carefully from the interface using a sterile Pasteur plastic pipet and wash initially in PBS containing 2% FCS (300*g*, for 10 min, at room temperature). At this stage and onwards, the centrifuge brake and acceleration are switched on. Count the cells in a hemocytometer and wash again in washing buffer (200*g*, for 10 min, at room temperature).

3. Resuspend the cell pellet using a volume of 80 µL of washing buffer per 1×10^7 based on counts between the two washing steps (*see* notes).

3.2. Magnetic Labeling of CD4$^+$ and CD8$^+$ T Cells

1. Take the primary hapten-conjugated MAb cocktail out of the fridge just before use and add to the cells (using 20 µL/1×10^7 cells that have been resuspended in 80 µL of washing buffer). Flick the tip of the tube a few times and place the tube on ice on a rocker for 20 min (*see* **Note 1**). Wash the cells twice in washing buffer using 20 times the volume of the cell suspension (*see* **Notes 2** and **3**). Resuspend the cells in washing buffer (1×10^7/80 µL). Add the secondary MAb (MACS paramagnetic MicroBeads coupled to antihapten MAb) (20 µL/1×10^7 cells) and treat as with the primary antibody, allowing 30 min of incubation. Wash the cells again as above in a 20× larger volume of washing buffer. Adjust the final resuspension of cells to give an optimum 1×10^8 cells/500 µL of washing buffer. At least 500 µL of buffer must be used even if fewer cells have been obtained. The cells must be well resuspended and should not contain aggregates. Remove any aggregates by passing the cells through a 30-µm filter supplied by the manufacturer (Miltenyi Biotec, München, Germany).

3.3. Magnetic Separation for the Isolation of CD4⁺ and CD8⁺ T Cells

3.3.1. Preparation of the Column

3.3.1.1. STERILIZATION WITH ETHANOL

Choose the depletion column and the appropriate MACS separator depending on the number of cells that will be processed (**Table 1**). The column needs to be prepared prior to passing the cells. This can be done in parallel with the preparation of cells. Place the column in the magnet. Remove the yellow cap from the tip of the column and attach the three-way stop-cock to the column as shown in **Fig. 3**. Fill the column from below (via a syringe attached to the side port (position one of the stop-cock) with 70% ethanol injected through the stop-cock using a 20 mL disposable syringe placed at 90° to the column. Turn the stop-cock into a run position (position 3) and allow the ethanol to run out.

3.3.1.2. COATING THE COLUMN

Take a separate syringe to inject cold PBS/2%FCS (stored on ice prior to injection) to fill up the column from below to the top. Close the tap and leave for 1 h. This allows the FCS proteins to coat the column and prevents nonspecific binding of cells. Allow to run off after 1 h. Remove the side syringe.

3.3.1.3. COOLING THE COLUMN

The column now needs to be cooled with ice-cold PBS/2%FCS. Take a 21G needle and cut the tip of the plastic sheath to avoid incidental prick injury. Attach the needle to the bottom end of the stop-cock and fasten to its bottom arm (**Fig. 3**). Add ice-cold PBS/2%FCS equivalent to 2–3 vol of the column from above and allow it to run slowly through the needle into a beaker. Make sure the fluid level does not fall below the top of the matrix. If this happens, fill the column from below with PBS/2%FCS using a side-syringe containing ice-cold PBS/2%FCS. This should expel any air bubbles in the matrix that would hamper subsequent binding of cells. Once the fluid level has come close to the top of the matrix close the stop-cock. The column is now ready for cell separation.

3.3.2. Separation of T-Cell Subsets

1. Depending on the type of column to be used, choose the appropriate needle that determines the flow (**Table 1**) and attach to the stop-cock. Close the stop-cock.
2. Place a 50-mL Falcon tube into a rack and around the needle to collect the eluted cells. Load the cell suspension from above into the column. Open the stop-cock and allow the fluid and unbound cells to run through. Keep topping up from above with ice-cold PBS/2%FCS to a total volume equivalent to 10 times the volume of the column. The eluted cells are collected for further analysis.
3. If desired, the bound cells can also be eluted by taking the column out of the magnet. Detach the stop-cock together with the needle and syringe from the column and place the yellow cap at the tip of the column. Remove the column

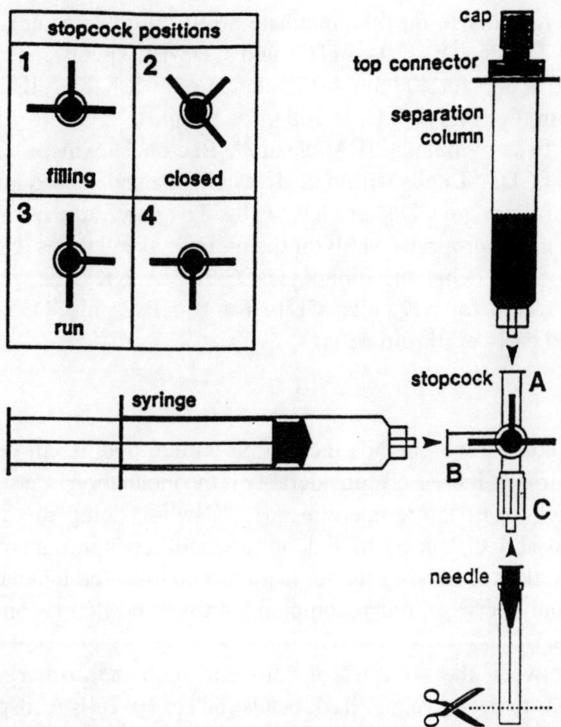

Fig. 3. The use of stop-cock and syringe to prepare the column and separate the cells. This is applied to columns that are used in conjunction with Vario or SuperMACS.

from the magnet and place above a suitable collection tube. Add ice-cold PBS/ 2%FCS from above and remove the stopper. Use PBS/2%FCS (up to five times the volume of the column) to flush the cells with short pulses. The plunger supplied with the column can be used for this. Note that this will give you positively selected cells that may have been activated by the separation procedure (*see* **Note 5**).

3.3.3. Assessment of Yield and Purity of the Negatively Selected T-Cell Subset

1. Spin the cells at 300*g* at room temperature for 10 min. Resuspend in 1 mL of culture medium. Take 90 µL of cell suspension and add 10 µL of trypan blue. Check the cell viability by trypan blue exclusion in a hemocytometer, which enables cell counting at the same time. The viability should be >98%. Adjust the cell concentration to 1×10^6 cells/mL of culture medium.
2. Evaluate the efficiency of the cell separation procedure by three-color flow cytometry using PerCP/FITC/PE-conjugated MAb (Becton Dickinson, Mountain

View, CA). In order to do this, incubate 50 µL aliquots of negatively depleted cells with CD3-PerCP, CD4-FITC, and CD8-PE specific MAb and isotype control MAb at 4°C for 30 min. After incubation, wash the cells in ice-cold PBS/ 2% FCS (spin the cells at 4°C, at 300*g*, for 10 min).

3. Analyse by flow cytometry (FACScan™, Becton Dickinson). First check the percentage of CD3$^+$ T cells within the live cell gate and subsequently assess what proportion of these are CD4$^+$ or CD8$^+$ cells. To analyze the non-T-cell contaminating cells, use appropriate MAb for the individual cell types (CD11b, CD14 for granulocytes, NK, cells, and monocytes; CD16 for NK cells, granulocytes, and monocytes; CD56 for NK cells; CD19 for B cells; and CD36 for monocytes, platelets, and early erythroid cells).

4. Notes

1. The manufacturer recommends incubation with antibodies in the fridge. In our hands, the purity is increased considerably if the incubation is assisted by rocking. If you cannot lower the temperature to 4°C while doing this (by keeping the whole rocker at 4°C), place the Falcon tube with cells into a container with ice and onto a rocker. Lowering the temperature doubles the incubation time (thus, the discrepancy between our recommended time and that recommended by the manufacturer).

2. The ratio between the volumes of cells and both the primary and secondary antibodies has to be 1:5 (e.g., 20 µL beads for 1×10^7 cells resuspended in 80 µL buffer). We recommend that after the first washing with PBS, the cells be counted to enable precise resuspension after the second wash (*see* **Subheading 3.1.3.**).

3. Use degassed washing buffer to avoid bubble formation in the column, which can decrease the flow and lead to clogging and impaired separation. You can degas the buffer by applying a vacuum or sonification for 10 min at room temperature. Alternatively, prepare the washing buffer the night before and store under sterile conditions. In our hands this does not increase the risk of contamination.

4. Storage conditions: keep the isolation kits at 4°C and the columns in a dark and dry place.

5. If you only have a MidiMACS in your laboratory, you can use columns designated for positive selection, such as MACS LS$^+$ separation columns, for cell depletion. This is now possible because of the high quality of the isolation kits such that high purities of eluted cells can be obtained. If using these systems, our suggestions are as follows:

    a. Attach the MidiMACS magnet to the MACS MultiStand and place the LS$^+$ separation column into the magnet.

    b. Place a collection tube under the column and wash the column by applying 3 mL of degassed buffer (or buffer which has been kept overnight at 4°C).

    c. Place the cell suspension processed as described above (containing up to a maximum of 2×10^9 total cells; 1×10^8 will be retained) onto the column.

    d. Collect the eluted cells, and rinse the column four times with 3 mL of washing buffer.

6. If you are not completely satisfied with the cell purity, pass the cells a second time over a new column. An alternative option is to reuse the same column provided the column has been thoroughly washed (using the method for eluting bound cells) and there are no bubbles in the column.

References

1. Stanciu, L. A., Shute, J., Promwong, C., Holgate, S. T., and Djukanović, R. (1996) Production of IL-8 and IL-4 by positively and negatively selected CD4$^+$ and CD8$^+$ human T cells following a four-step cell separation method including magnetic cell sorting (MACS). *J. Immunol. Methods* **189,** 107–115.
2. Stanciu, L. A., Shute, J., Promwong, C., Holgate, S. T., and , Djukanović, R. (1997) Increased levels of IL-4 in CD8$^+$ T cells in atopic asthma. *J. Allergy Clin. Immunol.* **100,** 373–378.
3. Oyaizu, N., Chirmule, N., Kalyanaraman, V. S., Hall, W. W., Good, R. A., and Pahwa, S. (1990) Human immunodeficiency virus type 1 envelope glycoprotein gp120 produces immune defects in CD4$^+$ T lymphocytes by inhibiting interleukin 2 mRNA. *Proc. Natl. Acad. Sci. USA* **87,** 2379–2383.
4. Goldman, F., Jensen, W. A. J., Johnson, G. L., Heasley, L., and Cambier, J. C. (1994) gp120 ligation of CD4 induces p56^{lck} activation and TCR desensitization independent of TCR tyrosine phosphorylation. *J. Immunol.* **153,** 2905–2917.
5. Ledbetter, J. A., June, C. H., Grosmaire, L. S., and Rabinovitch, P. S. (1987) Crosslinking of surface antigens causes mobilization of intracellular ionized calcium in T lymphocytes. *Proc. Natl. Acad. Sci. USA* **84,** 1384–1388.
6. Stumbles, P. and Mason, D. (1995) Activation of CD4$^+$ T cells in the presence of a nondepleting monoclonal antibody to CD4 induces a Th2-type response in vitro. *J. Exp. Med.* **182,** 5–13.
7. Jabado, N., Le Deist, F., Fischer, A., and Hivroz, C. (1994) Interaction of HIV gp120 and anti-CD4 antibodies with the CD4 molecule on human CD4$^+$ T cells inhibits the binding activity of NF-AT, NF-$_\kappa$B and AP-1, three nuclear factors regulating interleukin-2 gene enhancer activity. *Eur. J. Immunol.* **24,** 2646–2652.
8. Miltenyi, S., Muller, W., Weichel, W., and Radbruch, A. (1990) High gradient magnetic cell separation with MACS. *Cytometry* **11,** 231–238.
9. Böyum, A., Lovhaug, D., Tresland, L., and Nordlie, E. M. (1991) Separation of leukocytes: improved cell purity by fine adjustments of gradient medium density and osmolarity. *Scand. J. Immunol.* **34,** 697–712.

12

Isolation of T-Cell Antigens
by Retrovirus-Mediated Expression Cloning

Toshio Kitamura and Yoshihiro Morikawa

1. Introduction

Expression cloning is a powerful tool in isolating a cDNA for a protein when the protein is difficult to purify but can be detected by antibody staining or some biological activity, such as growth promoting activity. In this chapter, we focus on the cloning of cDNAs for surface proteins by expression cloning. Originally, expression cloning was performed in *Escherichia coli* (*E. coli*) transduced with cDNA libraries constructed in lamda phage-based vectors followed by screening using antibody staining. However, proteins produced in *E. coli* have no glycosylation, which is a disadvantage in detecting the expression of surface proteins by antibodies because significant numbers of monoclonal antibodies can only recognize glycosylated molecules, and sometimes proteins are not properly folded in *E. coli*. Therefore it was recommended to use polyclonal antibodies for the expression cloning using *E. coli*. Later, an expression-cloning method using mammalian cells was developed; plasmid vectors harboring the SV40 replication origin are amplified in COS cells expressing the SV40 large T antigens *(1,2)* such that cDNA products are detected and isolated efficiently. That is, the SV40 origin-bearing plasmids can replicate in COS cells *(2)*, allowing the plasmids to be recovered by transformation into *E. coli*. Amplification of the plasmid also greatly increases expression of the cDNA in the plasmid.

A notable modification was added to this method by Seed and Aruffo who used the panning procedure to collect COS cells expressing a cDNA of interest *(3–5)*. This modification was an enormous contribution to the cloning of cDNAs for many surface markers. The cell sorter has also been used for collecting COS cells expressing a cDNA of interest *(6)*. These strategies, how-

From: *Methods in Molecular Biology, Vol. 134: T Cell Protocols: Development and Activation*
Edited by: K. P. Kearse © Humana Press Inc., Totowa, NJ

ever, have some limitations as well; for example, we need to use specific cell lines such as COS cells that may sometimes give high staining backgrounds for antibodies of interest or already express endogenous molecules that react with the antibody. Another potential issue is that the expression of a particular molecule may require another molecule which is not expressed in COS cells. Therefore, it was important to develop an expression-cloning method in which a variety of target cells can be used depending on experimental purposes.

1.1. Usage of Retrovirus Vectors in Expression Cloning

Several groups have recently developed expression-cloning methods using retrovirus infection *(7–10)*. In contrast to transient transfection systems, retroviral gene transfer efficiently delivers genes stably into a wide range of target cells and is expected to overcome the limitations of the conventional expression-cloning method described in the introduction. In initial trials, NIH3T3-based packaging cell lines were used as retrovirus producers, and drug selection of packaging cells was usually required to establish transfected packaging cells in this method. However, it was difficult to cover large complexities of cDNA libraries using NIH3T3-based packaging cell lines because of the low efficiency of transient transfection in these cells. Moreover, the frequency of each cDNA in the library may change during the drug selection of stable packaging cell lines, and thus the resulting retrovirus stock may not represent the original cDNA library.

This current chapter, describes a method to isolate cDNAs for surface proteins using retrovirus cloning vectors and transient packaging cell lines such as BOSC23 *(11)* or Phoenix-Eco *(12)* which give high titers of retroviruses by transient transfection (**Fig. 1**) *(10,13)*. In this method, cDNA libraries are constructed in a simplified retroviral vector pMX or pMXI (**Fig. 2**). Retroviruses representing the cDNA library were generated using a transient retrovirus packaging system *(11,12)*. The supernatant of the packaging cell line, containing high-titer retroviruses (>3 × 10^6 plaque-forming units/mL), is then used to infect target cells, and infected cells are selected for expression of the cDNA of interest. Finally, the cDNA, which is responsible for the expression of the protein, is amplified by genomic PCR or RT-PCR using retrovirus vector primers.

2. Materials

2.1. cDNA Library Construction

1. FastTrack kit (Invitrogen, Carlsbad, CA).
2. SuperScript Choice System for cDNA Synthesis (Gibco-BRL, Grand Island, NY).
3. *Bst*XI adaptor (Invitrogen).
4. Phenol:chloroform:isoamyl alcohol (25:24:1) (Sigma, St. Louis, MO).
5. 7.5 *M* ammonium acetate (NH_4OAc).
6. 70% (v/v) ethanol (–20°C).

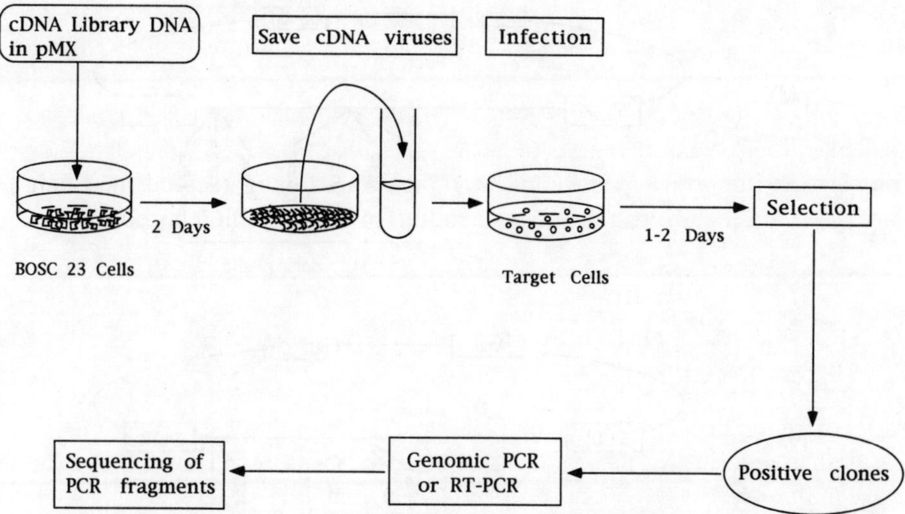

Fig. 1. Retrovirus-mediated expression cloning of cDNAs for cell surface markers. Flow diagram of cloning of a cDNA that encodes a surface protein of interest. Either sorting or panning can be used for the selection method. It is recommended to use single clones and not bulk populations for genomic or RT-PCR.

7. TE buffer: 10 mM Tris-HCl (pH 7.5), 1 mM EDTA.
8. TEN buffer: 10 mM Tris-HCl (pH. 7.5), 0.1 mM EDTA, 25 mM NaCl.
9. Mupid gel electroporesis aparatus (Advance, Tokyo, Japan).
10. Gene Pulser/*E. coli* Cuvet (Bio-Rad, Hercules, CA).
11. *E. coli* Pulser (Bio-Rad).
12. ElectroMAX DH10B cells (Gibco-BRL).
13. Qiagen Maxi prep kit (Qiagen, Santa Clarita, CA).

2.2. Production of Retrovirus Stock

1. BOSC23 *(11)* (*see* **Note 1**) or Phoenix-Eco *(12)* (*see* **Note 2**) packaging cells.
2. LIPOFECTAMINE Reagent (Gibco-BRL).
3. OPTI-MEM-I medium (Gibco-BRL).
4. GPT selection reagent (Specialty Media, Lavallette, NJ).
5. Dulbecco's minimal essential medium (DMEM).
6. Fetal calf serum (FCS).
7. Tissue culture dish.
8. Polystylene, round-bottom tube (Falcon2054, Becton Dickinson, Lincoln Park, NJ).

2.3. Infection and Transient Expression of Recombinant Retroviruses

1. Target cells (*see* **Note 3**).
2. Polybrene (hexadimethrine bromide, Sigma, St. Louis, MO).

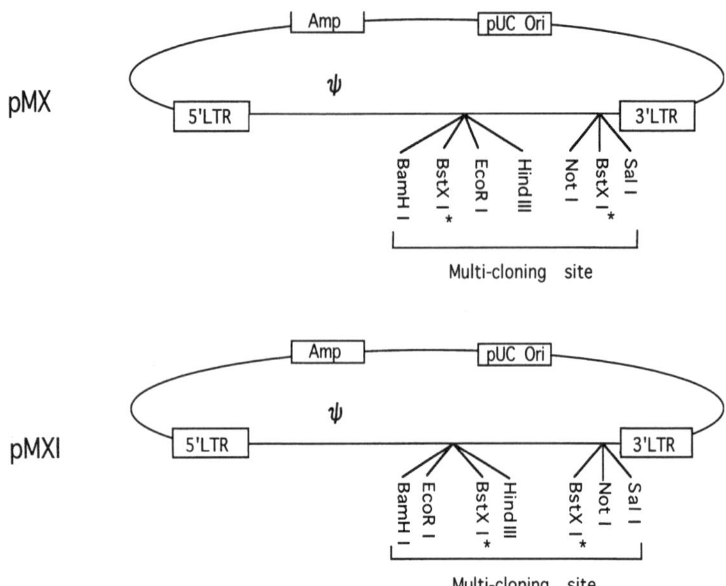

Fig. 2. Structure of the retrovirus vectors pMX and pMXI. The structure of pMXI (pMX improved, or pM eleven) is identical with that of pMX *(13)* except for the 5' and 3' multicloning sites which have different orders. For constructing nondirectional libraries in pMXI, cDNAs are inserted into *Bst*XI sites (*) so that *Bam*HI and *Eco*RI on the 5' cloning site and *Not*I and *Sal*I on the 3' cloning site can be utilized to cut out cDNA inserts. ψ: packaging signal; Amp: ampicillin resistance gene; ori: replication origin; LTR: long terminal repeat.

2.4. Sequencing of the Integrated Retroviruses

1. LA *Taq* polymerase (Takara, Shiga, Japan) (*see* **Note 4**).
2. Dye Terminator Cycle Sequencing Ready Reaction Kit (Perkin-Elmer, Warrington, Great Britain).
3. pMX and pMXI primers; 5' primer GGTGGACCATCCTCTAGACT, 3' primer CCCTTTTTCTGGAGACTAAAT.
4. 310 or 373A Genetic Analyzer (Applied Biosystems, Menlo Park, CA).
5. TA vector (Invitrogen).

3. Methods

3.1. cDNA Library Construction (Nondirectional, see Note 5) (Modified From the Protocol of SuperScript Choice System

3.1.1. cDNA Synthesis

1. Poly(A)⁺ RNA was prepared using FastTrack kit according to the manufacturer's protocol.

2. Add either 1 µg of oligo dT$_{12-18}$ primers, 0.1 µg of random hexamers or combinations of both primers (1 µg of oligo dT$_{12-18}$ primers and 0.1 µg of random hexamers) to a sterile 1.5-mL microcentrifuge tube (*see* **Note 6**).

3. Add 5 µg of mRNA and adjust the total volume to 8 µL using DEPC-treated water (*see* **Note 5**).

4. Heat the mixture at 70°C for 10 min, and quick chill on ice.

5. Collect the contents of the tube by brief centrifugation, and add 4 µL of 5X first strand buffer, 2 µL of 0.1 *M* dithiothreitol (DTT), and 1 µL of 10 m*M* dNTP mix.

6. Mix the contents of the tube by gently vortexing, and incubate the tube at 37°C for 2 min to equilibrate the temperature.

7. Add 5 µL of Superscript II reverse transcriptase (total volume of the reaction mixture is 20 µL), mix gently, and incubate the reaction mixture at 37°C for 1 h.

8. Place the tube on ice to terminate the reaction.

9. On ice, add 93 µL of DEPC-treated water, 30 µL of 5X second strand buffer, 3 µL of 10 m*M* dNTP mix, 1 µL of DNA ligase (10 U/mL), 4 µL of DNA polymerase I (10 U/mL), and 1 µL of RNase H (2 U/mL) in that order.

10. Vortex the tube gently to mix, and incubate the completed reaction for 2 h at 16°C.

11. Add 2 µL (10 U) of T4 DNA polymerase, and continue incubating at 16°C for 5 min.

12. Place the reaction on ice, and add 10 µL of 0.5 *M* EDTA.

13. Add 150 µL of phenol:chloroform:isoamyl alcohol (25:24:1), vortex throughly, and centrifuge at room temperature for 5 min at 14,000*g*.

14. Carefully remove 140 µL of the upper, aqueous layer and transfer it to a fresh 1.5-mL microcentrifuge tube.

15. Add 70 µL of 7.5 *M* NH$_4$OAc, followed by 0.5 mL of absolute ethanol (–20°C).

16. Vortex the mixture thoroughly, and centrifuge at room temperature for 20 min at 14,000*g*.

17. Remove the supernatant carefully, and wash the pellet with 0.5 mL of 70% ethanol (–20°C).

18. Centrifuge for 2 min at 14,000*g*, and remove the supernatant completely.

19. Dry the cDNA for more than 10 min to completely evaporate residual ethanol (*see* **Note 6**).

3.1.2. Adaptor Ligation

1. Hydrate the cDNA pellet prepared as above and set up a ligation reaction (final volume, 50 µL) as follows: 66 m*M* Tris-HCl (pH 7.6), 10 m*M* MgCl$_2$, 1 m*M* ATP, 14 m*M* DTT, 40 µg/mL *Bst*XI adaptor, 100 units/mL T4 DNA ligase.

2. Mix gently, spin briefly, and then incubate the reaction mixture at 16°C for 16 h (overnight).

3. Heat the reaction at 70°C for 10 min to inactivate the ligase, and chill on ice.

4. Add 50 µL of phenol:chloroform:isoamyl alcohol (25:24:1), vortex thoroughly, and centrifuge at room temperature for 5 min at 14,000*g*.

5. Carefully remove 45 µL of the upper, aqueous layer and transfer it to a fresh 1.5-mL microcentrifuge tube.

6. Add 5 µL of TE buffer, 25 µL of 7.5 *M* NH$_4$OAc, 5 µg of yeast tRNA and 150 µL of absolute ethanol (–20°C).
7. Vortex the mixture, and centrifuge at room temperature for 20 min at 14,000*g*.
8. Remove the supernatant carefully, and wash the pellet with 0.5 mL of 70% ethanol.
9. Centrifuge for 2 min at 14,000*g*, and remove the supernatant completely.
10. Dry the cDNA for 10 min to evaporate residual ethanol completely.

3.1.3. Column Chromatography (to Remove Unligated Adaptors)

1. Equilibrate the column supplied in the kit with TEN buffer four times according to the manufacturer's protocol.
2. Dissolve the cDNA in 100 µL of TEN buffer, and let the pellet hydrate on ice.
3. Apply the cDNA in TEN buffer to the center of the top frit of the equilibrated column and let it drain completely.
4. Add 100 µL of TEN buffer to the column top and let it drain completely.
5. Repeat **step 4** one more time.
6. Add 100 µL of TEN buffer and collect the effluent into a 1.5-mL microcentrifuge tube.
7. Repeat **step 6** one more time, and then add 150 µL of TEN buffer and collect the effluent into the 1.5-mL microcentrifuge tube that now contains 350 µL of the adaptor-ligated cDNA solution.

3.1.4. Insertion of cDNAs into the Vector After the Size Fractionation

1. Add 175 µL of 7.5 *M* NH4OAc, 5 µg of yeast tRNA and 700 µL of absolute ethanol (–20°C) to the effluent.
2. Perform ethanol precipitation according to **step 7–10** of **Subheading 3.1.2.**
3. Add 10 µL of TE buffer to the cDNA pellet.
4. Separate the cDNAs through a 0.9% agarose gel using a small gel electrophoresis aparatus, such as Mupid II. Cut out the gel fragment between 1 kbp and 10 kbp, and extract cDNA fragments using QiaexII according to the manufacturer's protocol.
5. Resuspend the size-separated cDNAs in 20 µL of TE buffer.
6. Ligate 2 µL (*see* **Note 7**) of the cDNA to the *Bst*XI sites of the pMX retrovirus vector (50 ng) in a 20 µL of the ligation reactions; 50 m*M* Tris-HCl (pH 7.6), 10 m*M* MgCl$_2$, 1 m*M* ATP, 5% (w/v) PEG 8000, 1 m*M* DTT, 50 ng of *Bst*XI-cut pMX, 2 µL of cDNA, and 50 units/mL T4 DNA ligase.
7. Vortex the reaction tube gently, spin it briefly, then incubate at 16°C overnight.
8. Heat the reaction at 70°C for 10 min to inactivate the ligase.
9. Add 2 µL of 3*M* NaOAc, 5 µg yeast tRNA, and then 60 µL of absolute ethanol (–20°C).
10. Perform ethanol precipitation according to **steps 7–10** of **Subheading 3.1.2.** (*see* **Note 8**)
11. Resuspend the pellet in 12 µL of TE buffer.

3.1.5. Transformation

1. Place two to three *E. coli* cuvets on ice.
2. Keep 1 mL of SOC medium in a sterile 10 mL culture tube at room temperature.
3. Remove ElectroMAX DH10B cells from –80°C freezer and thaw them on wet ice.
4. Add 2 µL each of the ligated DNA to each cuvets, and keep the unused portion at –20°C for future use.
5. Add 25 µL of DH10B cells to each cuvet containing the ligated DNA, and mix them by shaking the cuvets gently and briefly.
6. Electroporate the cuvets with 1.8 kV using an *E. coli* pulser.
7. Immediately add 0.2 mL of S.O.C. media directly to the cuvets, and keep them at room temperature for 10 min.
8. Collect the electroporated *E. coli* to a sterile 10 mL culture tube using SOC media (1 mL total for two or three cuvets).
9. Shake the tube at 150 rpm and 37°C for 45 min.
10. Amplify the culture in 200–500 mL of L broth with 50 µg/mL ampicillin for overnight at 37°C.
11. Simultaneouly with the large culture (200–500 mL), $1/10^4$ and $1/10^5$ of the culture is plated onto LB-agar plates to estimate the quality (total size and the average size of the insert) of the cDNA library.
12. Make 20 mL of glycerol stock and extract plasmid DNA from the rest of the overnight culture using a Qiagen maxi prep kit.

3.2. Production of Retrovirus Stock (see Note 9)

1. BOSC23 cells (2×10^6 cells) were seeded onto 60-mm dishes 1 d before the transfection and incubate the cells at 37°C in a CO_2 incubator (*see* **Note 10**).
2. Prepare the following solutions in polystyrene tubes: solution A, 3 µg of library DNA in 200 µL of OPTI-MEM-I medium, solution B, 18 µL of LIPOFECTAMINE Reagent in 200 µL of OPTI-MEM-I medium (*see* **Note 11**).
3. Add solution B to solution A slowly, mix gently, and incubate at room temperature for 30 min to allow DNA-liposome complexes to form.
4. While complexes form, rinse the cells once with 2 mL of serum-free OPTI-MEM I medium.
5. Add 1.6 mL of serum-free OPTI-MEM I medium to the tube containing the complexes, mix gently, and overlay the diluted complex solution onto the rinsed cells.
6. Incubate the cells with the complexes for 5 h at 37°C in a CO_2 incubator.
7. Add 2 mL of DMEM containing 20% of FCS without removing the transfection mixture.
8. Incubate the cells for 19 h at 37°C in a CO_2 incubator.
9. Replace the medium with 3 mL of fresh DMEM containing 10 % of FCS, incubate for another 24 h at 37°C in a CO_2 incubator, and then the retroviral supernatant is used for infection of target cells (*see* **Note 12**).

3.3. Infection of Recombinant Retroviruses and Collection of the Cells Expressing the Antigens of Interest

1. For infection of Ba/F3 cells, 4×10^6 cells are incubated with 10 mL of virus stock containing Polybrene (10 µg/mL) (*see* **Note 13**).
2. After 8 h, the cells are washed, resuspended in 20 mL fresh growth medium conatining 1 ng/mL murine IL-3, and cultivated for an additional 16 h.
3. The cells are then subjected to cell sorting (or panning).
4. The cell expressing the antigen of interest is cloned by single cell sorting or limiting dilution after several cycles of sorting or panning.

3.4. Cloning and Sequencing of the Integrated Retroviruses

Fifty nanograms of genomic DNA isolated from each clone is subjected to PCR. The PCR reaction is run for 35 cycles (1 min at 94°C, 2 min at 58°C, and 3 min at 72°C) using LA *taq* polymerase and pMX primers (*see* **Note 4**). The resulting PCR fragment is purified using Qiaex II and sequenced directly using *Taq* DyeDeoxy Terminator on an Applied Biosystems automatic sequencer.

When necessary, PCR fragments are cloned into the TA vector (Invitrogen) and then sequenced. Finally, the PCR fragment is inserted into the pMX vector, converted to retroviruses using BOSC23 cells, and the expression of the surface protein of interest is confirmed.

4. Notes

1. The Bosc23 cell line can be obtained from Dr. Warren S. Pear (e-mail address: wpear@mail.med.upenn.edu).
2. The Phoenix-Eco cell line can be obtained from Dr. Garry P. Nolan (e-mail address: gnolan@cmgm.stanford.edu).
3. Any infectable cell line can be used for the experiment. We usually use a mouse IL-3-dependent Ba/F3 cell line or a mouse thymoma cell line BW5147. A preferable infection efficiency of the target cells is 10–30%. When the infection efficiency is higher than 30%, infected cells tend to have multiple integration of proviruses. In some cell lines, such as BW5147 and NIH3T3, the infection efficiency is usually 100% and the average number of integration ranges from 5–10. In such a case, it is time consuming to examine which integration is responsible for the expression of the surface marker of interest. Therefore, it is recommended to dilute the cDNA viruses before use to adjust the infection efficiency to between 10 and 30%. The infection efficiency is estimated by a control experiment using pMX-EGFP.
4. Any *Taq* polymerase can be used. However, in our hands, LA-*Taq* polymerase worked most efficiently in these experiments.
5. It is also possible to make unidirectional libraries using Directional Cloning Tool Box (Invitrogen)(*10*). However, it is recommended to use nondirectional libraries because of the following reasons:

    a. Screening efficiency is very good in retrovirus-mediated expression cloning, and the presence of 50% antisense clones is not a big disadvantage.

    b. It's easier to make nondirectional libraries.

    c. For cloning of potentially large cDNA clones, it is recommended to use random hexamers or a combination of oligo dT and random primers to synthesize cDNAs, which are not possible for unidirectional libraries.

6. Half of the synthesized cDNA may be kept for future use.

7. Only a portion (1/10–1/2) of synthesized cDNA can give rise to a library whose size is large enough (containing about 1×10^6 independent clones). One microgram of mRNA is sufficient for making several good libraries.

8. At this step, it is very critical to dry up the pellet completely. The point is not to use more than 10 µL of QiaexII beads in one tube in DNA extraction. Inclusion of residual amounts of ethanol will greatly decrease the transformation efficiency.

9. The calcium phosphate transfection method can be used for producing retroviruses with similar efficiencies.

10. After long-term culture, titers of the retroviruses produced from BOSC23 cells tend to decrease. It is therefore recommended to use new batches of BOSC23 cells every 3–4 mo. BOSC23 cells are maintained in DMEM containing 10% FCS and GPT selection reagents. The cells are transferred into DMEM containing 10% FCS without GPT selection reagents 2 d before transfection. When you use Phoenix-Eco cells, cells that produce high titers of retroviruses can be selected by sorting for CD8 expression and diphtheria toxin resistance.

11. RPMI1640 medium or DMEM medium can be also used with slightly decreased efficiencies.

12. Do not add antibacterial agents to the media during transfection and virus production.

13. A control vector pMX-GFP is used to monitor infection efficiency.

Acknowledgment

The authors thank Ms. Chihiro Ozawa for her excellent help in preparation of this chapter.

References

1. Okayama, H. and Berg, P. (1983) A cDNA cloning vector that permits expression of cDNA inserts in mammalian cells. *Mol. Cell. Biol.* **3,** 280–289.

2. Gluzman, Y. (1981) SV40-transformed simian cells support the replication of early SV40 mutants. *Cell* **23,** 175–182.

3. Seed, B. and Aruffo, A. (1987) Molecular cloning of the CD2 antigen, the T-cell erythrocyte receptor, by a rapid immunoselection procedure. *Proc. Natl. Acad. Sci. USA* **84,** 3365–3369.

4. Aruffo, A. and Seed, B. (1987) Molecular cloning of a CD28 cDNA by a high-efficiency COS cell expression system. *Proc. Natl. Acad. Sci. USA* **84,** 8573–8577.

5. Aruffo, A. and Seed, B. (1987) Molecular cloning of two CD7 (T-cell leukemia antigen) cDNAs by a COS cell expression system. *EMBO J.* **6,** 3313–3316.

6. Yamasaki, K., Taga, T., Hirata, Y., Yawata, H., Kawanishi, Y., Seed, B., Taniguchi, T., Hirano, T., and Kishimoto, T. (1988) Cloning and expression of the human interleukin-6 (BSF-2/IFNβ2) receptor. *Science* **241,** 825–828.
7. Rayner, J. R. and Gonda, T. J. (1994) A simple and efficient procedure for generating stable expression libraries by cDNA cloning in a retroviral vector. *Mol. Cell. Biol.* **14,** 880–887.
8. Wong, B. Y., Chen, H., Chung, S. W., and Wong, P. M. (1994) High-efficiency identification of genes by functional analysis from a retroviral cDNA expression library. *J. Virol.* **68,** 5523–5531.
9. Whitehead, I., Kirk, H., and Kay, R. (1995) Expression cloning of oncogenes by retroviral transfer of cDNA libraries. *Mol. Cell. Biol.* **15,** 704–710.
10. Kitamura, T., Onishi, M., Kinoshita, S., Shibuya, A., Miyajima, A., and Nolan, G. P. (1995) Efficient screening of retroviral cDNA expression libraries. *Proc. Natl. Acad. Sci. USA* **92,** 9146–9150.
11. Pear, W. S., Nolan, G. P., Scott, M. L., and Baltimore, D. (1993) Production of high-titer helper-free retroviruses by transient transfection. *Proc. Natl. Acad. Sci. USA* **90,** 8392–8396.
12. Hitoshi, Y., Lorens, J., Kitada, S., Fisher, J., LaBarge, M., Ring, H. Z., Francke, U., Reed, J. C., Kinoshita, S., and Nola n, G. P. (1998) Toso, a cell surface, specific regulator of Fas-induced apoptosis in T cells. *Immun.* **8,** 461–471.
13. Onishi, M., Kinoshita, S., Morikawa, Y., Shibuya, A., Phillips, J., Lanier, L. L., Gorman, D. M., Nolan, G. P., Miyajima, A., and Kitamura, T. (1996) Applications of retrovirus-mediated expression cloning. *Exp. Hematol.* **24,** 324–329.

13

Flow Cytometric Analysis
of Murine T Lymphocytes

A Practical Guide

Melanie S. Vacchio and Elizabeth W. Shores

1. Introduction
1.1. General Considerations

As T cells develop in the thymus, they undergo distinct changes in their morphology and expression of cell surface antigens. Phenotypic changes in mature peripheral T cells also occur subsequent to T-cell activation, resulting from engagement of the T-cell antigen receptor (TCR) or exposure to specific biochemical reagents. The ability to objectively measure such changes has been greatly enhanced by the combined techniques of immunofluorescence and flow cytometry (FCM). Using these approaches, it is possible to detect cell surface antigens by staining cells with specific antibodies that are tagged with different fluorochromes. Moreover, a variety of different cellular parameters can be monitored simultaneously on an individual cell. Whereas the initial investiture in this technology can be expensive, it provides a powerful and rapid means of assessing states of T-cell development and activation.

The purpose of this current chapter is to familiarize scientists with the basic concepts and techniques in flow cytometry as it pertains to the analysis of T cells. The complexity of the technique can vary and will depend on the number and particular parameters that need to be assessed. Herein, the focus is on more straightforward applications of the procedure and providing specific examples. As the reader becomes familiar with the basic concepts and methods used in flow cytometry, the reader is encouraged to read more in-depth discussions in this area *(1–3)*.

From: *Methods in Molecular Biology, Vol. 134: T Cell Protocols: Development and Activation*
Edited by: K. P. Kearse © Humana Press Inc., Totowa, NJ

1.2. Importance of Cell Preparations

There are many things that contribute to the success of an FCM experiment. Of great importance are high quality cell preparations. It is impossible to over-emphasize the importance of careful cell preparation to the generation of clear, reproducible, and interpretable FCM data. Because of its importance, tips are provided for the preparation of lymphoid cell populations. Investigations of T-cell development, often involve phenotypic analysis of the thymus so thymus preparation is discussed. Although both the lymph node and spleen provide a source of mature T cells, the ratio of T to B cells is much higher in the lymph node than in the spleen and hence provides a very good source of mature T cells for ex vivo examination of T-cell populations.

1.3. Considerations and Approaches
to Immunofluorescent Staining

The most common cause of failed experiments is uninterpretable staining patterns resulting from lack of important controls. To avoid this problem, careful protocol design is essential, particularly in regard to inclusion of appropriate negative and positive controls. Determination of controls involves careful consideration of cell types to be used in the experiment and selection of appropriate control antibodies. (*see* **Note 1**).

Multicolor staining can be performed so that several different parameters can be examined on a single cell. Some investigators prefer to add each antibody separately, incubating and washing between each step. However, it is possible to add multiple antibodies simultaneously as long as each antibody is appropriately titered (*see* **Notes 2** and **3**). When choosing antibodies for multicolor analysis, it is important to make sure the antibodies do not cross block or sterically inhibit each other. Such would be the case if the determinants, to which the antibodies are directed, are located too near each other.

Cells can be stained directly (where the antibody is directly conjugated to fluorochrome) or indirectly. For direct staining, fluorochrome-labeled antibodies directed against cell surface determinants are added to the cells. Another option is to use antibodies coupled to biotin. Biotin coupled antibodies provide some flexibility since avidin is available tagged with a variety of different fluorochromes. Indirect staining can also be conducted. In this method, an unlabeled primary antibody directed to the antigen in question is added first, followed by the addition of a secondary anti-immunoglobulin reagent that is conjugated to a fluorochrome. The secondary antibody will vary depending on the isotype and species from which the primary antibody was derived. For example, if the primary antibody is a monoclonal IgG2a mouse anti-Thy1 antibody, the secondary antibody would need to recognize mouse IgG2a.

Selection of the secondary antibody is critical to data interpretation. Because B cells express surface Ig themselves (predominantly IgM and IgD), a secondary antibody that recognizes all mouse immunoglobulin isotypes would not only bind T cells coated with anti-Thy1, but also mouse B cells. Another possible pitfall to indirect staining stems from the use of the anti-FcR blocking antibody (*see* **Note 4**). If the secondary reagent detects this antibody, FcR will be detected if anti-FcR was used to block. In this circumstance it is advisable to either avoid an initial FcR block or to choose an isotype-specific labeled anti-IgG as a secondary antibody that does not detect the anti-FcR antibody. Finally, anti-rat Ig, or anti-hamster Ig antibodies will often crossreact with mouse surface Ig on B cells. This problem can be circumvented in some cases by absorbing secondary reagents against mouse Ig to minimize crossreactivity.

Sometimes it is important to combine indirect staining for one determinant with direct staining for another determinant. While it is possible to combine these approaches, the procedure needs to be carefully considered. The indirect staining should be performed first because the secondary anti-Ig reagent may bind to cell-bound conjugated antibodies. Also, because antibodies are multivalent, they can bind to primary antibodies with only one binding site, leaving the other site available to bind subsequently added directly conjugated antibodies (**Fig. 1**). To prevent the unbound site from reacting with subsequently added labeled antibodies, blocking the unbound site with unlabeled blocking antibody (either more of the primary antibody or an antibody of the same species and isotype of the primary antibody) is recommended prior to addition of other directly labeled antibodies.

1.4. Flow Cytometry: An Overview

The development of user-friendly flow cytometers has made it possible for an individual scientist to prepare cells, independently operate cytometers, and analyze data. Unlike more complicated cytometers that generally require dedicated operators, these new age cytometers provide a tremendous advantage to scientists who like to have complete and immediate control over their experiments. Such cytometers include the FACScan (Becton Dickinson, Cockeysville, MD) and the EPCS-XL (Beckman Coulter, Inc., Fullerton, CA). Other instruments combine analytical ability with the ability to actually separate or sort cell populations. For the purposes of this article, focus will be on the FACScan as it represents one of the most common flow cytometers used by scientists.

The principles behind FCM are relatively straightforward. Cells, stained with fluorochrome labeled antibodies directed against specific determinants, are directed under positive pressure (laminar flow) through a fluidics stream

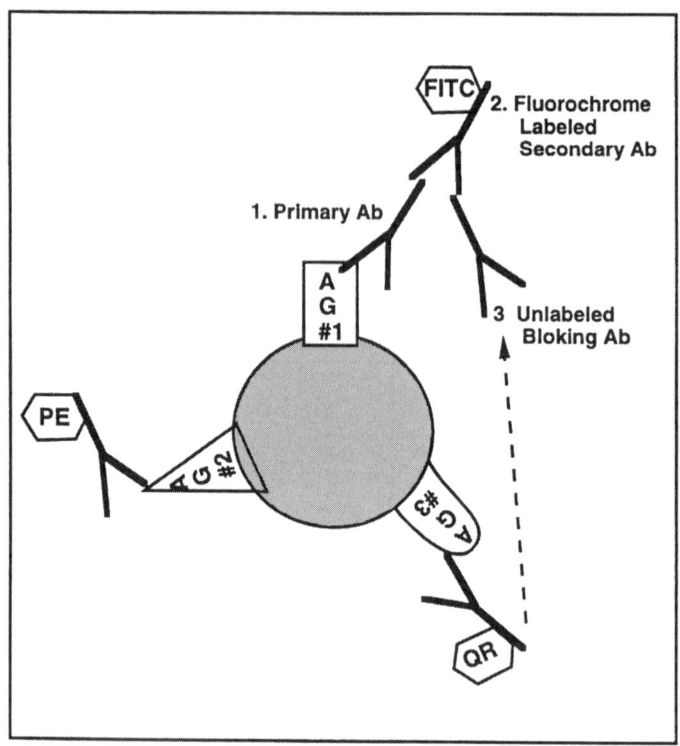

Fig. 1. Depiction of indirect staining in combination with direct staining. This picture represent cells that express antigen #1 (AG 1 square), antigen #2 (AG #2, triangle) and antigen #3 (AG #3, bullet). Unlabeled antibody directed against AG1 has been added. Cells were washed and an anti-Ig FITC labeled secondary antibody was added. The secondary antibody will bind to the primary antibody. If primary antibody is limiting relative to the secondary antibody, the secondary antibody will not have both binding sites engaged and potentially can bind subsequently labeled (PE or QR (Quantum Red, Red670, etc) antibodies. If AG #3 is not expressed on the cell surface, the cell may still appear to express AG#3 via binding to the free site of the secondary antibody (dotted line and arrow). To prevent this interaction, unlabeled free antibody is added to the staining reaction.

such that they are moving in "single file." As an individual cell passes through a laser beam emitting light at a defined wavelength (488 nm for the FACScan argon-ion laser), fluorochromes are excited and emit light at given wavelengths. Photomultiplier tubes are used to amplify signals from this emission. This analog signal is then converted to digital data and captured via specialized computer software. The computer stores multiple parameters on every event (cell) traversing the laser and this data can be analyzed at a later time. Although detailed data analysis occurs subsequent to data collection, flow cytometry can provide instant gratification to the anxious investigator as cellular phenotypes can be observed on the computer screen during data acquisition.

Depending on the particular cytometer, a number of different parameters can be assessed. The FACScan and its associated CellQuest software (Becton Dickinson, Cockeysville, MD) allows for simultaneous measurement of up to 5 different parameters on each individual cell. Two of these parameters are forward light scatter (FSC) and side (orthogonal) light scatter (SSC). Measurement of these parameters is not dependent on staining of cells with labeled antibodies but rather measures characteristics of cell morphology. FSC generally correlates with cell size whereas SSC correlates with cell granularity. The remaining parameters (FL1, FL2, and FL3) are used to measure the intensity of staining with fluorochrome-labeled antibodies and hence this intensity reflects the level of expression of a given cell surface antigen. FL1 measures signals coming from fluorescein isothiocyanate (FITC) labeled antibodies (green fluorescence) and detects emission optimally at 525 nm. FL2 measures signals generally coming from antibodies labeled with phycoerythrin (PE) (orange-red) and detects emission at 575 nm. FL3 is used to measure emission generally >613 nm and a number of new reagents have been designed to detect fluorescent emission at this range of wavelengths (violet), including Cychrome™ (Pharmingen), PerCP™ (Becton Dickinson), Red613™ (Life Technologies), Red670™ (made by Life Technologies) and quantum red™ (Sigma). Antibodies can also be coupled to biotin. Whereas biotin itself is not detectable by FCM, an avidin-fluorochrome conjugate can subsequently be added. Because avidin binds strongly to biotin and can be coupled to a variety of fluorochromes, this approach provides flexibility to experimental design, particularly for multicolor FCM.

Whereas a number of fluorochromes are available on the market, it is important to be aware that the applicability of these reagents to FCM with the FACScan is limited by their ability to be stimulated by the excitation wavelength of the FACScan's laser (488 nm). Therefore rhodamine-based dyes, allophycocyanin, and Texas Red are not suitable for use with the FACScan because they are not excited or only poorly excited at this wavelength.

Finally, a word of caution. Although flow cytometry is an extremely powerful and useful technique, inappropriate setup of the machine or lack of appropriate controls can lead to loss of valuable time, reagents, and/or misinterpretation of data. Therefore, this review emphasizes areas of critical concern so that common mistakes can be avoided.

1.5. Specific Applications of Flow Cytometry to Analysis of T Cells

Flow cytometry is an important technology for a number of scientific disciplines. The focus of this article is on T cells, so several specific applications to thymocyte and T-cell analysis are included.

1.5.1. CD4 vs CD8 Subset Analysis in the Thymus

A great deal can be learned about the state of thymocyte development by staining with antibodies against CD8, and CD4, with a third marker. This approach allows the investigator to analyze the expression of various markers at different stages of T-cell differentiation. In **Subheading 3.4.1.**, analysis of TCR expression on different thymocyte populations is exemplified.

1.5.2. Early Thymocyte Subsets

Subheading 3.4.2. will illustrate an approach by which CD4$^-$CD8$^-$ cells, which represent a relatively rare population of thymocytes, can be examined. Because it does not require physically removing the majority populations (such as by antibody and complement), it provides a means by which rare populations can be rapidly assessed. This approach involves using a combination of antibodies, all coupled to the same fluorochrome. In this example, thymocytes are stained with a cocktail of Red-670 labeled antibodies (including anti-CD4, anti-CD8, anti-CD3, anti-B220, anti-GR1, anti-MAC-1) *(4)*. Cells that are negative for these antigens represent the most immature CD4$^-$CD8$^-$ thymocytes. Expression of other cell surface antigens (CD25 and CD44) can be examined by also staining cells with FITC and PE-labeled antibodies and gating on cells that fail to stain with the FL3 antibodies.

1.5.3. Activated Peripheral T Cells (Live Gating on Activated Cells)

T cells become activated upon engagement of their TCR. The activation status of T cells can be monitored by assessing changes in their cellular morphology and expression of surface antigens. A means by which to track activated T cells in demonstrated in **Subheading 3.4.3.** In this example, increased cell size and surface expression of CD69 and CD25 demonstrate one approach by which to assess T-cell activation.

1.5.4. Analysis of Peripheral Blood Lymphocytes

Analysis of peripheral blood lymphocytes (PBLs) is a quick and rapid way to screen transgenic mice for expression of cell surface transgenic proteins. Small quantities of blood are obtained from mice, and cells can be stained with antibodies directed against transgenic molecules. This procedure is discussed in **Subheading 3.4.4.**

2. Materials

2.1. Cell Preparations

1. Media: Hanks balance salt solution (HBSS) or RPMI at pH 7.0 containing 5% fetal calf serum (FCS) at 4°C.

2. Ice bucket and ice.
3. Basic dissecting materials.
4. Small Petri dish.
5. 19-gage needles.
6. Gauze.
7. 100 µm nylon mesh.
8. ACK lysing reagent.

2.2. Immunofluorescent Staining

1. FCM buffer (for staining and washing): 0.1% BSA (fraction V), 0.1% NaN_3 in HBSS w/o phenol red maintained at 4°C (**Note 5**).
2. Appropriately titrated labeled antibodies (**Note 2**).
3. Anti-FcR antibody (**Note 4**).
4. Falcon 2052 tubes (12 × 75 mm). These tubes are specifically compatible with the FACScan.
5. 96 well U-bottom microtiter plates (optional, *see* **Notes 6**).
6. Cell suspensions at 10×10^6/mL
7. Pipeter: able to deliver 5–20 µL.
8. Pipet tips (2–200 µL).
9. Centrifuge.

2.3. Flow Cytometric Analysis

1. Cells, stained according to protocol, following the procedure above.
2. Compensation control tubes.
3. Flow cytometer with adequate supply of sheath fluid (as recommended by the manufacturer).
4. Computer associated with flow cytometer.
5. Data storage device.

3. Methods
3.1. Cell Preparation
3.1.1. Thymus Preparation

1. Sacrifice the animal. While cervical dislocation is a common means of sacrificing mice prior to removal of organs, it can cause extensive bleeding and hemorrhages in the thoracic region near the thymus. If this procedure is used, try to use an object with a defined edge (e.g., pencil, ruler) so as to quickly perform the procedure without causing extensive tissue damage. Dissect the animal as usual.
2. Remove the thymus quickly. Roll thymi on a piece of sterile gauze to remove associated fat, connective tissue, and RBC. Do not use RBC lysing agents on thymocytes as they are susceptible to damage.
3. Place thymi into a small Petri dish containing 1–2 mL of media and gently tease the thymus apart with needles or sharp forceps. Add 3–4 mL of cold media and pipet up and down several times to gently break up any cell clumps.

4. Pass cells through a small piece of 100 μm nylon mesh to remove clumps of tissue.
5. Dilute cell suspension with cold medium and centrifuge (250g, 10 min, 4°C). It is important to keep cells cold throughout staining.
6 Resuspend cell pellets with 1–5 mL medium. Count cells and dilute suspension to 10×10^6/mL.
7. For normal, 2–4-mo-old mice, $100–200 \times 10^6$ thymocytes are usually recovered from one thymus.

3.1.2. Lymph Node Preparation

1. Remove lymph nodes. Pooled lymph nodes usually include axial, inguinal, and popliteal nodes. Lymph nodes found within the peritoneal cavity, such a mesenteric nodes, may have some distinct properties and are often not used in standard pools of lymph nodes. However, such populations can be of interest and can be examined separately.
2. Gently tease cells from the node. Do not strenuously "mash" the cells as this approach results in high percentages of dead cells in the preparation.
3. Pass cell through 100 μm mesh. Dilute the cell suspension with cold medium, centrifuge (250g, 10 min, 4°C) and decant.
4. Resuspend the cell pellet with 5 mL cold medium, count and dilute suspension to 10×10^6/mL. Keep cells cold throughout the preparation procedure.
5. From a pool of 8 lymph nodes (excluding mesenteric nodes), a recovery of $5–20 \times 10^6$ cells can be expected.

3.1.3. Spleen Preparation

1. Remove spleen from sacrificed mouse and place it in a petri dish with small amount of media.
2. Tease cells from spleen.
3. Add ACK lysing reagent (5 mL per 1–2 spleens) for 1 min. Because this organ contains large numbers of RBC, use of this RBC lysing agent is recommended.
4. Add additional cold media (5–10 mL) to dilute the lysing reagent and centrifuge (250g, 10 min, 4°C).
5. Decant and repeat **step 4.** Resuspend the cells. Because RBC lysis often results in clumps, pass splenocytes through small piece of 100 μm nylon mesh prior to FCM.
6. Count and dilute suspension in cold media to 10×10^6/mL. Keep cells cold throughout the preparation procedure.
7. A normal spleen usually yields $50–100 \times 10^6$ cells.

3.2. Staining of Cells for FCM

3.2.1. Procedure for Direct Staining

1. Add 100 μL of cell suspension (10×10^6/mL) to tube or well. This will result in 1×10^6 cells/vessel. Add FCM buffer to fill the vessel. Keep the cells at 4°C.

2. Centrifuge in standard table top centrifuge at 4°C. For staining in plates, centrifuge for 1–2 min at 300*g*. For tubes, centrifuge 5–10 min at 250*g*.

3. Decant. Resuspend cells in FCM buffer, centrifuge as **step 2**, and decant.

4. Add 5 µL 2.4G2 (anti-FcR antibody). This antibody should have been previously titered (*see* **Note 2**).

5. Without washing, add 10 µL of directly labeled (FITC, PE, Biotin, Red 670, etc) antibodies. If the working concentration of antibodies is maintained at 5X, 5 different antibodies can be added simultaneously. If less antibody is added, q.s. to the final volume with FCM buffer. As discussed in **Notes 2** and **3** using appropriately titered antibodies is essential to the generation of clear flow cytometry data.

6. Carefully mix the cells and antibodies. This can be done by raking the test tube against the side of a bumpy surface, such as a test tube rack. When staining in wells, a multichannel pipetman can be used to pipet and mix the suspension several times. Be careful not to overflow and mix the contents of the wells when staining in microtiter plates. This mixing step is important. If cells are not thoroughly mixed with antibodies, artificial subpopulations of cells will be observed upon analysis with the cytometer.

7. Cover vessel with light shielding material (e.g., aluminum foil) and place cells in 4°C refrigeration for 30–40 min.

8. Wash cells 3 times with FCM buffer. Washing is important because unbound biotinylated antibodies will act as a sink when fluorochrome-tagged avidin is subsequently added, thus reducing staining efficiency. For staining in tubes, add 3 mL for each wash. When staining in wells, add 200 µL of FCM buffer to the wells for each wash. Decant after last centrifuge.

9. If a biotin labeled antibodies was used, add 10 µL of avidin conjugate (5X) and 40 µL of FCM buffer and mix. If an avidin-conjugate is not required, progress to **step 12**.

10. Cover and place in 4°C refrigerator 10 min. Do not leave in longer than 10 min as the cells can aggregate.

11. Wash and centrifuge cells as in **step 2.**

12. Transfer cells to 12 × 75 plastic tube. Add additional FCM buffer so the final volume is between 400–500 µL. Cover tubes with aluminum foil and store at 4°C until you are ready to analyze them on the FACScan (*see* **Note 7**).

3.2.2. Procedure for Indirect Staining: Single and Multicolor Staining

1. Perform **steps 1–3** from **Subheading 3.1.2.**

2. If the secondary antibody binds to 2.4G2, do not add 2.4G2. If this is not a problem, add 5 µL of 2.4G2 as in **Subheading 3.2.1.**

3. Add the primary antibody. The antibody can be in the form of a B cell hybridoma supernatant or purified antibody. However, it should have been titered prior to use.

4. Mix well and place in a 4°C refrigerator for 30–40 min.

5. Wash the cells 3 times with FCM buffer. It is important to wash out residual primary antibody before adding the secondary antibody as any residual unbound

antibody can serve as a sink for the secondary antibody and reduce the intensity of staining.

6. Add 10 µL of the labeled secondary antibody.
7. Mix well. Cover with foil and place in 4°C refrigerator for 30–40 min.
8. Wash 3× as described in **Subheading 3.2.1., step 8**.
   Note: If single-color analysis is being performed, you are now done and can proceed to **Subheading 3.2.1., step 12** above.
9. If multicolor-analysis is to be performed subsequent to indirect staining, add additional unlabeled primary antibody and place in 4°C refrigerator for 10–15 min (to block unbound binding sites, **Fig. 1**).
10. DO NOT WASH! Add directly labeled antibodies. Mix the mixture carefully, cover with foil, and place in 4°C refrigerator for 30–40 min.
11. Wash cells 3× and transfer to fresh Falcon tubes as described above in **Subheading 3.2.1, step 12** in a volume of 400–500 µL.

3.3. Flow Cytometric Analysis: General

The following instructions will assume some basic knowledge of the flow cytometer being used. The proper set up of the cytometer is critical to the generation of interpretable data and it is emphasized that investigators should take time in preparing controls and setting up the instrument.

3.3.1. Initial Cytometer and Computer Setup

1. Start up the flow cytometer as described in the instruction manual. (Make sure the reservoir is full and waste is empty) and allow the machine to warm up.
2. Launch the acquisition program. (For the FACScan, this is the CELLQuest program.)
3. For the purpose of this description, we will assume three-color analysis. Therefore, call up histogram panels showing:
   a. Two-color plots of (FSC vs SSC), (FL1 vs FL2), (FL1 vs FL3), and (FL2 vs FL3) and
   b. Single-color histograms of FL1, FL2 and FL3.
4. As per usual procedure, set up information regarding data storage and connect to the cytometer.
5. Display instrument control panels, i.e., the "detector/amps" and "compensation" windows.

3.3.2. Parameter Setting

1. Adjust parameter setting so cells can be viewed on the computer screen. The optimal settings will vary with the particular cytometer, labeled antibodies being used, and cell population being examined. Guideline settings for analysis of cultured or ex vivo murine T cells are provided in **Table 1**. These setting will allow visualization of most murine T-cell populations. FSC and SSC profiles for lymphocytes are best visualized on linear settings using E00. However, T cell

Table 1
Guidelines Settings for Analysis of Murine Thymocytes/T Cells

Detector/amp setting

Parameter	Voltage	Amp	Mode
FSC	E00	1.2–1.6	Linear
SSC	31–400	1–3	Linear
FL1 (FITC)	500–600	NA	Log
FL2 (PE)	500–550	NA	Log
FL3 (Red670/QR)	600–700	NA	Log

Compensation

Parameter	Setting (X)
FL1- (X)% FL2	0.4–0.6
FL2- (X)% FL1	28–40
FL2- (X)% FL3	2–6
FL3- (X)% FL2	10–26

lines are often significantly larger than normal T cells and require a FSC setting of E-1. Moreover, as described in **Subheading 3.3.4.**, each experiment requires adjustment of parameter settings using proper control populations, including unstained cells and cells stained separately with single fluorochrome labeled antibodies.

3.3.3. FSC and SSC Gating
to Exclude Dead Cells, RBC, and Debris (Live Gating)

A live cell gate can be applied to exclude dead cells, RBC, and debris (demonstrated in **Fig. 2**).

1. While in setup mode, begin to acquire data on unstained cells, observing data in the FSC vs SSC panel.
2. Adjust the voltage and amplifier gain for FSC and SSC, so the major population of cells appears in the middle of FSC vs SSC panel.
3. Adjust FSC threshold to approx 52 to exclude cell debris.
4. In the FSC vs SSC histogram, draw a region around the cells on which you wish to collect data. This should be called "R1" (similar to the gate **Fig. 2G, I**).
5. Set the desired gate for acquisition, collection, and storage.
6. Sometimes, forward and side scatter gating may not adequately exclude dead or dying cells. In this case, cells can be stained with dyes to help better discriminate live and dead cells (*see* **Note 9**).

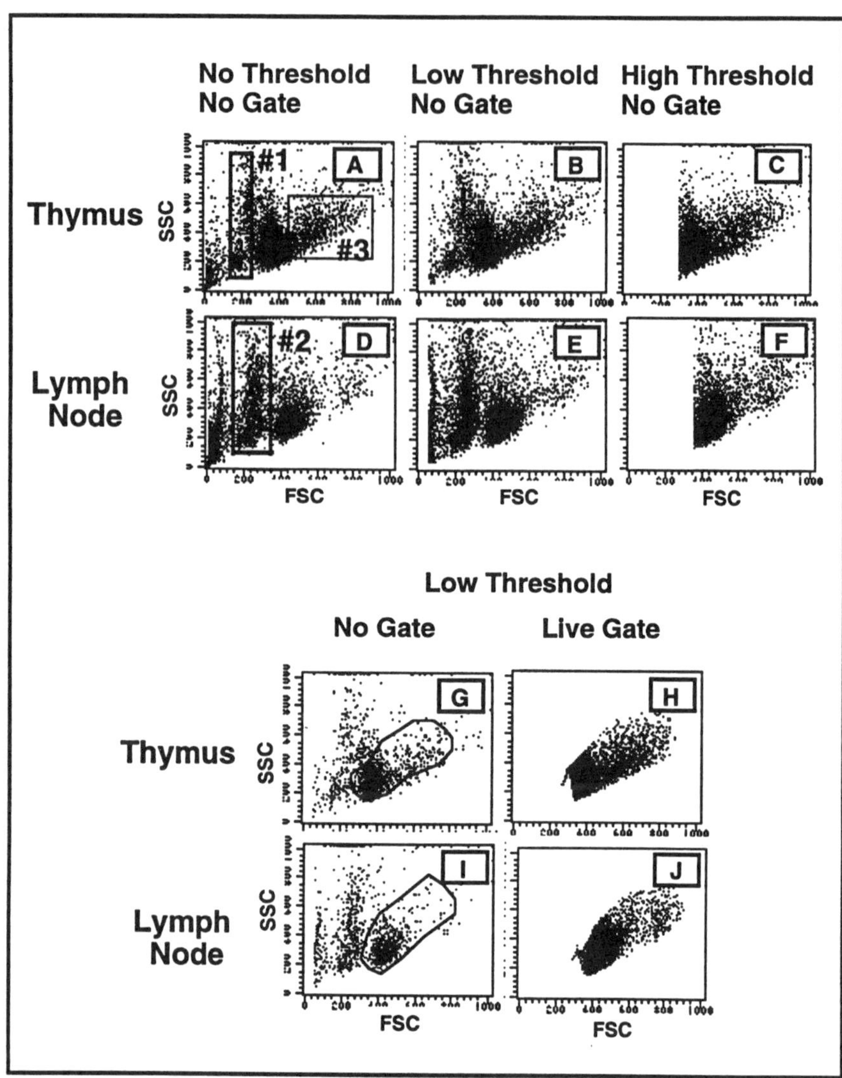

Fig. 2. Collection of live cells. This figure represents different approaches to acquiring and collecting data on live cells. FSC vs SSC is shown for thymocytes and lymph node cells. Panels **A** and **D** show results when neither a threshold nor a gate is applied. **B** and **E** show results when a relatively low FL2 threshold *(52)* is applied to just gate out small material and debris. **C** and **F** show results when a high threshold is applied (320–364) in order to remove debris and dying cells from data viewing and collection. Dead and dying cells fall into box #1 (thymus) and #2 (lymph node cells) and data on these cells is not viewed using the high threshold used in **C** and **F**. Panels **G–J** show results when a low threshold is applied and a gate is applied during data analysis (subsequent to data collection **(G,I)** or during data acquisition **(H,J)**. Box #3 shown in Panel **A** represents the region in which immature CD4⁻CD8⁻ thymocytes are located.

3.3.4. Optimize Settings for Fluorescence Parameters

1. In "Set up" mode, run unstained cells.
2. Adjust the detector/amp for each fluorescence parameter so that the peak is close to the *y*-axis but is still clearly visible.
3. Run each tube stained with individual antibodies to make sure the FL1, FL2, and FL3 are on scale.

3.3.5. Compensation

For multicolor experiments, correct compensation is critical (*see* **Note 10**). **Fig. 3** is provided as an example to demonstrate correct and incorrect compenstation.

1. Still in set up mode, run unstained cells. Note the fluorescence intensity for each of the fluorescence parameters.
2. Run cells that have been stained with FITC alone. A positive and negative peak should be observed. For example, when staining peripheral T cells with anti-CD3-FITC, B cell /macrophages will be negative and T cells will be positive.
3. Look at the two parameter histogram of FL1 vs FL2. While FL2 should be negative (no PE-labeled antibody was added), unless compensation is applied, $FL1^+FL2^+$ cells (double positive) are generally observed (**Fig. 3C, E**). Adjust the FL2-FL1 compensation until FL2 signal is no longer observed (**Fig. 3A**). The single color histogram of FL2 and FL3 with cells stained with FL1 alone, should be comparable to that of unstained cells (**Fig. 3B**).
4. Run cells that have been stained with PE-labeled antibody alone. Similarly adjust compensation in FL1-FL2 so no signal is observed in FL1 channel. Also adjust the FL3-FL2 compensation so that no signal is observed in the FL3 channel. Sometimes it is not possible to "compensate" the signal in FL1 and FL2. This finding is often because of autofluorescence, a situation discussed in **Note 10.**
5. Run cells that have been stained with FL3 alone. Adjust FL2-FL3 so that no signal is observed in the FL2 channel. Because the spectral overlap between FL1 and FL3 is generally negligible, an option for adjusting this compensation is not provided. If the compensation required to adjust FL2-% FL3 becomes very large (or impossible), it is likely caused by the unstable nature of the fluorochromes used to detect signals in the FL3 channel (*see* **Note 12**).

3.3.6. Data Collection

1. With the flow cytometer properly set up, experimental samples can now be collected. Place tube in the sampling probe and collect data. The number of events collected will vary with the purpose of the experiment *see* **Note 13**).

3.4. Flow Cytometic Analysis: Specific Applications

3.4.1. CD4 vs CD8 Subset Analysis of Thymocytes (*Fig. 4*)

1. Stain thymocytes as shown below.

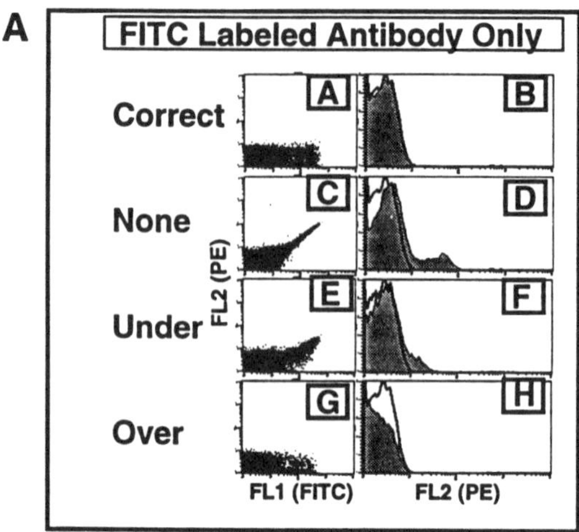

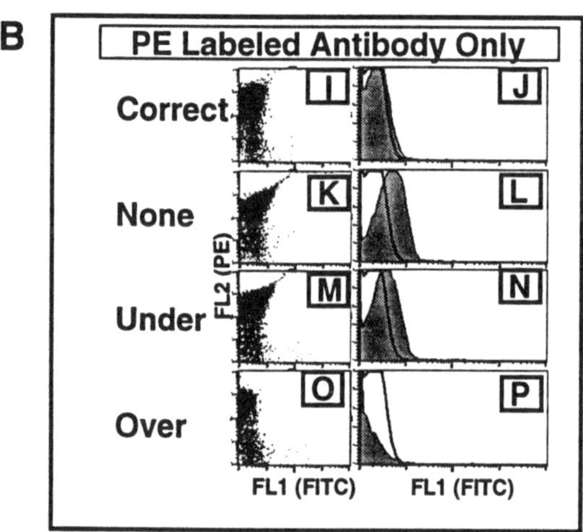

Fig. 3. Compensation. Thymocytes were stained with FITC and PE labeled antibodies. Top panel shows cells stained with FITC labeled antibodies alone and the lower panel represents cells stained with PE-labeled antibody alone. For the single parameter histograms in the top panel, shaded areas represents FL2 signal from FITC labeled cells and the solid line represent FL2 signal from cells that were unstained. For the single parameter histograms in the lower panel, shaded areas represents FL1 signal from PE labeled cells and the solid line represent FL1 signal from cells that were unstained. If the signal is not adequately compensated in FL2-%FL1, **(C–F)** or FL1-%FL2 **(K–N)** cells will appear positive for both FITC and PE even though only FITC or PE labeled antibody was added. Conversely, over compensation results in the inappropriate loss of signal, below that of unstained cells **(G,H,O,P)**.

Tube	Purpose	2.4G2	FITC Ab	PE-Ab	QR-Ab
1	Compensation	+	None	None	None
2		+	Anti-CD3	None	None
3		+	None	Anti-CD8	None
4		+	None	None	Anti-CD4
5	Experimental	+	Control	Control	Control
6		+	Control	Anti-CD8	Anti-CD4
7		+	Anti-CD3	Anti-CD8	Anti-CD4

2. In set up mode, run unstained thymocytes.
3. Adjust settings as in **Table 1**.
4. Draw an FSC vs SSC gate (R1) as shown in **Fig. 2.** The larger cells contain many of the precursor CD4⁻CD8⁻ thymocytes (**Fig. 2A, Box #2**).
5. Under acquire, set the collection gate to collect 10–15,000 event in R1.
6. Perform compensation as described above, using the thymocyte stained separately with each individual antibody, i.e., tubes 1–4.
7. If the compensation has been performed correctly, examination of FL2 vs FL3 on tube 7 (CD8 vs CD4), should give you a picture resembling a bird. (*see* **Fig. 4**).
8. Change to acquistion mode and acquire data from tubes 5–7.
9. The acquisition phase of the experiment is now complete.
10. Open up data analysis program.
11. Select a dual parameter histogram of FL2 vs FL3
12. Display the file for tube 7 (CD3 vs CD8 vs CD4).
13. Draw regions as shown in **Fig. 4**.

   R1= CD4⁻CD8⁺, R2 = CD4⁺CD8, R3 = CD4⁻CD8⁺, R4 = CD4⁺CD8⁻.

14. Draw 4 histograms of FL1 (CD3), but use a different region/gate for each histogram. As shown in **Fig. 4**, each histogram shows the intensity of TCR staining on that thymocyte subpopulation. Compare staining with CD3 (filled peaks) to that observed with the isotype control (open peaks) (**Fig. 4**). The comparison of staining in tube 6 and 7 allows one to compare control and experimental staining on subpopulations of thymocytes defined by expression of CD4 and CD8.

3.4.2. Examination of Early Thymocyte Subsets (*Fig. 5*)

1. Stain thymocytes as shown below:

Tube	Purpose	2.4G2	FITC-Ab	PE Ab	Red670-Ab
1	Set up	+	None	None	None
2		+	Anti-CD4	None	None
3		+	None	Anti-CD8	None
4		+	None	None	Anti-CD4, CD8, CD3,B220, GR1,MAC-1
5	Experimental	+	None	None	None

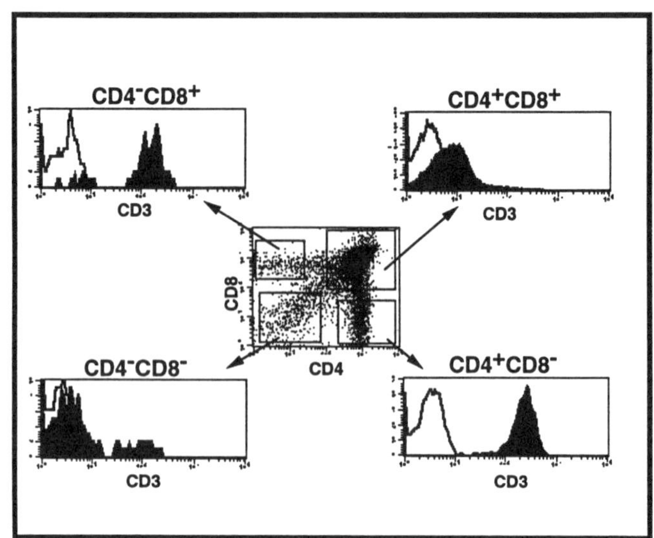

Fig. 4. Differential gating to reveal expression of determinants on subpopulations of T cells. Thymocytes were stained with anti-CD3-FITC or control-FITC. The cells were also stained with anti-CD8-PE and anti-CD4-Red670. Expression of CD3 on defined population of thymocytes was examined by software gating (subsequent to data acquisition) on CD4⁻CD8⁻, CD4⁺CD8⁺, CD4⁺CD8⁻, and CD4⁻CD8⁺ thymocytes. Shaded areas show staining with anti-CD3 and solid lines depict negative control staining on the same subpopulation of thymocytes.

| 6 | + | None | None | Anti-CD4,CD8, CD3,B220, GR1,MAC-1 |
| 7 | + | Anti-CD44 | Anti-CD25 | Anti-CD4,CD8, CD3,B220, GR1,MAC-1 |

2. Set up the cytometer and compensation settings with control tubes as described in **Subheading 3.4.1.**
3. Use a large FSC gate as immature thymocytes are large (**Fig. 2**)
4. Using tube 4 above, examine the FL3 histogram. Define a gate (R2) that defines cells negative for Red670 antibodies (anti-CD4,CD8,CD3,B220,GR1,MAC-1). Under data acquisition, collect 3–5000 cells in the R2 gate. The investigator can now either save all data (which will require a lot of memory) or just data on cells in the R2 gate. Either way, this gating/acquisition approach will allow for the generation of histograms showing significant numbers of events representing relative rare CD4⁻CD8⁻ thymocytes (*see* **Note 13**).
5. Change to acquisition mode and collect data from tubes 5–7.
6. Data acquisition is now complete.

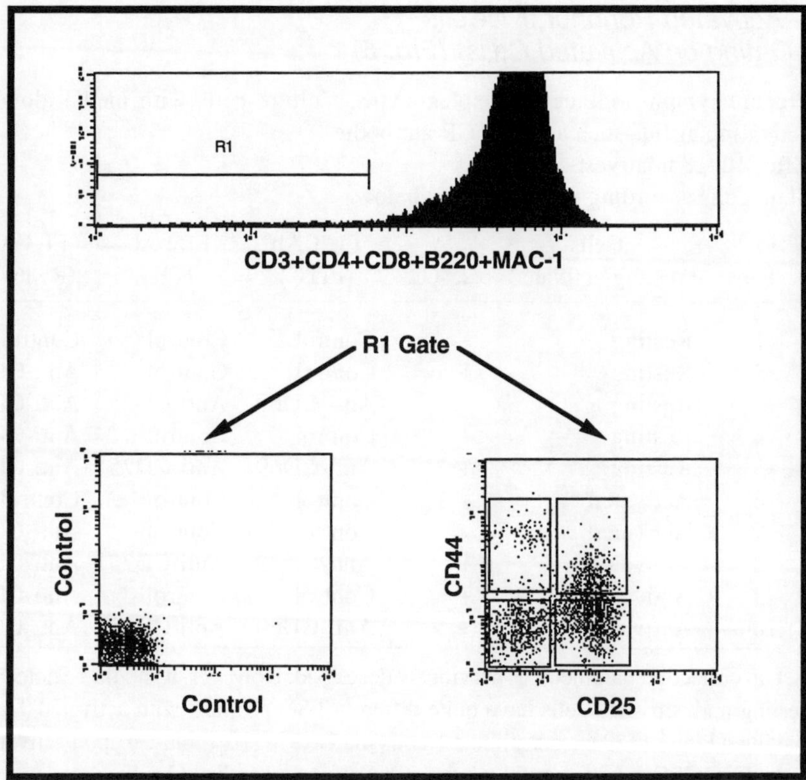

Fig. 5. FCM analysis of rare subpopulations without physical enrichment. Thymocytes were stained with either control FITC- and control PE- labeled antibodies or anti-CD44-FITC and anti-CD25-PE. Cells were also stained with a cocktail of biotin-labeled antibodies directed against CD3, CD4, CD8, B220, and MAC-1. Avidin Red670 was subsequently added to reveal binding of the biotin-labeled antibodies. Data acquisition was set up so as to acquire 3000 events in the R1 gate (top histogram). For data analysis, the same R1 gate was applied and dual color histograms are shown. The pattern of expression of CD44 and CD25 is typical of early CD4$^-$CD8$^-$ thymocytes.

7. To analyze data, open up data analysis program
8. On the palette, select a histogram of FL3.
9. Display the file for tube 6, and draw region on the FL3-negative cells as illustrated in **Fig. 5**. The analysis gate should be similar to that used for acquisition (R2 above). This gating step will not be necessary if only data on FL3-negative cells was saved
10. Select a dot plot of FL1 vs FL2 showing those cells that fall in the R1 gate. Compare this dot plot to that from tube 7. CD25 and CD44 expression on the CD4$^-$CD8$^-$ cells that fall in R1 should resemble the populations in **Fig. 5**.

3.4.3. Activated Peripheral T Cells
(Live Gating on Activated Cells) (**Fig. 6**)

1. Prepare lymph node cells or splenocytes. Culture cells with media alone or activating agents such as anti-TCR antibodies.
2. After 12–18 h harvest cells.
3. Stain cells according to the protocol below.

Tube	Cells resting/activated	2.4G2	FL 1 Ab (FITC)	FL2 Ab (PE)	FL3 Ab (Red670)
1	Resting	+	Control	Control	Control
2	Resting	+	Control	Control	Anti-CD4
3	Resting	+	Anti-CD69	Anti-CD25	Anti-CD4
4	Resting	+	Control	Control	Anti-CD8
5	Resting	+	Anti-CD69	Anti-CD25	Anti-CD8
6	Activated	+	Control	Control	Control
7	Activated	+	Control	Control	Anti-CD4
8	Activated	+	Anti-CD69	Anti-CD25	Anti-CD4
9	Activated	+	Control	Control	Anti-CD8
10	Activated	+	Anti-CD69	Anti-CD25	Anti-CD8

4. Set up collection parameter as previously described. However, it should be noted that resting and activated cells have quite different FSC profiles, with activated T cells having a larger FSC intensity since T cells increase in size ("blast") upon activation. Set a FSC/SSC gate that will include both resting and activated cells.
5. Under data acquisition, collect data on 5000–10,000 cells in the R1 gate for all tubes.
6. Data acquisition is now complete.
7. To analyze data, open up data analysis program.
8. On the palette, select a dual parameter histogram of control FL1 vs CD4 (QR) for tube 2. Draw an analysis gate (R1) of CD4-positive cells (**Fig. 6**).
9. Choose a single parameter histogram and display CD69 (FL1 (tube 3) on resting (unactivated) CD4$^+$ cells (R1).
10. Overlay with data from tube 8 (representing activated T cells stained with CD69 in FL1). Use the same CD4+ (R1) gate. Levels of CD4 and CD8 may change slightly after activation but gates can be drawn to include both resting and activated CD4 or CD8 cells.
11. Extend this analysis to CD8 cells, drawing a new gate to include CD8 cells (R3). A similar approach can be used to examined changes in CD25 expression. Together, this approach allows for the comparison of activation antigens on activated and resting T-cell subpopulations.

3.4.4. Analysis of Peripheral Blood Lymphocytes

1. Heparinized mouse blood is obtained by tail-bleeding a mouse into a tube containing 10 µL of heparin (3000 U/mL).

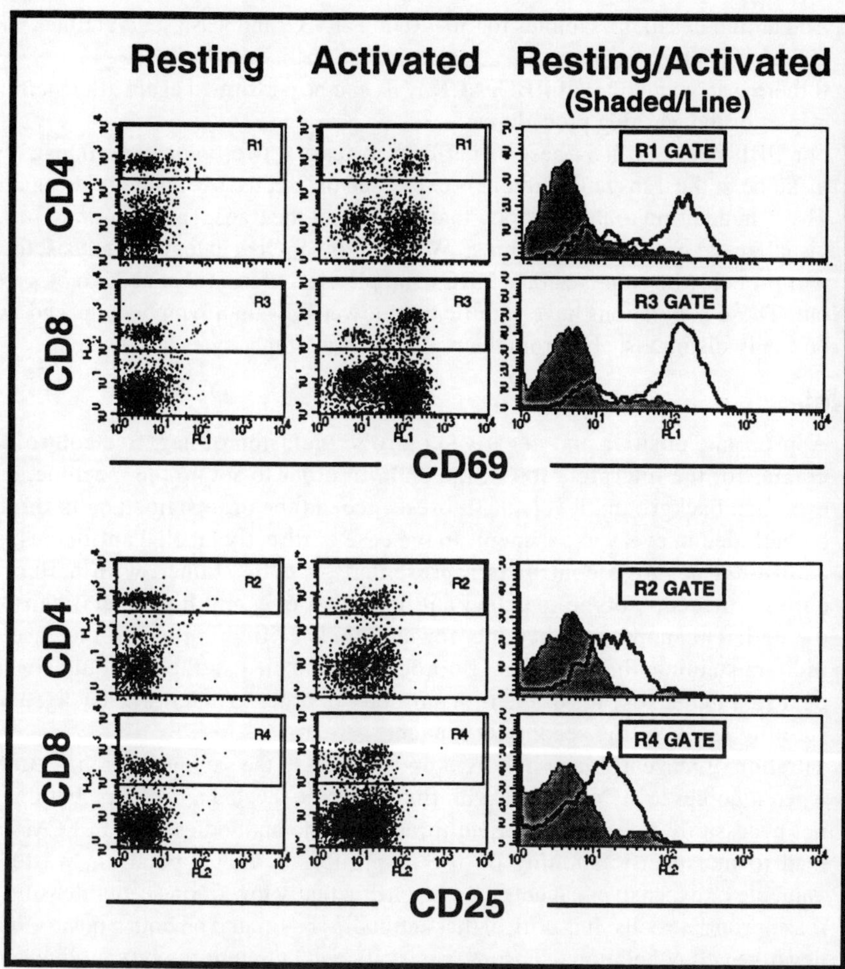

Fig. 6. Application of FCM to assessment of T cell activation. Splenocytes were cultured for 12 h in the presence of media alone or anti-CD3. Cells were harvested and stained with control antibodies or anti-CD69-FITC and anti-CD25-PE. Both CD69 and CD25 levels increase upon T cell activation. Cells were subsequently stained with anti-CD4 Red670 or anti-CD8 Red670. Gates R1, R2, R3 or R4 were applied to examine cell surface expression of CD69 or CD25 on CD4-positive or CD8-positive cells. For single color histograms, shaded areas represent staining on unactivated cells and solid lines represent staining on activated cells.

2. Place 10–25 µL of blood into each of two wells (one for control and one for experimental) in a 96-well U-bottom plate.
3. Add 200 µL of ACK lysing buffer/well for 2 min.
4. After this time, the samples are centrifuged, media flicked off, then washed with 200 µL of FCM buffer, and centrifuged again.

5. Add antibodies to the samples for 30–40 min at 4°C, and wash several times with 200 µL of buffer.
6. If there is large number of RBC, ACK lysis can be performed again after staining as part of the washing procedures.
7. For PBL analysis, it is best to perform at least a two-color experiment. For instance, if the transgenic protein is expressed on T cells, use an antibody against Thy-1 in addition to the antibody that will detect the transgenic protein to better visualize the population of interest. When setting up live gates for analysis, there will probably be some residual RBCs and platelets present that need to be gated out. These populations have significantly lower FSC than lymphocytes and will be easily distinguishable from the region where lymphocytes are located.

4. Notes

1. Appropriate positive and negative controls: Inclusion of negative controls is crucial for the interpretation of the data. In order to set up the machine, and establish background levels of fluorescence, a tube of unstained cells should be included in every experiment. In the case of directly labeled antibodies, an additional negative control is represented by cells stained with a fluoro-chrome-tagged, isotype-matched antibody that does not bind specifically to the cell. This approach accounts for any nonspecific binding. In the case of indirect staining, the secondary-fluorochrome-labeled antibody should always be tested in the absence of the first antibody in order to determine background staining levels of the secondary reagent.
2. Titration of reagent: Many investigators fall prey to the saying "More is better!" when it comes to staining cells with fluorochrome labeled antibodies, but this is not necessarily true. Inappropriate titration of the antibodies used in FCM can lead to nonspecific staining on the inappropriate cell population, waste of valuable or expensive reagents, or even artifactually low fluorescent intensity on the appropriate cells. It is critical that antibodies be titrated on both a positive and negative cell population to ensure specificity and optimum fluorescent intensity. Often investigators will use antibodies at concentrations recommended by the manufacturer. The appropriateness of that concentration should always be veri-fied by the investigator in their particular situation by titration on positive and negative cells. Optimal concentrations will lead to a fluorescence intensity simi-lar to unstained cells for negative cells and high intensity on positive cells. As mentioned in **Note 3**, stocks of antibodies can be maintained at 5× such that mul-tiple antibodies may be added at the same time without overdiluting the optimal concentration for each antibody. For example, if optimum staining is observed at 1:1000, the stock solution is maintained at 1:200 and 10 µL is added to 1×10^6 cells along with 40 µL of other antibodies or FACS buffer.
3. Antibody working dilutions: It is useful to maintaining a working stock of antibodies at a concentration five times higher than their optimally titered concentration. This approach allows for the addition of multiple antibodies if the final volume is approx 50 µL.

4. FcR block: Whereas the reaction of cells with labeled antibodies can reveal the cell surface expression of molecules to which those antibodies are directed, Fc regions on antibodies can also react with cells (B cells and macrophages) bearing Fc receptors (FcR). Hence a cell may stain positively with an antibody even though it does not express the antigen to which the antibody is directed. The addition of an unlabeled antibody against the murine FcR (FcRII/III) provides one mechanism to prevent this problem when staining murine lymphocytes. Therefore, addition of anti-FcR antibody (2.4G2) is added to cells first and followed by subsequent staining steps. When using a secondary antibody specific for rat Ig, cells expressing FcR will be detected if 2.4G2 was used to block (2.4G2 is rat IgG2b antibody). In this circumstance it is advisable to either avoid an initial FcR block or to choose an isotype specific labeled anti-IgG as a secondary antibody that does not detect 2.4G2.

5. Staining buffer: It is important to wash the cells in the FCM buffer as the buffer contains sodium azide that blocks the metabolic activity of the cells and will inhibit the down modulation of surface determinants during reaction with antibody. It is also important to keep the cells at 4°C during the procedure for the same reason. Although 1% BSA is used by some investigators, 0.1% BSA is usually sufficient. Use of FCS should be avoided because it contains biotin, which can compete for binding to fluorochrome-tagged avidin.

6. Reaction vessel: Cells are typically stained in tubes for FCM experiments. Alternatively, for large experiments or when cell number is limiting, cells can be stained in wells of round bottom microtiter plates. Procedures performed in microtiter plates can be more rapid and use less reagents. However, antibodies must be appropriately titered (*see* **Note 2**). Some investigators think the microtiter plate method does not allow for adequate wash volumes. However, this is generally not a significant problem. Another advantage is that there is less cell loss during the staining and washing procedures which becomes an important consideration when cell numbers are limiting (for example, RAG$^{-/-}$ and SCID mice have very small thymi). Individual scientists should compare the two approaches themselves. The procedure discussed in this article has been optimized for staining 1×10^6 cells per reaction. However, fewer cells can also be stained. When $>2 \times 10^6$ cells are to be stained, it may be advantageous to perform staining in tubes; amounts of antibodies will also have to be adjusted.

7. Time to analysis: Although not the optimal approach, freshly isolated murine T cells can be stained and held over night at 4°C for analysis the next morning without paraformaldehyde fixation. If samples will not be analyzed within 18 h of staining (for fresh cells) or 4 h (for activated cells), samples should be fixed *(5)*. However, fixing the cells results in alteration of cell size, affecting the ability to discriminate between live and dead cells, and may make live gating difficult.

8. Live gating: Forward and side scatter parameters can be used to help exclude dead cells, RBC, and debris from data collection and analysis. This live gating can be approached by two diffferent methods. On one hand, the threshold value for FSC can be adjusted to exclude debris and most of the dying cells. The diffi-

culty with this approach is that cells falling below this value will not be viewed. The inability to evaluate such data could lead to the loss of valuable and unexpected information. For example, a high threshold setting as shown in **Fig. 2C** and **F** would exclude most of the dying cells (**Fig. 2A,D, box #1,2**). Large amounts of cell death or apoptosis can be an important parameter of which the investigator should be aware. Another useful approach, is to set the threshold at relatively low level (FSC 52) to just exclude cell debris (**Fig. 2G–J**). A live cell gate can then be applied as shown (**Fig. 2G–J**). This approach allows the investigator to decide to either collect and store all data (**Fig. 2G,I**) or view all data during acquisition and only store the data in the live gate (**Fig. 2H,J**). When data on live cells is to be collected, set gates similar to the one shown in **Fig. 2G** and **I** for either thymocytes or peripheral T cells. For analysis of immature thymocytes and activated T cells, it is important not to limit the gate too stringently since both CD4$^-$CD8$^-$ immature thymocytes (**Fig. 2A, box #3**) and activated T cells (not shown) are larger than most thymocytes (CD4$^+$ and/or CD8$^+$) and resting T cells. FSC and SSC characteristics will differ for macrophage and other nonlymphoid cells. Therefore such cells may fall outside of this lymphocyte gate.

9. Elimination of dead cells by propidium iodide gating: If fresh cell preparations are prepared carefully, there are relatively few dying or dead cells. These can easily be gated out when setting the live gate because they are usually smaller in the FSC profile (*see* **Figs. 2A, box #1** and **2D, box #2**). The presence of a significant number of dead cells from freshly isolated tissues may indicate a problem in preparation. However, in some cases in which the cells have been cultured in vitro, there may be dramatically more dead cells and it may be desirable to ensure that these cells are not collected for analysis (**Fig. 2D,E** contains relatively large numbers of dying cells). One option is to pass cells over cell separation media (e.g., Ficoll or Percoll) in order to remove dead cells prior to staining. This may not be possible with limiting numbers of cells. Alternatively, propidium iodide (PI) staining can be performed. In dead and dying cells, membrane permeability allows PI to reach the nucleus and bind the DNA, whereas this does not occur in live cells with intact membranes. Excitation at 488 nm causes PI to fluoresce in FL3. Ten microliters of PI (100 µg/mL) is added to the sample tube (containing 400–500 µL of cell suspension) prior to collection and cells staining very brightly in FL3 are excluded from collection by gating for the PI-negative population. The problem with this approach is that it can only be performed with a 1- or 2-color experiment since the FL3 is required to gate out the dead cells. Also, in setting up the machine, a single tube with PI must be used for setting the compensation in FL3 to avoid overlap between FL2 and FL3.

10. Compensation controls: Before getting started, it is necessary to consider which fluorochromes will be used in the experimental staining. This issue is important so that the control or "compensation" populations will be appropriately stained and available for the correct set up of the cytometer. Because the emission spectrum of some fluorochromes overlap (FL1 and FL2, FL2 and FL3), it is critical to

electronically "subtract" or compensate the overlapping portion of the signal. This prevents the appearance of artifactual "double positive" populations. In order to perform electronic compensation, one must have prepared cells that are stained singly for each of the fluorochromes used in the experiment. For example, if cells are to be stained and analyzed for the simultaneous expression of CD3 (FITC, FL1), CD8 (PE, FL2), and CD4 (FL3, Red 670), compensation controls would consist of cells stained with

a. Nothing,
b. Anti-CD3-FITC alone,
c. Anti-CD8-PE alone, and
d. Anti-CD4-Red670 alone.

If the protocol calls for several different antibody specificities coupled to a given fluorochrome, it may be necessary to set up several different compensation tubes with the different antibodies. For example, if both anti-Thy1.2- FITC and anti-CD3-FITC are to be used in the experiment and if their fluorescent intensity are significantly different, then different amounts of compensation can be required. Therefore, it is helpful to set up two FITC compensation tubes (i.e., one with anti-Thy1.2 FITC and one with anti-CD3-FITC). Data on experimental groups stained with anti-Thy1.2 FITC (high fluorescence intensity) can be collected with one compensation value. The compensation can then be changed and data on experimental groups stained with anti-CD3-FITC (moderate fluorescence intensity) can be collected. Finally, if an antigen is expressed on a rare population of cells, it is difficult to use antibody staining for this antigen for compensation. For example, if CD25 expression by thymocytes is to be experimentally examined with anti-CD25-PE, anti-CD25-PE would not be a good compensation conrol as the thymus contains few ($\leq$1%) $CD25^+$ cells. In this case, thymocytes stained with anti-CD8-PE could provide a reasonable PE compensation control. The staining of cells for compensation is performed just as described for single color experimental staining (**Subheading 3.2.1.**)

11. Autofluorescence: Dead or dying cells will often display autofluorescence that results in signal in the FL1 and FL2 channels that cannot be compensated. For example, activated T cells often display autofluorescence. This fluorescence signal cannot be compensated and will need to be evaluated in the context of the experimental staining. This is why unstained controls are important.

12. Tandem conjugates: Many of the fluorochromes used for FL3 staining are tandem conjugates. For example, "Red670" and "quantum red" are tandem conjugates of PE and Cy5. These reagent can be unstable when exposed to light (*6*). This instability results in the generation of the PE signal alone. The hallmark of this problem is the inability to compensate and remove FL2 signals when cells are stained with a FL3-fluorochrome alone. (*see* **Note10**).

13. Collection and storage of data: For large populations, generally collection of 10,000 events is sufficient. If small populations of cells are the focus of the experiment, it is important to take into account the number of cells that

need to be analyzed to make the data reliable. Therefore, larger numbers of events (25,000–100,000) should be collected. Alternatively, a useful trick is to instruct the machine to collect a specific number of events of the population of interest by counting events within a gate drawn around those cells. In this manner, all events will be collected until the desired population reaches a number that facilitates analysis.

14. Intracellular staining: Although this chapter has concentrated on cell surface markers, it is also possible to examine expression of some intracellular proteins by flow cytometry. In this case cells are generally fixed lightly, permeabilized by gentle detergents, and stained with labeled antibodies that have been properly titrated (*see* **ref.** *7* for details).

References

1. Otten, G., Yokoyama, W., and Holmes, K. (1994) Immunofluorescence and cell sorting in *Current Protocols in Immunology* (Coligan, J. E., Kruisbeek, A. M., Margulies, D. H., Shevach, E. M., and Strober,W., eds.), John Wiley and Sons, Inc., New York.

2. Shapiro, H. M. (1988) *Practical Flow Cytometry*, 2nd ed. Wiley-Liss, New York , Section 5.4..

3. Darzynkiewicz, Z., Robinson, J. P., and Crissman, H. A., eds. *Flow Cytometry*, 2nd ed. Academic, San Diego, CA.

4. Godfrey, D. I., Kennedy, J., Suda, T., and Zlotnik, A. (1993) A developmental pathway involving four phenotypically and functionally distinct subsets of CD3-CD4-CD8- triple-negative adult mouse thymocytes defined by CD44 and CD25 expression. *J. Immunol.* **150,** 4244–4252.

5. Lanier, L. L. and Warner, N. L. (1981) Paraformaldehyde fixation of hematopoietic cells for quantative flow cytometry (FACS) analysis. *J. Immunol. Methods* **47,** 25–30.

6. Steward, C. C. and Steward, S. J. (1994) Cell preparation for the identification of leukocytes, in *Flow Cytometry*, 2nd ed. *Academic Press Inc.*, (Darzynkiewicz, Z., Robinson, J. P., and Crissman, H. A., eds.), San Diego, CA.

7. Levelt, C. N., Ehrfeld, A., and Eichmann, K. (1993) Regulation of thymocyte development through CD3. I. Timepoint of ligation of CD3ε determines clonal deletion of induction of developmental program. *J. Exp. Med.* **177,** 707–716.

14

Production and Characterization
of Immature Murine T-Lymphoma Cell Lines

Ellen R. Richie and Dawn A. Walker

1. Introduction

Intrathymic T-cell differentiation proceeds through a series of discrete stages in which developmental changes in gene expression modify cell surface phenotype and functional potential (reviewed in *1–3*). Thymocyte progenitors in the $CD4^-8^-$ double negative (DN) compartment give rise to the predominant $CD4^+8^+$ double positive (DP) subset which is subjected to positive and negative selection pressures within the cortical microenvironment. The majority of DP thymocytes undergo apoptosis as a result of negative selection or failure to receive a positive selecting signal. Only a minority of DP cells that express T-cell receptors (TCRs) with appropriate affinity/avidity for self-peptide/ major histocompatibility complex (MHC) complexes undergo positive selection. Positively selected DP thymocytes down-regulate CD4 or CD8 coreceptors and migrate to the medulla where additional maturation events occur prior to the peripheral emigration of $CD4^+8^-$ and $CD4^-8^+$ single positive (SP) cells. The establishment of continuously growing SP cell lines has greatly facilitated investigations of surface receptor expression, signal transduction pathways, and cytokine production by mature T cells. In contrast, it has not been feasible to establish long-term cultures of DN or DP thymocytes, a limitation that is likely because of the short half-life of these immature subsets *(1,4)*. As an approach to circumvent this obstacle, thymic lymphomas that correspond to immature thymocyte subsets arrested at an early maturation stage, have been adapted to continuous in vitro culture. This chapter describes a method for establishing and maintaining long-term cell lines of transformed immature T cells derived from primary spontaneous or induced thymic lymphomas.

From: *Methods in Molecular Biology, Vol. 134: T Cell Protocols: Development and Activation*
Edited by: K. P. Kearse © Humana Press Inc., Totowa, NJ

1.1. T-Cell Lymphoma Cell Lines as Models of Immature T-Cell Subsets

There are both advantages and disadvantages to utilizing T-lymphoma lines as representative counterparts of normal immature thymocyte subsets. Perhaps the most obvious benefit is the uniformity afforded by clonally-derived transformed cell lines as opposed to the heterogeneity characteristic of normal polyclonal thymocytes. In addition, in vitro propagation of continuously replicating cell lines facilitates procurement of relatively large numbers of cells for subsequent structural or functional analysis. For example, DN and DP lymphoma lines have been employed to isolate and immunochemically characterize immature CD3/TCR complexes *(5,6)*. In this regard, a DN lymphoma line was used to initially identify and characterize the pre-TCRα (gp33) peptide that associates with TCR-β to form the pre-TCR heterodimer *(7)*.

Lymphoma cell lines also have served as useful models for investigating the functional consequences of activating immature thymocytes by various stimuli. In contrast to functionally and phenotypically heterogeneous normal thymocyte suspensions, cloned lymphoma lines provide a homogeneous source of immature T cells in which studies of the molecular events induced by activation with various stimuli can be evaluated in the absence of contaminating cells that may enhance or interfere with signaling pathways *(8–10)*. In this regard, the CD4⁺8⁺ DPK cell line derived from a spontaneous thymic lymphoma of a TCR transgenic mouse differentiates to express a CD4⁺8⁻ phenotype after activation with cognate peptide/MHC class II expressing accessory cells *(11)*. Subsequent work investigating signaling pathways that impact this process showed that differentiation is blocked in the absence of NF-κB activity and is potentiated by expression of a constitutively activated Ras construct *(12,13)*.

One disadvantage in studying lymphoma cell lines is the possibility that unknown aberrations resulting from the transformed nature of these cells may influence the phenotypic and/or functional parameters under investigation. Therefore, it is important to verify the conclusions obtained with thymic lymphoma cell lines in experiments performed with corresponding normal T-cell subsets. Another disadvantage associated with some, but not all, lymphoma cell lines, is a tendency for phenotypic instability to occur during long-term culture. This may be due, in part, to the ability of a small fraction of primitive progenitors to continue to differentiate even in the absence of exogenously added cytokines or accessory cells *(10,14)*. Finally, the fact that lymphoma cell lines are constantly proliferating may preclude certain types of studies such as analyses of events involved in the activation of G_0 cells. Nevertheless, despite these potential disadvantages, studies from numerous laboratories have shown that immature thymic lymphoma cell lines are valuable models of immature thymocyte subsets.

2. Materials

1. Standard equipment for tissue culture including laminar flow tissue culture cabinet, humidified 37°C, 5% CO_2 incubator.
2. Sterile instruments including forceps, scissors and/or scalpel.
3. Falcon or Costar disposable tissue culture dishes, flasks, pipets—Fisher Scientific (Pittsburgh, PA).
4. Nunc 1.2 mL cryovials-Fisher Scientific (Pittsburgh, PA).
5. Sterile Hank's balanced salt solution (HBSS): 0.14 g of $CaCl_2$, 0.4 g of KCl, 0.06 g of KH_2PO_4, 0.1 g of $MgCl_2{\cdot}6H_2O$, 0.1 g of $MgSO_4{\cdot}7H_2O$, 8.0 g of NaCl, 0.35 g of $NaHCO_3$, 0.06 g of $Na_2HPO_4{\cdot}2H_2O$ and 0.01 g of phenol red per 1 liter of distilled water. The final pH should be 7.2–7.4. HBSS can be purchased as a 10X stock from Gibco-BRL (Grand Island, NY).
6. Fetal calf serum (FCS): FCS is available from several commercial sources. However, each batch must be pretested to determine if it is suitable for supporting optimal cell growth (*see* **Note 4**). The FCS is heat inactivated for 30 min at 56°C and added to the medium to give a final concentration of 10%.
7. Dulbecco's modified Eagle's minimum essential medium (DMEM)-Gibco-BRL. The DMEM is supplemented with 2 mM L-glutamine, 0.1 mM MEM nonessential amino acids, 1 mM sodium pyruvate, 5×10^{-5} M 2β-mercaptoethanol. These reagents are available from Gibco-BRL. Heat-inactivated FCS is added to a final concentration of 10%. The supplemented media containing FCS is referred to as DMEM-10.
8. Freezing media: 90% (v/v) DMEM-10 and 10% dimethyl sulfoxide (DMSO) Sigma (St. Louis, MO).

3. Methods

3.1. Establishment of Lymphoma Cell Lines

Adaptation of primary thymic lymphomas to continuous in vitro culture can be readily accomplished, but requires familiarity with basic tissue culture techniques *(15,16)*, (*see* **Note 1**). A flow diagram briefly outlining the procedure is shown in **Fig. 1**.

1. Sacrifice thymic lymphoma bearing mice according to IACUC approved procedure and cleanse the ventral surface with 70% ethanol. Make a 1 cm incision just rostral to the point of the sternum and retract the skin rostrally and caudally. Using sterile instruments and aseptic technique, cut the sternum. Remove the lymphoma and place it in a tissue culture dish containing 10 mL of sterile HBSS.
2. Rinse the lymphoma several times by gentle swirling in successive tissue culture dishes with fresh HBSS. Using a fine scissors and forceps, carefully remove parathymic lymph nodes and any connective tissue or debris clinging to the outer capsule.
3. Mince all, or a portion of (*see* **Note 2**), the lymphoma into 1–2 mm fragments using a scalpel or scissors. Transfer the fragments to a new dish with 5 mL of DMEM-10 media and mince as finely as possible.

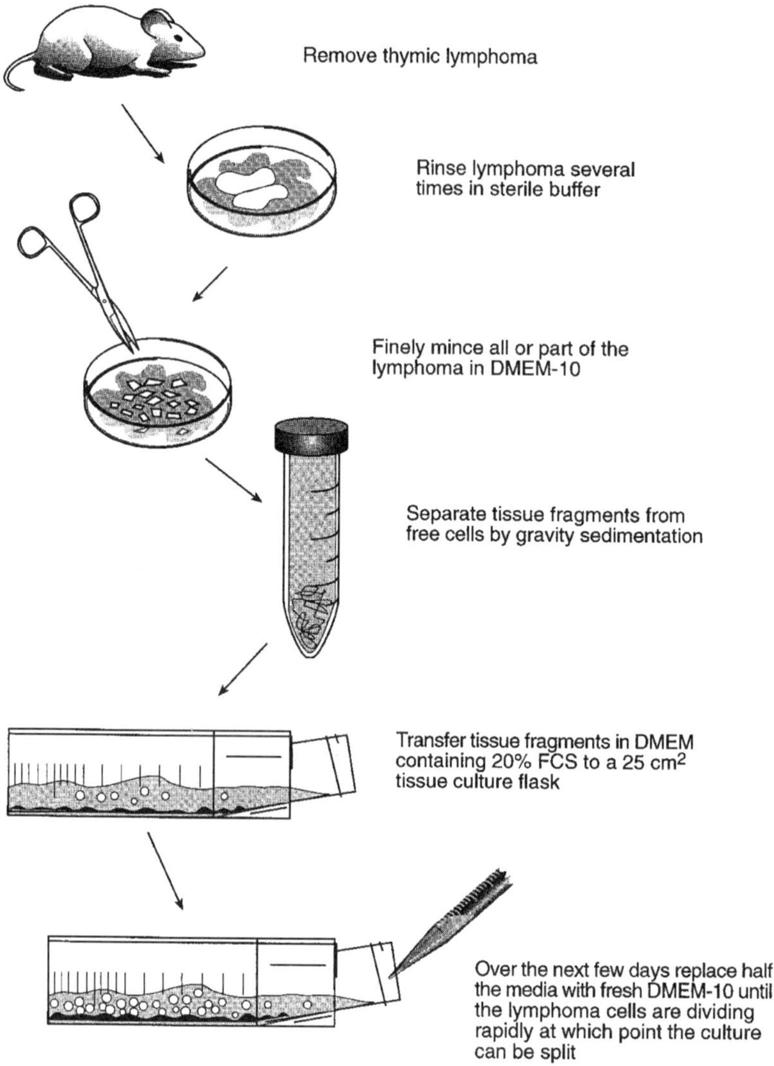

Fig. 1. Flow chart of the major steps in establishing a continuous cell line from a primary thymic lymphoma.

4. Transfer the resulting small tissue fragments to a sterile 15 mL centrifuge tube and bring the volume up to 13 mL, replace the cap and swirl gently. Allow the crude suspension to settle for 5–10 min until small fragments are visible in the bottom of the tube while the suspension still appears turbid.

5. Remove and discard the cells remaining in suspension and add 13 mL of fresh media. Repeat **step 4** until the suspension appears clear, indicating removal of the majority of free floating cells.

6. Add 3 mL of DMEM-10 to the remaining small fragments at the bottom of the centrifuge tube and transfer the entire contents to a 25 cm^2 tissue culture flask. Rinse the centrifuge tube with 3 mL of DMEM-10 and add to the tissue culture flask. Repeat rinse procedure once.

7. Add 1 mL of FCS to the tissue culture flask to bring the final serum concentration to 20% and incubate the tissue culture flask at 37°C in a humidified 5% CO_2 incubator.

8. The following day, there should be a layer of adherent cells with some clumps of lymphoma cells remaining in suspension. On each of three successive days, remove one half of the media and replace it with fresh DMEM-10.

9. For the next several weeks, monitor the flask daily and replace spent media as needed when the media becomes acidic (yellow in color). If the adherent cells become rapidly confluent and the media is depleted quickly, it may be necessary to split the cells into two flasks.

10. After a variable period of time, usually 1–4 wk, lymphoma cells will appear to dislodge from the substratum. These large transformed cells will proliferate rapidly in suspension (*see* **Note 3**).

11. When the lymphoma cells are dividing and rapidly depleting the media within 2–3 d, the culture can be split. Tighten the cap and tap the flask briskly several times to dislodge adherent cells. After gently swirling the flask, transfer 5 mL of the suspension to a new 25 cm^2 tissue culture flask containing 5 mL of fresh media.

12. To "wean" the lymphoma cell line from the adherent cells, repeat **step 11**, but do not attempt to dislodge the adherent layer when the cells in suspension are passaged. After repeating this process several times, the lymphoma cell line will become independent of the adherent layer. Different lymphoma lines vary in the length of time required for cocultivation with the adherent monolayer. In most cases, lymphoma cells can be "weaned" from the adherent cells after 4–6 wk in culture.

13. The parent cell line may be cloned by a standard limiting dilution procedure. An aliquot of the parent cell line is resuspended in DMEM-10 at a final concentration of 5 cells/mL. One–tenth of a milliliter is plated into each well of a 96-well tissue culture plate containing an additional 0.1 mL of DMEM-10. The plates are incubated at 37°C in a humidified 5% CO_2 incubator for 10–14 d or until cell growth is observed. The contents of each positive well are transferred to a 25 cm^2 tissue culture flask containing 5 mL of fresh DMEM-10 media. After the cells are expanded in culture, they can be subcloned by repeating the procedure. Alternatively, if a flow cytometer with cell sorting capability is available, cell lines can be cloned using the single-cell deposition feature.

14. Established lymphoma cell lines generally have a 12–24 h generation time. To maintain the cells in log phase, split the cultures at a 1:10 or 1:20 ratio of existing cell suspension to fresh DMEM-10 three times per week.

3.1. Characterization and Freezing of Lymphoma Cell Lines

1. Different lymphoma lines vary in their growth characteristics and viability is greatly reduced when the cells are grown to high density (usually >4 × 10^6/mL)

Therefore, growth curves must be established for each cell line to determine the doubling time and saturation density.

2. After the parent and clonal cell lines are established, aliquots should be frozen to preserve cells at early passage. It is best to cryopreserve the lymphoma line when the cells are in log phase. Transfer the contents of a tissue culture flask to a sterile centrifuge tube and spin at 200*g* for 10 min at 4°C. Gently resuspend the cells in 1 mL of freezing media and transfer to a 1.2 mL cryovial. Place the cryovial at –20°C (in a nonself-defrosting freezer) for 1 h prior to transfer to a liquid nitrogen storage freezer. To thaw the cells, twirl the cryovial in a 37°C water bath. Immediately after thawing, wipe off the outside of the vial with 70% EtOH. Using a 1 mL pipet add the cell suspension drop-wise to a 15 mL centrifuge tube containing 12 mL of prewarmed DMEM-10, mix gently and centrifuge at 200*g* for 5 min at 4°C. Resuspend the cells in 10 mL of DMEM-10 and transfer the suspension to a 25 cm^2 tissue culture flask.

3. Characterization of surface marker expression (CD4, CD8, CD3, etc.) by immunofluorescence staining and flow cytometric analysis will verify whether the lymphoma cell line maintains the phenotypic profile of the primary lymphoma. Additional characterization such as immunochemical analysis of surface or metabolically labeled cells, functional studies, gene expression, growth in syngeneic animals, etc. can be performed depending on the specific objectives of the investigator (*see* **Note 5**).

4. Notes

1. This method for establishing continuous lymphoma cell lines is a modification of an earlier report emphasizing the importance of including adherent cells in the initial stages of adapting lymphoma cells to continuous in vitro culture *(17)*. Using this approach, we have established lymphoma cell lines from spontaneous, carcinogen-induced and radiation-induced murine thymic lymphomas with a success rate exceeding 70%.

2. Since thymic lymphomas are frequently quite large, it is not necessary to use the entire tumor for establishing a cell line. Instead, a portion of the primary lymphoma can be processed through a wire mesh to obtain single-cell suspensions as is routinely done for preparing normal thymocyte suspensions. The primary lymphoma cells can then be used for flow cytometric (or other types of) analysis and excess cells cryopreserved for future comparison with the established cell line. For example, one can compare the surface marker phenotype of early passage cell lines with that of the original lymphoma to determine whether the in vitro adapted cells represent the major population of neoplastic cells that comprised the primary tumor.

3. A crisis period often occurs within the first few weeks of culture during which there may be substantial death of the cells in suspension and partial sloughing of the adherent layer. However, if the cultures are maintained and the media is replaced as needed, a proliferative population of lymphoma cells will usually emerge to produce a continuously growing cell line.

4. Since different batches of FCS vary in their ability to support optimal cell growth, it is essential to pretest samples of different FCS lots on previously established lymphoma cell lines before switching to a new lot. After identifying a FCS lot that supports propagation of several cell lines, it is convenient to order a relatively large number of bottles if storage space is available. Alternatively, it may be possible for the vendor to reserve a number of bottles of the selected batch for the investigator.

5. Although the cell surface phenotype of some lymphoma lines is stably maintained after months of continuous in vitro growth, the expression of certain markers, such as CD4 or CD8, may diminish with time in other cell lines. Therefore, it is useful to monitor surface marker expression on lymphoma cell lines at regular intervals. If phenotypic drift does occur, one can thaw early passage cells and/or use flow cytometric sorting to isolate the desired subsets for continued propagation.

Acknowledgments

The authors thank Carla Carter for valuable suggestions and Carrie McKinley for help in manuscript preparation. This work was supported by NIH grant CA37912 and a grant from the Bruce McMillan, Jr. Fdn.

References

1. Robey, E. and Fowlkes, B. J. (1994) Selective events in T-cell development. *Annu. Rev. Immunol.* **12,** 675–705.
2. von Boehmer, H. (1994) Positive selection of lymphocytes. *Cell* **76,** 219–228.
3. Zuniga-Pflucker, J. C. and Lenardo, M. J. (1996) Regulation of thymocyte development from immature progenitors. *Curr. Opin. Immunol.* **8,** 215–224.
4. Kishimoto, H., Surh, C. D., and Sprent, J. (1995) Upregulation of surface markers on dying thymocytes. *J. Exp. Med.* **181,** 649–655.
5. Punt, J. A., Kubo, R. T., Saito, T., Finkel, T. H., Kathiresan, S., Blank, K. J., and Hashimoto, Y. (1991) Surface expression of a T cell receptor beta (TCR-β) chain in the absence of TCR-α, -δ, and -γ proteins. *J. Exp. Med.* **174,** 775–783.
6. Mombaerts, P., Terhorst, C., Jacks, T., Tonegawa, S., and Sancho, J. (1995) Characterization of immature thymocyte lines derived from T-cell receptor or recombination activating gene 1 and p53 double mutant mice. *Proc. Natl. Acad. Sci. USA* **92,** 7420–7424.
7. Groettrup, M., Ungewiss, K., Azogui, O., Palacios, R., Owen, M. J., Hayday, A. C., and von Boehmer, H. (1993) A novel disulfide-linked heterodimer on pre-T cells consists of the T cell receptor β chain and a 33kD glycoprotein. *Cell* **75,** 283–294.
8. Riegel, J. S., Richie, E. R., and Allison, J. P. (1990) Nuclear events after activation of CD4$^+$8$^+$ thymocytes. *J. Immunol.* **144,** 3611–3618.
9. Richie, E. R., McEntire, B., Phillips, J., and Allison, J. P. (1988) Altered expression of lymphocyte differentiation antigens on phorbol ester-activated CD4$^+$8$^+$ cells. *J. Immunol.* **140,** 4115–4122.

10. Lazo, P. A., Klein-Szanto, A. J. P., and Tsichlis, P. N. (1990) T-cell lymphoma lines derived from rat thymomas induced by Moloney murine leukemia virus: phenotypic diversity and its implications. *J. Virol.* **64,** 3948–3959.

11. Kaye, J. and Ellenberger, D. L. (1992) Differentiation of an immature T cell line: a model of thymic positive selection. *Cell* **71,** 423–435.

12. Shao, H., Rubin, E. M., Chen, L.-Y., and Kaye, J. (1997) A role for Ras signaling in coreceptor regulation during differentiation of a double-positive thymocyte cell line. *J. Immunol.* **159,** 5773–5736.

13. Ochoa-Garay, J., Kaye, J., and Coligan, J. E. (1998) Nuclear factor κB is required for peptide antigen-induced differentiation of a CD4$^+$CD8$^+$ thymocyte line. *J. Immunol.* **160,** 3835–3843.

14. Richie, E. R., McEntire, B. B., Coghlan, L., and Poenie, M. (1991) Murine T-lymphomas corresponding to the immature CD4$^-$8$^+$ thymocyte subset. *Develop. Immunol.* **1,** 255–264.

15. Freshney, I. R. (1994) *Culture of Animal Cells: A Manual of Basic Technique,* Wiley-Liss, New York, NY.

16. Celis, J. E. (Ed.) (1998) *Cell Biology, A Laboratory Handbook,* Academic Press, New York, NY.

17. Hiai, H., Nishi, Y., Miyazawa, T., Matsudaira, Y., and Nishizuka, Y. (1981) Mouse lymphoid leukemias:symbiotic complexes of neoplastic lymphocytes and their microenvironment. *J. Natl. Canc. Inst.* **66,** 713–722.

15

Production and Characterization of T Cell Hybridomas

Janice White, John Kappler, and Philippa Marrack

1. Introduction

T-cell hybridomas were first produced some 20 yr ago (*1*). They have been used for research in almost all aspects of T-cell biology ranging from experiments on T-cell receptors and their specificity to the cytokines produced by T cells and the factors that lead to T-cell death. For biological studies, T-cell hybridomas have several advantages over normal T cells and T-cell lines. T-cell hybridomas grow rapidly in tissue culture. Their proliferation does not require components other than those of normal medium and serum. The cells divide spontaneously. Normal resting T cells do not divide in culture and must be freshly isolated from animals immediately before use. T-cell lines and clones do divide in vitro, however they require stimulation in the form of antigen and antigen presenting cells and/or cytokines such as interleukin 2 (IL-2). These nontransformed cells are therefore more trouble and more expensive to culture than hybridomas are and there is always the danger that inappropriate cells from the antigen presenting population will contaminate the specific T-cell preparation. There is also the danger that T-cell lines will senesce, a phenomenon which does not apply to hybridomas. T-cell hybridomas are usually easy to clone and may have plating efficiencies approaching the ideal. Finally, because they grow so well in culture, T-cell hybridomas, unlike their untransformed counterparts, can be selected for mutants, infected and transformed, thus allowing genetic manipulations that are not possible in normal T cells.

T-cell hybridomas have their disadvantages of course. Because they contain greater than 2N chromosomes, they are liable to shed chromosomes and are thus much less genetically stable than normal cells. This property may lead to

From: *Methods in Molecular Biology, Vol. 134: T Cell Protocols: Development and Activation*
Edited by: K. P. Kearse © Humana Press Inc., Totowa, NJ

loss of chromosomes coding for, for example, the T-cell receptors of the incoming normal T cell. The tumor parent of most T-cell hybridomas is a mouse thymoma, BW5147 *(2)*. This tumor has properties that are not always desirable and are expressed in the hybridomas produced from it. For example, BW5147 derived cells never express **CD8** in a stable way unless the cells have been transfected with an exogenous and expressible **CD8** gene *(3–5)*. BW5147 derived cells have a tendency to extinguish expression of CD4 and are not cytotoxic unless incubated in IL-2 containing supernatants *(6,7)*. Finally genetic programs expressed in BW5147 may mask those of the normal T-cell parent and affect the properties of the hybridoma. For example, very few hybridomas made with BW5147 secrete interferonγ (IFNγ, *8*), although this cytokine is made by many normal T cells after stimulation *(9)*. Also, T-cell hybridomas divide constitutively, of course, and normal T cells do not. Thus T-cell hybridomas are probably not good models for normal T cells in studies on T-cell proliferation or even death.

1.1. Choice of Tumor Cell Parents for T-Cell Hybridomas

Production of hybridomas requires a tumor cell parent. Many transformed mouse T-cell lines, and a few human and rat T-cell tumors, are candidates for this role. However, experience of the last 20 yr has taught us that one cell line above all others is by far the best for use. This cell line, BW5147, was produced from a spontaneous thymoma isolated from AKR mice at the Jackson Laboratory in the 1950s. It was selected for resistance to azaguanine and, hence, sensitivity to hypoxanthine aminopterin thymidine (HAT) selection, and also for sensitivity to ouabain by Hyman *(2)*. Kontiainen et al., the first group to describe production of T-cell hybridomas, made a good choice when they selected BW5147 as the tumor cell parent *(1)*. BW5147 and its hybridomas divide rapidly in culture with doubling times of 12–16 h. BW5147, which readily fuses to yield hybridomas, has a very stable genotype.

The cell line does have its disadvantages, however. Like most mouse cell lines it yields few hybridomas with human cells. Human-mouse hybridomas produced with this cell line lose human chromosomes rapidly and, in the presence of HAT medium, usually retain only the selected human X chromosome. As previously mentioned above, BW5147 hybrids do not usually express **CD8** and are relatively unstable for expression of **CD4**. For all these reasons many other cell lines have been tested for their suitability as parents.

Nearly all have completely failed the test because, despite attempts with many different fusion conditions, nearly all other cell lines fail to yield T-cell hybridomas at a useful frequency. For example, the human T-cell tumor, JURKAT only rarely gives rise to hybridomas regardless of the fusion conditions. Likewise other mouse cell lines such as EL4 and S49 do not produce hybrid progeny. Of all the tumors which are not BW5147 derived only one, a rat tumor, C58, has been at all useful *(6)*.

We have no idea what distinguishes BW5147 from other cell lines. Whatever it is, the property of frequent fusion is inherited by the progeny of BW5147 since hybridomas produced from this cell line can be used with great success in further fusions to produce double or even triple hybridomas *(8)*.

At the moment several derivatives of BW5147 are often used as the tumor cell parents for hybridomas. These cell lines and their properties are listed in **Table 1**.

2. Materials

2.1. Culture Medium and Salts Solutions

1. BW5147 and its hybridomas grow in standard laboratory tissue culture medium supplemented with 10% fetal bovine serum (FBS) and $2 \times 10^{-5} M$ 2-mercaptoethanol. For example, Dulbecco's medium or an enriched minimal essential medium (MEM) can be used. If MEM is the medium of choice it should be enriched with essential and nonessential amino acids, at final concentrations of ×0.3 and ×1.1 respectively, 292 mg/L glutamine and 2.86 gm/L sodium bicarbonate. The antibiotics penicillin, streptomycin and gentamycin can also be added. It is not a good idea to add other buffering agents such as HEPES and certainly not additional phosphate.
2. Hybridomas are selected in medium containing 0.1 mM hypoxanthine, 0.4 μM aminopterin and 0.016 mM thymidine.
3. Normal T cells are grown in Click's medium to which 1% fresh normal mouse serum and antigen have been added. The mixture is sterilized through a 0.2 μM filter prior to use.
4. All cultures are performed at 37°C in an atmosphere of 90% air, 10% CO_2.
5. Cells are isolated and washed in Earle's balanced salts solution (BSS) or MEM without other additions.
6. Dead cells are removed using a step gradient of Ficoll Hypaque (LSM, Organon Teknika, Durham, NC).
7. Fusions are performed in MEM without FBS or enrichment or additional glutamine or antibiotics.
8. Cells are fused with a 50% w/w mixture of polyethylene glycol 1450 (PEG, Sigma Corp., St Louis, MO, P-5402) and MEM without any other additions. Serum must not be present. To make this, 1450 PEG is melted in a boiling water bath taking care that the water bath does not boil dry during this procedure. 10 g aliquots of the PEG are then weighed into 50 mL sterile conical polypropylene centrifuge tubes and kept for future use. On the day of fusion the PEG in one of these tubes is melted in a boiling water bath or a microwave oven. 10 mL of MEM is added and the contents of the tube mixed. The mixture is then sterilized through a 0.2 mM filter. The first 8 mL of mixture through the filter is discarded and the

Table 1
Cell Lines Which are Candidates for the Production of T cell Hybridomas

Line	Sensitivity	Properties	Ref
BW5147	HAT, Oua	Expresses its own functional TCR α and β chain genes (coding for Vα1 and Vβ1). Does not express CD3δ.	2
BW5147 α-β-	HAT	Contains no functional TCR genes. Does not express CD3δ.	11
BW Lyt2-4	HAT	Like BW5147α-β- except expresses CD8α.	4
58	HAT	Contains no functional TCR genes. Expresses all CD3 proteins.	12
C58	HAT	Rat T cell tumor.	6
CEM		Human T cell lymphoma	13

remainder kept for the fusion in a sealed tube, gassed with 90% air, 10% CO_2 to maintain the pH of the mixture. The tube is stored at 37°C.

2.2. T Cell Priming In Vivo

1. T cells are primed in animals by the method preferred by the investigators. In our laboratory this procedure usually involves an emulsion of antigen in complete Freund's adjuvant.

3. Methods

3.1. Preparation of Priming Antigen

1. T cells are primed in vivo by the investigator's method of choice. In our laboratory this is achieved by injection of an emulsion of a 50% v/v mixture of 5 mg/mL antigen dissolved in BSS and complete Freund's adjuvant. This mixture is emulsified using a sonicator or with emulsifying syringes. The quality of the emulsion is judged by its thickness. The emulsion should not flow freely and a drop of the emulsion in water should not readily disperse.

3.2. Immunization of Mice

1. Again, this can be done in many ways. In our laboratory animals are immunized with 0.04 mL of the emulsion described in **Subheading 3.1., step 1** administered

from a 1 mL syringe using a 25G needle. Mice are immunized in the base of the tail. The needle of the syringe is inserted under the tail skin about 0.5 cm from the animal's body, and the needle slid under the skin towards the animal until the tip of the needle is level with the beginning of the body. 0.04 mL of the emulsion is then slowly squeezed from the syringe. Care should be taken to avoid injecting the animal intravenously (this will immediately kill the animal) and that the injected emulsion does not leak out of the hole at the insertion point of the needle.

2. Hamsters are immunized with similar amounts of emulsion, delivered subcutaneously in the scruff of the neck.

3. Rats are immunized with 0.2 mL of the emulsion at several subcutaneous sites in the scruff of the neck.

3.3. Preparation of Antigen Activated T Cells

1. Seven to nine days after administration of antigen, animals are sacrificed and lymph nodes draining the sites of injection harvested. For mice immunized in the base of the tail these lymph nodes are the inguinals and periaortics. For animals immunized in the scruff of the neck these lymph nodes are the brachial and axillary and, possibly, the submandibular.

2. The lymph nodes are dispersed with two pairs of forceps and resuspended to 4×10^6 cells/mL in Click's medium containing 1% fresh normal mouse serum, additional sodium bicarbonate to a final concentration of 863 µg/mL, 5×10^{-5} M 2-mercaptoethanol and antibiotics.

3. The suspension is plated at 1.5 mL/well in the wells of 24-well tissue culture plates and the cells incubated for 4 d under an atmosphere of 90% air, 10% CO_2.

4. After this culture the cells are harvested, spun down for 10 min at 1000g and resuspended in 5 mL BSS 15% FCS.

5. This is layered on top of 2 mL Ficoll Hypaque in a 15 mL sterile tissue culture tube and the tube spun at 1500g at room temperature for 15 min.

6. After this spin, live cells will be at the interface between the BSS and Ficoll, and dead cells and red cells in the pellet. The live cell layer is recovered and washed once in BSS.

7. Cells are then resuspended at 1×10^5/mL in complete tumor medium (CTM) containing 3 IU/mL IL-2.

8. The suspension is cultured in flat tissue culture flasks under 90% air, 10% CO_2 for 3 d.

9. Cells are harvested and washed in BSS. If necessary, dead cells may again be removed using a Ficoll Hypaque step gradient.

3.4. Preparation of BW5147 Cells

1. Cultured in CTM, BW5147 divides nearly twice a day. Cell lines derived from BW5147, such as the TCR α- β- variant *(10)*, divide somewhat more slowly. *See* **Note 1** about the density at which this and other cell lines can be grown.

2. In preparation for fusion, the tumor cell parent is harvested while it is still clearly in log phase, i.e., before it has reached 7×10^5/mL.

3. Immediately before fusion the tumor cells are harvested from culture and washed once in BSS.

3.5. Fusion

1. 10^7 parent tumor cells are added to a 50 mL sterile conical polypropylene centrifuge tube (*see* **Note 2**).
2. Add up to 5×10^7 T-cell blasts to this tube.
3. Spin the mixture of cells down.
4. Pour off supernatant.
5. Wash once with BSS.
6. Pour off supernatant.
7. Spin the tube at 1000g for 3 min to collect residual moisture in the bottom of the tube.
8. Remove residual moisture carefully with a Pasteur pipet without disturbing the cell pellet.
9. Hold the tube sideways and tap it gently to disperse the pellet slightly.
10. Place the tube in a 37°C water bath (usually a small beaker) in a sterile culture hood.
11. Add 1 mL of a 1:1 W/W mixture of PEG 1450 and MEM to the pellet over the course of 45 s.
12. Partially resuspend the pellet by one titration using a 10 mL sterile pipet. The goal is to keep the cells in clumps, and yet make the clumps small enough to allow complete penetration of the PEG:MEM mixture.
13. Stand the mixture in the 37°C water bath for 45 s.
14. Dilute the PEG by addition of 37°C MEM as follows: 1 mL MEM is added over the course of 30 s, then 2 mL for the next 30 s, 3 mL for the next and 4 mL for the next. The remaining 40 mL of MEM is then added gently by running it down the side of the tube. After each addition the PEG and MEM are mixed by very gentle swirling of the tube.
15. Incubate the cells and MEM for 5 min at 37°C.
16. Spin the cells down.
17. Pour off supernatant.
18. Wash the pellet once with BSS without resuspension of the cell pellet.
19. Add 10 mL CTM to the washed cell pellet and resuspend the cells by very gentle titration with a 10 mL pipet.
20. Add a further 40 mL CTM added to the tube.
21. Pour the mixture into a sterile basin and aliquot at 0.1 mL/well into four 96-well tissue culture plates, using a 12 channel pipetman.
22. Add a further 40 mL CTM to the remaining 10 mL mixture of cells and plate this into another four 96-well plates.
23. Repeat this procedure once more. This serial dilution of plated cells is used because it is difficult to predict how many hybridomas will appear and it is desirable to avoid plating the hybrids at a density of more than 1/well. The plating conditions will vary, however, depending upon the operator's experience and the number of input T-cell blasts.

3.5.1. Growth and Selection of Hybridomas

1. The fusion plates are cultured at 37°C.
2. Add 0.05 mL CTM containing 3× concentration of HAT when the parent tumor cells cover 20–25% of the surface area of the wells. BW5147 and its hybrids make factors, such as IL-6, which help their own growth. We therefore allow the BW5147 cells to grow in the fusion plates before adding HAT. Depending upon the initial density of plating this is between 1 and 3 d after fusion. HAT is never added to the fusion wells earlier than 24 h after fusion.
3. Every 5 d change the medium completely by gently dumping the supernatants of the wells into a sink and adding, using a 12 channel pipetman, 0.1 mL fresh CTM + HAT to each well.
4. Beginning at day 7 after fusion inspect the 96-well tissue culture plates daily for hybridoma growth. Transfer the hybridomas into 1.5 mL CTM + HAT to the wells of 24 well tissue culture plates when they reach a density such that their growth is visible to the naked eye.
5. Do not wean the hybridomas from HAT until 15 d or more after fusion. At this point all the parent tumor cells should be dead (**Note 3**).

3.6. Assay of T Cell Hybridomas

1. The assay used will depend on the purpose of the fusion. Antigen specific T-cell hybridomas are screened as follows. When the hybridomas cover about 1/3 the area of the 24-well plates, place 0.2 mL of each hybridoma cells in duplicate in the wells of a 96-well tissue culture plate.
2. Allow the cells to settle, or spin them down.
3. Remove the supernatant by gentle dumping.
4. Rapidly add 10^5 tumor cells or 10^6 normal spleen cells to act as antigen presenting cells in 200 μL CTM.
5. Add antigen to one of the two duplicate wells.
6. Incubate the mixture overnight at 37°C.
7. Remove 80 μL supernatant from each mixture and place in the first of a series of wells.
8. Serially dilute another 80 μL of the same superantants below the first well using CTM + HAT or HT.
9. Add 4000 IL-2 dependent cells (e.g., HT-2 or CTLL).
10. Incubate overnight at 37°C.
11. Assess survival or proliferation of the IL-2 dependent cells.
12. Standardize the titer against a dilution of IL-2 of known activity.
13. Clone desirable hybridomas and freeze them in liquid nitrogen.

4. Notes

1. Like most cell lines in tissue culture, BW5147 dies when its concentration in medium exceeds 10^6/mL. We always grow it up to concentrations lower than this. T-cell hybridomas also die at concentrations higher than 10^6/mL. Moreover the stress of high cell concentrations tends to select for faster growing variants, variants that have often lost some of the chromosomes of

the hybridoma, including chromosomes that code for the normal T-cell parent TCR α and β chains. It is therefore inadvisable to culture hybridomas at cell concentrations higher than 7×10^5/mL.

2. It is important to use a minimum of 10^7 parent tumor cells even if very few T-cell blasts are to be used in the fusion. This ensures that the cell pellet is detectable and easy to manipulate.

3. Because of the dangers of an imbalance between concentrations of the poison, aminopterin, and its substitutes, hypoxanthine and thymidine, do not move the hybridomas directly from medium containing HAT to normal CTM. Instead use CTM containing HT only as an intermediate medium.

References

1. Kontiainen, S., Simpson, E., Bohrer, E., Beverly, P. C. L., Herzenberg, L. A., Fitzpatrick, W. A., Vogt, P., Torano, A., McKenzie, I. F. C., and Feldmann, M. (1987) T cell lines producing antigen-specific suppressor factor. *Nature (London)* **274,** 477–479.

2. Hyman, R. (1973) Studies on surface antigen variants. Isolation of two complementary variants for Thy 1.2 *J. Nat Cancer Inst.* **50,** 415–425.

3. Carbone, A. M., Marrack, P., and Kappler, J. W. (1988) Remethylation at sites 5' of the murine Lyt 2 gene in association with shut down of Lyt 2 expression. *J. Immunol.* **141,**1369–1378.

4. Burgert, H.-G., White, J., Weltzein, H.-U., Marrack, P., and Kappler, J. W. (1989) Reactivity of Vb17a$^+$ CD8$^+$ T cell hybrids: Analysis using a new CD8$^+$ T cell fusion partner. *J. Exp. Med.* **170,** 1887–1904.

5. Kanagawa, O., Nakauchi, H., Sekaly, R. P., Maeda, K., and Takagaki, Y. (1990) Expression and function of the transfected CD8 alpha chain in murine T cell hybridomas. *Int. Immunol.* **2,** 957–964.

6. Kanagawa, O. and Chiller, J. M. (1985) Lymphokine-mediated induction of cytolytic activity in a T cell hybridoma. *J. Immunol.* *134,* 397–403.

7. Nabholz, M., Cianfriglia, M., Acuto, O., Conzelmann, A., Haas, W., von Boehmer, H., MacDonald, H. R., Pohlit, H. and Johnson J. P. (1980) Cytolytically active, murine T-cell hybrids. *Nature (London)* **287,** 437–439.

8. Zlotnik, A., Roberts, W. K., Vasil, A., Blumenthal, E., LaRosa, F., Leibson, H. J., Endres, R. O., Graham, S. D., Jr., White, J., Hill, J., Henson, P., Klein, J. R., Bevan, M. J., Marrack, P., and Kappler, J. W. (1983) Coordinate production by a T cell hybridoma of gamma interferon and three other lymphokine activities. Multiple activities of a single lymphokine? *J. Immunol.* **131,** 794–810.

9. Mossmann, T. R. and Coffman, R. L. (1989) TH1 and TH2 cells: Different patterns of lymphokine secretion lead to different functional properties. *Adv. Immunol.* **7,** 145–173.

10. Kappler, J., Skidmore, B., White, J., and Marrack, P. (1981) Antigen-inducible, H-2-restricted, interleukin-2 producing T cell hybridomas: Lack of independent antigen and H-2 recognition. *J. Exp. Med.* **153,** 1198–1210.

11. White, J., Blackman, M., Bill, J., Kappler, J., Marrack, P., Gold, D.P., and Born, W. (1989) Two better cell lines for making hybridomas expressing specific T cell receptors. *J. Immunol.* **143,** 1822–1825.

12. Letourneur, F. and Malissen, B. (1989) Derivation of a T cell hybridoma variant deprived of functional T cell receptor alpha and beta chain transcripts reveals a nonfunctional alpha-mRNA of BW5147 origin. *Eur. J. Immunol.* **19,** 2269–2274.
13. Hgiuchi, M., Nakamura, N., Tsuchiya, S. I., and Osawa T. (1984) Macrophage-activating factor for cytotoxicity produced by a human T-cell hybridoma. *Cell Immunol.* **87,** 626–636.

III

OVERVIEW FOR CHAPTERS 17–29

16

Something Happens;
A Brief History of TCR Signal Transduction

John J. O'Shea

1. Introduction

If truth be told, when asked to write this chapter my first reaction was not positive; I thought "I am too young! (aren't I?)." However, when I considered the Editor's request, I realized that I had been fortunate to have had my formative scientific years coincide with extraordinary advances in our understanding of the T-cell receptor (TCR) signaling and to have been part of a laboratory that contributed to this field in a major way. First though, a disclaimer: this is a personal and biased view of this field; I was not an experienced scientist witnessing these discoveries, I was just a "post-doc." So the perspective may be idiosyncratic, and I apologize at the outset for my "Bethesda-centricity." Nonetheless, to begin Part IV, I would like to review what I viewed as the major breakthroughs that led to our present comprehension of TCR signal transduction, including how the understanding of the structure of the TCR came about and how that, in turn, led to insights into signaling.

2. The Nature of the TCR

I was an Internal Medicine resident in 1981. I had decided to come to the NIH to try to make my scientific fortune and become an immunologist. It dawned on me, however, that if I was going to the NIH, I really needed to re-learn immunology, given its rapid advances. Although I was not enrolled as a graduate student, Dr. Bertie Argyris kindly consented to my taking her immunology seminar series. She wisely insisted though, that I present along with the graduate students. Ironically, the subject she gave me to discuss was the nature of the TCR.

From: *Methods in Molecular Biology, Vol. 134: T Cell Protocols: Development and Activation*
Edited by: K. P. Kearse © Humana Press Inc., Totowa, NJ

No doubt, it comes as no surprise that our understanding of the TCR in the early 1980s was primitive, at best. Equally, however, our understanding of other immunologic issues, like immunoglobulin structure and gene rearrangement, was very sophisticated. Indeed, rereading these chapters from my old textbooks, the discussion these topics bring about seem quite "au courant"; we were by no means in the immunological dark ages. In contrast though, the discussions of TCRs in these texts is either very terse or very confusing. The point is that in the 1980s, immunology was hardly primitive. The understanding of many immunological molecules and processes was very detailed, but the understanding of the TCR was not.

Unfortunately, I did not save my notes from this presentation, but what I discussed in the seminar were the controversies surrounding the nature of the TCR. Another personal irony is that in preparing this talk, one of the textbooks I used was *Medical Immunology (1)*. What a shock it was to me a few years later when I began working with Rick Klausner to realize that he had been a medical student when he wrote this text!

It was quite clear already that B and T cells recognized antigen differently, namely that whereas B cells reacted to free antigen, T cells reacted to antigen only when other cells were present. It was also well established that Major Histocompatability Complex (MHC) genes strongly influenced antigen recognition. Indeed the notion that T cells "see" antigen in the context of MHC was appreciated. However, it was not clear whether one or more than one receptor recognized antigen and MHC. Some cartoons from that era depict an MHC receptor and a separate antigen receptor (such a configuration served as cover art for another text I used — **ref.** *2*). Alternatively, though, it had been considered that a single receptor might bind both antigen and MHC. How diverse antigens were recognized by the TCR was completely unknown. Thus, some investigators looked for immunoglobulin on T cells and because of the vagaries of some of the reagents, it was found. Another view of the receptor was that it comprised immunoglobulin V genes. It was further hypothesized that the IgV domains associated with other domains encoded by MHC genes. Support for this idea came from experiments in which mice were immunized with a particular antigen and anti-idiotype antibodies were produced that reacted with both T and B cells. Immunoprecipitation experiments revealed a 35 kDa polypeptide on T cells but not B cells *(2)*. Indeed it was considered unlikely by some that organisms would have two entirely different sets of genes for antigen recognition, their argument being that it would be unlikely and inefficient that this problem would be solved twice in evolution *(3)*. But when T cells were probed for Ig genes or analyzed for Ig gene rearrangement, this was not found, of course. A third idea was simply that the TCR was Ig-like. Although in retrospect this suggestion is entirely sensible, it should be pointed out that in the early 1980s a number of genes (MHC molecules for instance) were known to be members of the Ig supergene family *(3)*. Thus, being Ig-like alone was unlikely to facilitate the discovery of the TCR.

Despite my efforts in preparing this talk, I remember thinking that this was a hopelessly complex subject. What was so confusing? In retrospect, it now seems so simple and straightforward.

3. The Discovery of the TCR

There were a number of key building blocks that led to the discovery of the TCR. One fundamental step was the development of the technology of growing T-cell clones either with antigen and IL-2 or through immortalization by fusion with a T lymphoma, analogous to the production of hybridomas (ca 1979–1980). This allowed the production of large numbers of T cells with a single antigen receptor. This led directly to the production of monoclonal antibodies that recognized the TCR (ca 1983) by several groups, including those led by John Kappler and Pippa Marrack, Stuart Schlossman and Ellis Reinherz, and Jim Allison (reviewed in **ref. 4**). These antibodies immunoprecipitated a complex of about 90 kDa, which upon reduction migrated with a molecular weight of 45 kDa.

At about the same time, the stunning achievement of the cloning of TCR chains was being accomplished by the groups led by Tak Mak and Mark Davis in 1984. Their strategy relied on the cloning of mRNAs expressed in T cells but not B cells. The resultant selectively expressed cDNAs were screened for those that were products of genes that were specifically rearranged in T cells. The TCR β chain was thus initially found and the α chain cloned shortly thereafter. It was then shown that the polypeptides encoded by these genes reacted with the anti-TCR monoclonal antibodies. The loop was definitively closed when TCR genes were transfected into a T-cell clone and conferred both antigen and MHC specificity. With the solution of the structure of MHC molecules bound to antigen *(5)*, it became relatively easy to understand how antigen could be recognized by TCRs.

4. The TCR: A Multichain Complex

Although the identification of TCR genes readily provided an explanation of how diverse antigens could be recognized, another problem became very clear. The intracellular domain of the TCR was diminutive. How could the TCR transmit signals? **Fig. 1** is a depiction of how the TCR transmits signals that Rick and I prepared on my brand new Macintosh computer in 1985. This was a popular depiction used by various members of the lab to introduce their seminars.

Recall that at the time the TCR was discovered, we knew precious little about the structure of receptors in general. Carbohydrate receptors and the

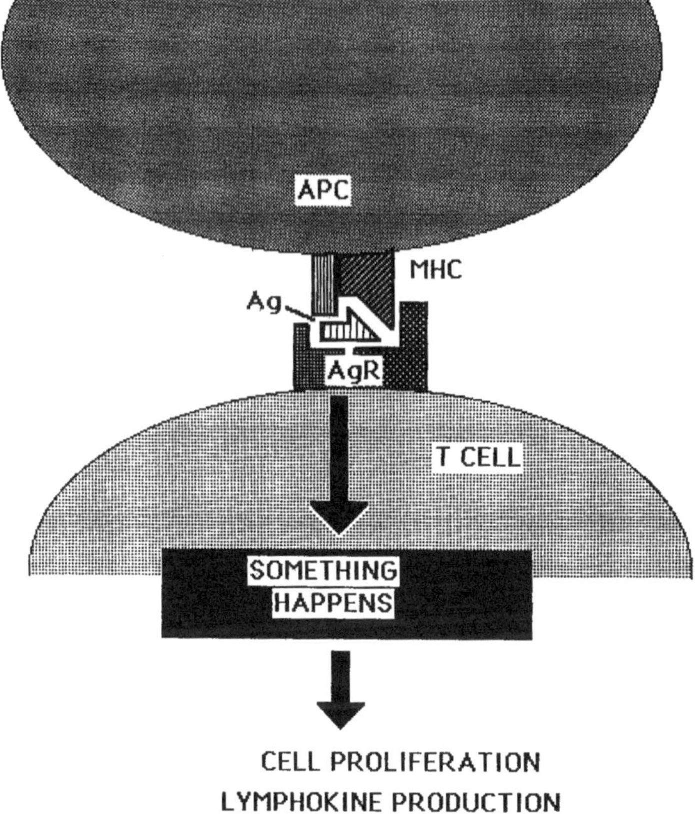

Fig. 1. The black box model of TCR signaling. In 1985, we knew that occupancy of the TCR activated T cells and we also knew that perturbation of the receptor triggered phosphoinositide turnover and calcium mobilization, but we had no idea how the receptor might trigger these events.

acetylcholine receptor had been purified in the mid 1970s *(6)*. Endocytosis of receptors was intensively studied. Fc receptors were characterized in vitro and in vivo. However, because of their relatively small amounts, their large size, and their hydrophobicity, biochemical approaches, in general, did not permit the elucidation of the primary structure of receptors, in contrast to other more abundant and soluble polypeptides, like insulin or immunoglobulins. Thus, although the primary structure of a carbohybrate receptor had been determined by biochemical means, we were generally ignorant of the primary structure of eukaryotic transmembrane receptors until the advent of molecular cloning techniques. The first receptor whose sequence we knew was the acetylcholine receptor from Torpedo; this was cloned in 1982.

Shortly thereafter, the low-density lipoprotein receptor and the transferrin receptor were cloned (1983). The next year, IL-2 receptor α chain (CD25), the asialoglycoprotein, and epidermal growth factor receptor were cloned. Given this limited information though, there were no clear ideas on how these different receptors signaled and how this might relate to the TCR. For the IgE receptor, it was envisioned early on that crosslinking the receptor was an essential aspect in initiating signaling *(7)*. But there was little way to foresee what this meant biochemically. At this time, work on signaling emphasized the idea of second messengers. Much was being learned about how G-protein coupled receptors signaled but it was also unclear if this had any relationship to receptors like the TCR. Also, other receptors had been shown to alter intracellular calcium concentration; indeed the importance of calcium as a second messenger had been noted since the 1940s. During the 1980s, more receptors were being found to mobilize calcium in large measure because of improvements in detecting alterations of the intracellular levels of this ion. The generation of TCR antibodies permitted investigators like Art Weiss and John Imboden to do some of the earliest experiments showing that TCR crosslinking led to calcium flux *(8)*. At this time, the role of phosphoinositide (PI) metabolism in regulating calcium mobilization was also being sorted out. Thus, it was shown that TCR crosslinking leads to PI hydrolysis. It was also shown that T cells could be activated pharmacologically by the combination of calcium ionophore and phorbol ester. All that was left then was to link the TCR with the PI pathway. A good candidate for such a linkage would be a G-protein, as this is important for other receptors. Experiments investigating the role of G-proteins in TCR signaling were therefore undertaken and the results were inconclusive.

A major advance in understanding T-cell signaling, however, came when the complete structure of the TCR was elucidated, in particular the discovery of the invariant chains of the receptor, CD3 molecules, and the ζ chain. I have a vivid recollection of this because at the time, I was working on a completely different group of receptors, complement receptors. I was having problems doing clean immunoprecipitations of metabolically labeled receptor, and it was suggested that I talk to Larry Samelson. Samelson was among the first to produce anti-TCR monoclonal antibodies. He showed me data in which he immunoprecipitated with his TCR-α chain antibody and pulled down the disulfide linked α and β chains of the receptor. But in addition, he also consistently pulled down low-molecular-weight material. He was able to "clean up" his blots by using more stringent detergents. Fortunately, Samelson and others quickly realized the importance of these other proteins; it was discovered that these proteins were the so-called CD3 proteins. Monoclonal antibodies against mouse and human T cells produced by Ellis Reinherz, Jeff Bluestone, and others facilitated this discovery. Reinherz recognized that when cells were lysed with the appropriate detergents the same complex of proteins were immuno-precipitated with both anti-TCR and anti-CD3 antibodies. Serendipitously though, the solubilized mouse TCR complex was less fragile than the human complex. It was therefore through the analysis of the mouse TCR complex that Rick Klausner, Larry Samelson, and Joe Harford discovered yet another receptor subunit, the TCRζ chain, which was then cloned by Allan Weissman. TCRζ subunit, of course, turned out to also be part of the human complex and to be pivotally important in the conception of signaling.

The picture that emerged was that the TCR comprised products of rear-ranging antigen receptor genes associated with CD3 proteins and the ζ chain (ca. 1985). But why on earth should this gamish be called a receptor? It is relatively easy to get dirty immunoprecipitates, so these other putative subunits could be artifactual. Thus, although these polypeptides were consistently observed in TCR immunoprecipitates, this complex picture of the TCR was initially met with some skepticism. However, what members of Klausner's and Terhorst's labs were able to show was that without all of these chains, the receptor is not expressed optimally on the cell surface. The other piece of information, which was by no means overlooked at the time, was that the TCR components had charged residues in their transmembrane domains. Though relatively few receptors had been cloned at this point, this finding alone was striking. Thus, despite this unlikely configuration, it became clear that it was appropriate to conceive of the TCR as a complex. Subsequently, we now know that the TCR was the prototype of a family of receptors that has been termed the multichain immune recognition receptors, which also includes the B-cell antigen receptor and Fc receptors *(8)*. Indeed, we now know that the situation is even more complex in that other forms of the receptor are produced during T-cell ontogeny.

5. TCR Phosphorylation and the Birth of ITAMs

The good news provided by the more complicated TCR was that unlike the α and β chains; that have mere nubbins of intracellular domains, CD3 proteins and the ζ chain have more substantive intracellular segments. Indeed, ζ is the opposite of the α and β chains; it has a diminutive extracellular domain and a relatively large cytoplasmic segment. Unfortunately, though, there was nothing revealing about the sequence of the intracellular domains.

In 1980, it was discovered that the v-src oncongene encoded a protein kinase that phosphorylated tyrosine residues. Around this time, it was also discovered that growth factor receptors were tyrosine kinases and were phosphorylated in response to ligand *(10)*. Larry Samelson therefore set out to see if the TCR was phosphorylated in an analogous manner. Again, I vividly remember another pivotal experiment that Samelson presented at Klausner's lab meeting (which parenthetically was held a few yards from where Gil Ashwell had purified one of the first receptors *[5]*). This was a phosphorylation experiment in which Samelson was able to show that upon ligand binding, the TCR coprecipitated a variety of phosphoproteins. Later, Samelson was able to show that the phosphorylation occurred on phosphoserine, phosphothreonine, and importantly, phosphotyrosine residues. He later confirmed this result using an exciting new reagent, anti-phosphotyrosine antibodies (1986). Subsequently, it was shown that the major phosphotyrosine-containing protein was none other than ζ itself. In addition, CD3 proteins were tyrosine and serine phosphory-lated. An obvious but important conclusion of these studies was that TCR crosslinking resulted in activation of tyrosine and serine kinases.

In 1985, the Perlmutter and Sefton labs cloned a new src family tyrosine kinase expressed in T cells that was ultimately called Lck. Work from Veillette, Bolen, and Rudd in 1988–1989 showed that Lck was associated with CD4 and CD8, and that it phosphorylated the TCR. In contrast, Fyn, another src family tyrosine kinase, was shown to be associated with CD3ϵ by Samelson. These discoveries solved, in large measure, the question of which kinases are responsible for phosphorylating the TCR. Later, the importance of Fyn and Lck in TCR signaling was shown by genetic manipulation of cells and mice. Still later another key tyrosine kinase, Zap-70, was cloned by Art Weiss and Andy Chan.

In 1989, a brief letter by Michael Reth was published in which he drew attention to the fact that the ζ chain contained 3 motifs ($YXXLX_{7/8}YXXL$) that were also present in CD3 subunits, Igα and Igβ, of the B cell antigen receptor and FcϵRγ and FcϵRβ *(12)*. He proposed that the precise spacing of these residues was important and these sites could be bound by signaling molecules. Reth speculated that the sites were likely important for the propagation of signals leading to proliferation and differentiation. These motifs, of course, are now termed immunoreceptor tyrosine-based activation motifs (ITAMs) and their central importance in signaling by the TCR and related receptors is well established, but we still did not understand why these motifs were so important and how they served to transmit signals.

The pressing question for many receptors, then, was how did receptor tyrosine phosphorylation effect signal transduction? The importance of tyrosine phosphorylation in regulating critical cell processes was quite evident based on the discovery of various oncogenes, but these findings begged the question, how? It was clear that a major substrate phosphorylated in response to growth factors and antigen was the receptor itself, but this did not get us very far; we were still at the cell membrane. The hunt, therefore, was on to find the critical phosphotyrosine substrates but the initial search was not very fruitful.

It was not until about 1990 that the importance of receptor phosphorylation came into sharp focus with the understanding that phosphotyrosine residues are recognized by specialized modules, SH2 domains, contained within a large number of signaling proteins *(11)*. This led to the current view that ligand induces dimerization of receptor tyrosine kinases, activating their enzymatic activity, which results in receptor autophosphorylation. This, in turn, results in the recruitment of proteins with SH2 domains, some of which are signaling molecules and some of which are adapter proteins. This is how tyrosyl phosphorylation can serve as a molecular switch. With the understanding of the function of SH2 domains, it was now apparent how TCR phosphorylation could initiate signaling. The finding that Zap-70 bound the ITAMs in ζ fit well with a larger view of SH2-phosphotyrosine interactions. The TCR, of course, became the paradigm by which other receptors in the MIRR family functioned. Thus in seven years (1982–1989), we went from being entirely ignorant of the structure of the TCR to having a rather detailed conceptual understanding of how signaling originates upon recognition of antigen. Moreover, a number of tyrosine-phosphorylated substrates have now been identified and their contribution to signaling is now being assessed (**Fig. 2**).

6. Conclusions

For me, it was wonderful to see this story unfold. But the more pressing question now is, what are the important issues that lie ahead of us and what, if any, lessons can be learned from the discovery of the TCR that might help us in our future quests?

One obvious lesson is that biological processes can be both simpler and more complicated than we initially envision. Certainly, no one proposed that the structure of the TCR was as complex as it actually is. Many did think that the TCR was likely to be immunoglobulin-like and the idea that antigen and MHC were recognized by a single receptor was one of the models that was entertained. But none of the models I came across proposed a modular receptor comprising antigen recognition and signaling components, encoded as separate gene products. Still, despite this complexity, the idea that phosphorylated receptors recruit signaling molecules is a remarkably simple solution to the problem of how receptor occupancy is sensed by the cell. Overall, signal transduction seems far more straightforward now than when we talked about various second messengers in the early 1980s.

Another lesson exemplified by the elucidation of the TCR, then, is that knowing the structure greatly facilitates the understanding of function. This is true both in terms of understanding the primary (the recognition of ITAMs) and three-dimensional structure (the crystal structure of MHC). There was really no plausible hypothesis for signaling that preceded the

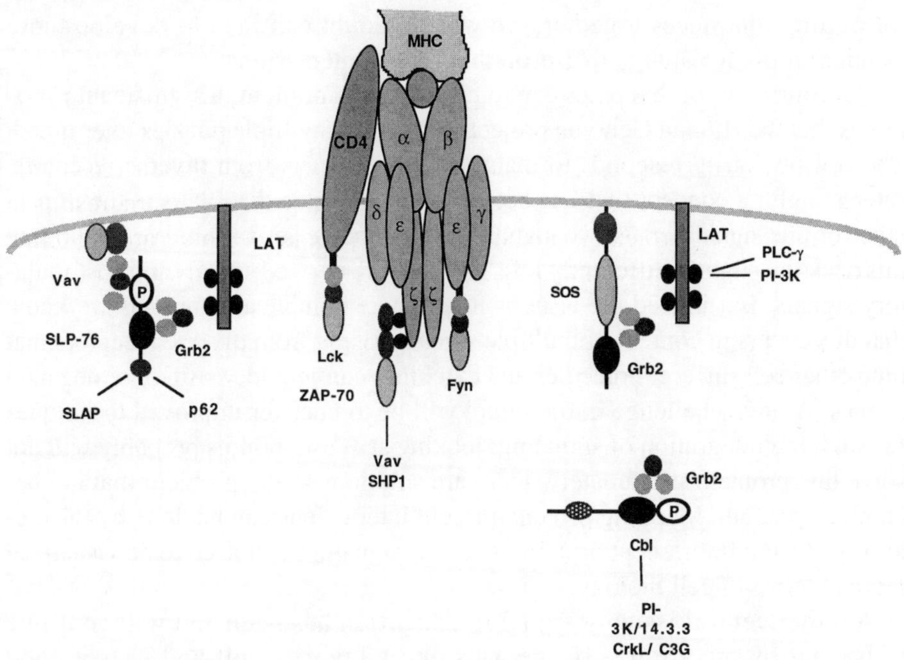

Fig. 2. TCR signaling in 1999. Great strides have been made in our understanding of TCR-dependent signal transduction both in terms of the kinases activated and their substrates. Additionally, much more emphasis is now placed on the formation of signaling complexes and less on the production of second messengers.

knowledge of the structure. This principle will probably continue to hold true as we dissect out the other pieces in the signaling puzzle; knowing the structure of different intermediates will no doubt simplify pathways that now seem hopelessly complex.

The completion of the Human Genome Project will facilitate our understanding of signal transduction because in the future we will at least have all the pieces of the puzzle in front of us and we will know their shapes. A useful strategy for starting a jigsaw puzzles is to find edge pieces; finding the middle pieces is often harder. We have put the edge pieces in place by identifying receptors and the proteins they interact with. The other edge of the puzzle, if you will, is DNA, and great progress has been made in identifying transcription factors. As our notions of signal transduction have evolved from second messenger models to protein–protein interaction schemes, a remaining challenge now is to completely fill in the middle part of the puzzle. This may seem more complicated now that we have more pieces to play with. However, we also have more robust tools like the yeast two-hybrid system for putting the pieces together; we will no doubt continue to develop more efficient tools for analysis of protein–protein interactions.

Continuing with this puzzle metaphor for the moment, a significant problem is that the Human Genome project will give us multiple puzzles intermixed. The cell obviously responds to many different signals from diverse receptors. Interestingly, a concept that has been considered since the 1960s is the importance of one signal versus two signals in lymphocyte activation. We now frame this question slightly differently referring to TCR-derived signals and costimulatory signals. But indeed the issue is much more complicated now as we know that this occurs in context of multiple signals arising from diverse receptors that bind other cell surface molecules and cytokines can provide positive or negative signals. A great challenge in the future will be to uncover improved techniques for studying integration of signaling; looking at Western blots probably will not solve this problem. Fortunately, there are solutions to the problem that are becoming apparent. Mapping protein–protein interactions can be done by the creation of fusion fluorescent proteins. Clearly, signaling will need to be visualized more in terms of cell biology.

Another central issue in signal transduction has been and will continue to be that of specificity. If one uses one's favorite cell and uses a good reagent, involvement of a particular player can often be demonstrated. But is it an important or essential piece? Early studies of calcium and phosphoinositide turnover demonstrated that this was pertinent to lymphocyte activation. But it is also true of many other cells; how does this event explain the great specificity that can be achieved by a given receptor? Morever, even if a given event can be shown to occur for a variety of receptors, how do we know that is it essential and for what pathways? The completion of the Human Genome Project will not help us with this problem; more likely than not it will exacerbate it. Fortunately, these issues can be nicely addressed with genetically engineered mice and cells. The importance of verifying the physiologic function of different intermediates in vivo will continue to be an essential issue in signal transduction. Equally interesting will be the contribution of these different intermediates to the pathogenesis of disease, as will the role of modifier genes on disease severity. Mouse genetics should be invaluable in attacking these problems.

References

1. Thaler, M. S., Klausner, R. D., and Cohen, H. J. (1977) *Medical Immunology.* J. B. Lippincott Co., Philadephia, PA.
2. Golub, E. S. (1981) *The Cellular Basis of the Immune Response,* 2nd ed. Sinauer Associates, Inc., Sunderland, MA.

3. Jensenius, J. C. and Williams, A. F. (1982) The T lymphocyte antigen receptor-paradigm lost. *Nature* **300,** 583–589.

4. Hedrick, S. M. and Eidelman, F. J. (1993) T lymphocyte antigen receptors in *Fundamental Immunology,* 3rd ed. (Paul, W., ed.), Raven, New York.

5. Bjorkman, P. J., Saper, M. A., Samraoui, B., Bennett, W. S., Strominger, J. L., and Wiley, D. C. (1987) Structure of the human MHC class I histocompatibility antigen, HLA-A2. *Nature* **329,** 506–512.

6. Harford, J. and Ashwell, G., (1985) Chemical and physical properties of the hepatic receptor for asialoglycoproteins, in *Endocytosis* (Pastan, I. and Willingham, M. C., eds.), Plenum Publishing, New York, pp. 69–83.

7. Metzger, H. (1977) The cellular receptor for IgE, in *Receptors and Recognition* (Cuatracasas, P. and Greaves, M. F., eds.), Wiley, New York, pp. 75–102.

8. Weiss, A. (1998) T lymphocye activation, in *Fundamental Immunology* 3rd ed. (Paul, W., ed.), Raven, New York, pp. 411–448.

9. Keegan, A. and Paul, W. E., (1998) Multichain immune recognition receptors: similarities in structure and signaling pathways. *Immunol. Today* **13,** 63–68.

10. Alberts, B., Bray, D., Lewis, J., Raff, M., Roberts, K., and Watson, J. D. (1994) *Molecular Biology of the Cell,* 3rd ed., Garland Publishing, New York.

11. Koch, C. A., Anderson, D., Moran, M., Ellis, C., and Pawson, T. (1991) SH2 and SH3 domains: elements that control interactions of cytoplasmic signaling proteins. *Science* **252,** 668–674.

12. Reth, M. (1989) Antigen receptor tail clue. *Nature* **338,** 383,384.

IV

T-CELL ACTIVATION

17

Measurement of Phosphatidylinositol (PI) Hydrolysis in Activated T Lymphocytes

Seth Mark Berney and T. Prescott Atkinson

1. Introduction

T-cell activation by antigen-receptor ligation results in rapid activation of phospholipase-Cγ1 (PLC). Activated PLC hydrolyzes membrane inositol phospholipids (PIP$_2$) generating two second messengers: inositol(1,4,5)tris phosphate (IP$_3$) and diacylglycerol (DG) *(1)*. IP$_3$ stimulates release of intracellularly stored Ca^{2+} resulting in the initial intracellular Ca^{2+} peak whereas, DAG activates protein kinase C (PKC) with an accompanying shift in that enzyme from cytosol to membrane **(Fig. 1)** *(2–5)*.

Previous techniques in the measurement of T-cell receptor-mediated activation of PLC have included estimation of the intracellular calcium concentration using fluorescent probes, such as Indo-1 (an indirect measure of IP$_3$ generation), or quantitation of IP$_3$ release using either anion exchange chromatography or high performance liquid chomatography (HPLC) *(7)*. However, IP$_3$ measurement by the above methods has low sensitivity, and poor labeling efficiency, and is relatively labor intensive. An additional IP$_3$ assay is available commercially in the form of a competitive radioligand binding assay (Amersham Life Science, Arlington Heights, IL). In this assay, unlabeled IP$_3$ (isolated from stimulated cells) competes with a known amount of ^{3}H-IP$_3$ for a fixed number of sites on bovine adrenal IP$_3$-binding proteins. The amount of ^{3}H bound to the binding protein is compared to a standard curve and the amount of cellular IP$_3$ is determined. However, this technique requires the investigator to isolate the IP$_3$ from the activated cells. This limits the utility of the assay in evaluating cell–cell interactions because of the difficulty isolating IP$_3$ from only the reacting cell, not the stimulating cell.

From: *Methods in Molecular Biology, Vol. 134: T Cell Protocols: Development and Activation*
Edited by: K. P. Kearse © Humana Press Inc., Totowa, NJ

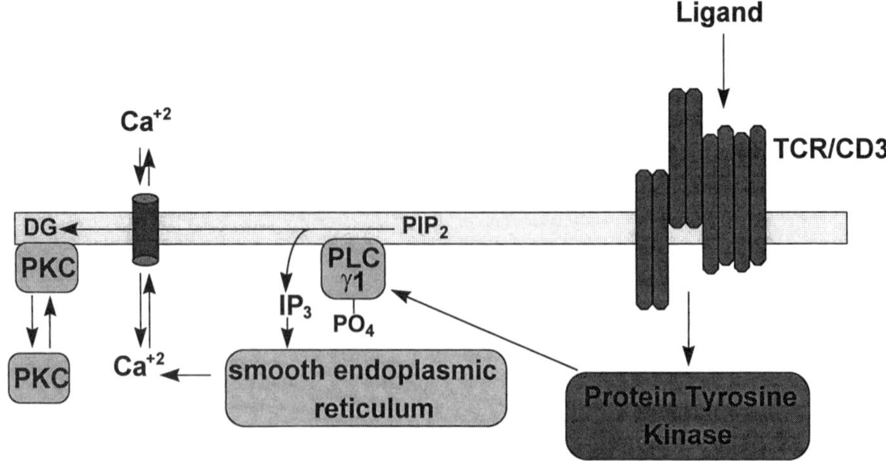

Fig. 1. T-cell receptor signaling begins with the ligand–receptor interaction, resulting in activation of protein tyrosine kinases that phosphorylate PLC-γ1, resulting in PIP$_2$ turnover, increased intracellular calcium [Ca^{2+}]$_i$, and protein kinase C (PKC) activation. PKC and [Ca^{2+}]$_i$ participate in the regulation of interleukin 2 (IL-2) gene transcription and IL-2 receptor gene transcription in T cells *(5,6)*.

Staphylococcal alpha hemolysin (α-toxin) is a protein that inserts into cell membranes forming 2–3 nm transmembrane pores. These pores only allow passage of molecules less than about 1000 Daltons in mol wt. Cells permeabilized with α-toxin generally exclude Trypan blue (mol wt = 960.8) and do not release large intracellular components, such as cytoplasmic LDH *(8)*. The inositol labeling step previously took 20 h by passive uptake, making prolonged cell culture a necessary step. Further, some cells, such as human T lymphocytes, label rather poorly by this method (unpublished observations, T. P. Atkinson). However, T cells permeabilized with α-toxin efficiently incorporate ^{3}H-myoinositol into membrane phospholipids over a period of 50 min. Lymphocytes labeled by this method remain fully capable of receptor-mediated PI hydrolysis, making this technique a useful and rapid means of analyzing the early signaling cascade.

In this chapter, we describe a method for the measurement of phosphatidylinositol hydrolysis by rapid incorporation of labeled inositol in α-toxin permeabilized cells *(9)*. Although this technique does not specifically measure IP$_3$, it measures total inositol phosphates released by receptor-mediated PI hydrolysis.

The procedure is divided into four steps:

1. T-cell purification.
2. Permeabilization and intracellular labeling with ^{3}H-myoinositol.

3. Cellular activation.
4. Measurement of PI hydrolysis.

2. Materials
2.1. T-Cell Purification

1. Phosphate-buffered saline (PBS), pH 7.2, without Ca^{2+} with 5% heat-inactivated fetal calf serum (CFS) (wash buffer).
2. Ficoll-Hypaque.
3. Cocktail containing antihuman CD14, CD19, and CD56 MAbs sufficient to brightly stain peripheral blood mononuclear cells (PBMCs) in dose response (*see* **Note 1**).
4. Goat antimouse IgG-magnetic beads (Miltenyi Biotech, Auburn, CA).
5. BS magnetic sorting column (Miltenyi Biotech).
6. 25-gage flow regulating needle (Miltenyi Biotech or any 25-gage sterile hypodermic needle).
7. Magnetic sorting magnet (Miltenyi Biotech).
8. Trypan blue (0.4% in PBS).
9. 70 or 95% ethyl alcohol (ETOH).
10. Hemocytometer (or other cell counting device).

2.2. Intracellular Labeling with ^{3}H-Myoinositol

1. 12×75 mm polypropylene tubes (Falcon, Franklin Lakes, NJ).
2. Permeabilization buffer (PB): 20 mM potassium PIPES (dipotassium salt), 50 mM potassium glutamate, 5 mM glucose, 7 mM magnesium acetate, and 1 mM EGTA in 500 mL ddH_2O, pH to 7.1. Filter and store at 4°C. (may be made as a 10X stock).
3. 1 M $CaCl_2$ in ddH_2O; filter and store at 4°C.
4. Heat inactivated FCS (Hyclone, Logan, UT).
5. Staphylococcal α-toxin stock (1.9 µg/mL) (Accurate Chemical and Scientific Corporation, Westbury, NY): Reconstitute one vial (0.25 mg) in 0.5 mL of 1X PB. Aliquot (25 µL) and freeze at –20°C.
6. 100 mM ATP (Boeringer Mannheim, Indianapolis, IN): Dissolve 5 g in 70 mL 0.2 N NaOH, adjust pH to 7.0 and adjust volume to 82.6 mL. Aliquot (500 µL) and freeze at –20°C.
7. ^{3}H-myoinositol (myo[2-^{3}H]inositol [19.1 Ci/mmol] [TRK 911 B27]) (Amersham Life Sciences, Arlington Heights, IL): **Radiation hazard**. Store at 4°C.

2.3. Cell Activation

1. 12×75 mm polypropylene tubes (Falcon).
2. 1X PB containing 0.1% heat-inactivated FCS and 0.24 mM $CaCl_2$ (0.1 µM free Ca^{2+}) *(10–12)*.
3. Goat-antimouse IgG (Southern Biotechnology Associates): 1 mg/mL (azide free).
4. Cell stimulus, e.g., anti-CD3 MAb.

5. LiCl (lithium chloride) (Fisher Chemicals, Houston, TX) (*see* **Note 2**).
6. Na_3VO_4 (sodium orthovanadate) (Fisher): 100 m*M* solution in PB (make fresh for each experiment) (made after cells are labeled because activity is not stable in solution). (*see* **Note 3**).
7. Stop solution:methanol: 4 *N* HCl:chloroform (200:2:100) (**toxic–keep covered**) (Fisher).

2.4. Measurement of PI Hydrolysis

1. Scintillation tubes (snap cap Bio Vials) (Beckman Instruments, Fulton, CA).
2. Scintillation counter.
3. Scintillation fluid (e.g., Ecolume, ICN, Costa Mesa, CA).
4. 0.1 *N* HCl.
5. Chloroform (**toxic–store in a ventilation hood**).

3. Methods

3.1. T Cell Purification

The following method has served in our laboratories as an efficient and reproducible way to isolate large numbers of human peripheral blood T lymphocytes at a high level of purity. Other methods may be equally satisfactory, the main objective being the isolation of the cells with as little prior activation as possible. Further, several tumor lines, including Jurkat and RBL-2H3, load and trigger well using this method.

1. Following standard (formerly known as universal precautions [*see* **Note 4**]) draw blood from donor (anticipate approx 10^6 PBMC/mL blood after Ficoll-Hypaque). Isolate PBMC by Ficoll-Hypaque density centrifugation and wash twice with wash buffer. Resuspend cells with approx 75–100 µL of the cocktail of anti-CD14, anti-CD19, and anti-CD56 MAb (to fully resuspend the cell pellet) and incubate on ice for 15 min.
2. Wash cells twice with ice-cold wash buffer, resuspend in 40 µL ice-cold wash buffer/10^7 cells and incubate 15 min on ice with 10 µL/10^7 cells of goat antimouse IgG-magnetic beads.
3. Wash cells once and resuspend in 500 µL cold wash buffer. Wash a BS magnetic sorting column with 50 µL of 70–95% ethanol followed by 100 mL wash buffer (to purge the column of air bubbles, which can slow the separation). Attach a three-way stop-cock to the column and a 25-gage needle to the stop-cock and flush the stop-cock and needle with wash buffer (to purge air bubbles). Apply the cell suspension to the top of the column and allow the cell suspension to run into the column. Wash the column with 25 mL wash buffer and collect the effluent from the needle at the bottom.
4. For care of column *see* **Note 5**.

3.2. Intracellular Labeling with ^{3}H-Myoinositol

1. Wash the T-cell-enriched column effluent three times with PB containing 0.1% heat inactivated FCS and 0.24 m*M* $CaCl_2$ (0.1 µ*M* free Ca^{2+}) and count. Resus-

pend the cells in a 12×75 mm polypropylene tube with 1 mL of same PB containing 50 µL ATP, 10 mL ^{3}H-myoinositol, and 15.6 µL α-toxin per 3×10^7 cells.
2. Incubate the cells in a 37°C water bath for 50 min.
3. Gently wash the cells three times with PB containing 0.1% heat-inactivated FCS and 0.24 mM CaCl$_2$ to remove all unincorporated [^{3}H]-myoinositol and count with a hemocytometer with Trypan blue to assess viability. Remember the wash buffer is now radioactive and must be discarded appropriately.

3.3. Cell Activation

The technique used to activate the cells obviously depends on the cell type and the receptor(s) being studied. We describe a method below that has provided reproducible and easily measured PI hydrolysis by aggregation of the T-cell receptor CD3 complex.

1. A dose-response experiment is useful to identify the optimal final concentration of the primary and secondary (crosslinking) antibodies. Dilute the anti-CD3 MAb (we use OKT3) and isotype control MAb in working PB to 22X the desired final concentration. We use a final concentration of approx 2 ng/mL anti-CD3 antibody and at least a fivefold molar excess of the secondary antibody.
2. Resuspend the cells in either a 15 mL conical tube or a 50 mL conical tube (depending on the final cell volume needed) at $1–5 \times 10^6$ cells/mL PB containing 50 µL ATP/ mL (final concentration 5 mM) and 10 mM LiCl. Each sample tube will receive 200 µL of cell solution.
3. Place 10 µL of each diluted MAb into the bottom of 12×75 mm polypropylene tubes in triplicate.
4. Place 10 µL of the tyrosine phosphatase inhibitor sodium orthovanadate (Na$_3$VO$_4$) (final concentration 4.8 mM) into the bottom of triplicate 12×75 mm polypropylene tubes.
5. Add room temperature cell suspension (200 µL) to each tube at timed intervals, vortex gently, and incubate in a 37°C water bath for total of 10 min (*see* **Note 6**). After 2 min incubation, add 10 µL goat antimouse IgG to each tube to further crosslink the surface receptors. Gently vortex and replace into the water bath for the remainder of the 10 min incubation.
6. After the 10 min incubation add 750 µL stop solution to each tube, gently vortex, cap, and place in rack at room temperature.

3.4. Measurement of PI Hydrolysis

1. Add 250 µL 0.1 N HCl and 250 µL chloroform to each tube, cap tightly, vortex, and centrifuge at 51g for 5 min.
2. Decant 750 µL of the aqueous phase (upper phase containing soluble inositol phosphates) and quantitate using a scintillation counter.
3. Transfer the entire organic phase (lower phase containing inositol phospholipids) to empty scintillation vials, place a in chemical/ventilation hood until all solvent has evaporated (overnight), then quantitate using a scintillation counter.

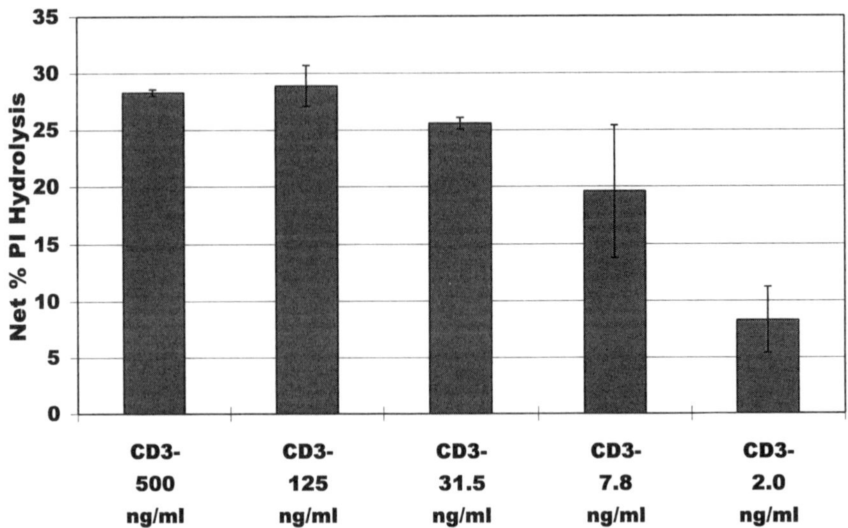

Fig. 2. Freshly isolated human T cells were incubated with either negative isotype control MAb for anti-CD3 MAb, or anti-CD3 MAb (labeled CD3) at varying concentrations or orthovanadate (labeled VO4) for 10 min at 37°C. After 2 min of incubation, goat antimouse IgG antibody (15 µg/mL) was added to each sample. Each datapoint represents the mean of triplicate samples + SD. The *y*-axis is labeled net % PI hydrolysis.

4. Percent PI hydrolysis = aqueous DPM/(aqueous DPM + organic DPM) × 100%. Aqueous DPM = measured aqueous × 915/750 (total aqueous volume is approx 915 µL and only 750 µL was decanted). Net percent PI hydrolysis is obtained by subtracting the PI hydrolysis measured in the isotype control tubes (*see* **Note 7**) (**Fig. 2**) (**Table 1**).

4. Notes

1. Prior to sorting, the optimal concentrations of anti-CD14, anti-CD19, and anti-CD56 MAb need to be determined. The optimal concentration saturates the monocyte's, B cell's, and NK cell's surface receptors (respectively) by flow cytometry. This will prevent wasting the antibody and minimize the chance of cell contamination.
2. Lithium chloride acts to prevent cellular recycling of the inositol phosphates into phospholipid *(13)*.
3. Sodium orthovanodate is used as a positive control because its phosphatase inhibition results in unopposed kinase activity and therefore maximal PLC-γ1 activation and PI hydrolysis *(14)*.
4. Standard precautions refer to the precautions employed when handling human body fluid and tissue samples. "Standard precautions synthesize the major features of Universal (Blood and Body Fluid) precautions (designed to reduce

Table 1
PI Hydrolysis Data and Calculations

	Aqueous DPM	Aqueous corrected DPM	Organic	Total DPM	% PI hydrolysis	Average	SD	Net % PI hydrolysis
G2a	578	705	3972	4678	15.1	14.5	0.7	0.0
	559	682	4371	5053	13.5			
	635	775	4450	5224	14.8			
CD3-	2201	2685	3544	6229	43.1	42.8	0.3	28.3
500 ng/mL	2258	2755	3676	6431	42.8			
	2262	2760	3750	6510	42.4			
125 ng/mL	2266	2765	3309	6073	45.5	43.4	1.8	28.9
	2182	2662	3456	6118	43.5			
	1954	2384	3412	5796	41.1			
31.5 ng/mL	1769	2158	3310	5468	39.5	40.1	0.5	25.6
	1862	2272	3389	5661	40.1			
	1866	2277	3320	5597	40.7			
7.8 ng/mL	1499	1829	5238	7067	25.9	34.1	5.8	19.6
	1563	1907	3089	4996	38.2			
	1568	1913	3096	5009	38.2			
2 ng/mL	1300	1586	4351	5937	26.7	22.7	2.9	8.3
	1089	1329	5424	6753	19.7			
	1183	1443	5172	6615	21.8			

the risk of transmission of bloodborne pathogens) and Body Substance Precautions (designed to reduce the risk of transmission of pathogens from moist body substances)." Gloves are recommended for anticipated contact with blood and specified body fluids, and hands are to be washed immediately after gloves are removed *(15)*.

5. After each sort attach a 60-mL syringe to the stop-cock and vigorously aspirate 300–400 mL of tap water followed by 120 mL of soapy water through the column. Soak the column in soapy water for at least 30 min and rinse out the soap by reaspirating the column with 300 mL of water using the syringe. Last, to minimize the chance of rust formation, aspirate the column with 50–100 mL of 70% EtOH, dry it using wall suction, and store it in a desiccator. This will help preserve the column for multiple uses. However, if rust forms on the metal meshwork within the column the efficiency will change and the column should be discarded. We have used a single column for 15–20 sorts.

6. A repeating pipeter allows for rapid, consistent delivery of the cell suspension. We typically dispense the cell suspension to 4 tubes every 15 s.

7. If increased background occurs (PI hydrolysis with the isotype control MAb) the cells could be already partially stimulated (as seen in sick individuals, roughly handled cells, or some cell lines). High background can also result from too long a stimulation time, stimulation at a high temperature (e.g., 39–40°C), or possibly from stimulation of contaminating B cells or monocytes via their Fc receptors (which nonspecifically bind the isotype control antibody). Low signal could result from too short a triggering time, a water bath that is too cold, insufficient labeling, insufficient ATP during the labeling or triggering step, or problems related to the primary or secondary antibody concentrations. The extent of PI hydrolysis is directly related to the number of receptors per cell and the extent of crosslinking.

This method is potentially applicable to any surface receptor that signals via PI hydrolysis and may be useful in investigating the integrity of normal receptor signaling pathways and the disorders brought about by defects in those pathways.

References

1. Weiss, A. (1993) *Fundamental Immunology*, 3rd ed.: *T Lymphocyte Activation* (Paul, W. E., ed.) Raven, New York, p. 467.
2. Imboden, J. and Stobo, J. D. (1985) Transmembrane signaling by the T cell antigen receptor. Perturbation of the T3 antigen receptor complex generates inositol phosphates and releases calcium ions from intracellular stores. *J. Exp. Med.* **161,** 446.
3. Nishizuka, Y. (1984) The role of protein kinase C in cell surface signal transduction and tumour promotion. *Nature* **308,** 693.
4. Farrar, W. L. and Ruscetti, F. W. (1986) Association of protein kinase C activation with IL-2 receptor expression. *J. Immunol.* **136,** 1266.
5. Manger, B., Weiss, A., Imboden, J., Laing, T., and Stobo, J. D. (1987) The role of protein kinase C in transmembrane signaling by the T cell antigen receptor complex. *J. Immunol.* **139,** 2755.

6. Imboden, J. B. and Weiss, A. (1987) The T-cell antigen receptor regulates sustained increases in cytoplasmic free Ca^{2+} through extracellular Ca^{2+} influx and ongoing intracellular Ca^{2+} mobilization. *Biochem. J.* **247,** 695.

7. Imboden, J., Shoback, D. M., and Inokuchi, S. (1993) *Current Protocols in Immunology, Vol. 2, Analysis of Inositol Phospholipid Turnover During Lymphocyte Activation.* (Coligan, J. E., Kruisbeek, A. M., Margulies, D. H., Shevach, E. M., and Strober, W., eds.), Wiley, New York, p. 11.1.1.

8. Ahnert-Hilger, G., Bhakdi, S., and Gratzl, M. (1985) Minimal requirements for exocytosis. A study using PC12 cells permeabilized with staphylococcal α-toxin. *J. Biol. Chem.* **260,** 12,730.

9. Berney, S. M. and Atkinson, T. P. (1995) Phosphatidylinositol hydrolysis in freshly isolated human lymphocytes. *J. Immunol. Methods* **186(1),** 71–77.

10. Hohman, R. (1988) Aggregation of IgE receptors induces degranulation in rat basophilic leukemia cells permeabilized with alpha-toxin from *Staphylococcus aureus. Proc. Natl. Acad. Sci. USA* **85,** 1624.

11. Hohman, R., Hultsch, T., and Talbot, E. (1990) IgE receptor-mediated phosphatidylinositol hydrolysis and exocytosis from rat basophilic leukemia cells are independent of extracellular Ca^{++} in a hypotonic buffer containing a high concentration of K^+. *J. Immunol.* **145,** 3876.

12. Atkinson, T. P., Kaliner, M. A., and Hohman, R. J. (1992) Phospholipase C-γ1 is translocated to the membrane of rat basophilic leukemia cells in response to aggregation of IgE receptors. *J. Immunol.* **148,** 2194.

13. Majerus, P. W. (1992) Inositol phosphate biochemistry. *Annu. Rev. Biochem.* **61,** 225–250.

14. Atkinson, T. P., Lee, C., Rhee, S., and Hohman, R. (1993) Orthovanadate induces translocation of phospholipase c-γ1 and -γ2 in permeabilized mast cells. *J. Immunol.* **151,** 1448.

15. Hospital Infection Control Practices Advisory Committee, Part 1. Evolution of Isolation Practices. February 18, 1997. From Center for Disease Control; Internet Homepage.

18

Fluorescence Polarization as an Early Measure of T-Lymphocyte Stimulation

Mordechai Deutsch, Naomi Zurgil,
Menachem Kaufman, and Gideon Berke

1. Introduction

Transmembrane stimulation of lymphocytes at the G_o-G_1 resting phase, induced by specific antigens, mitogens, or by antibodies to certain cell surface molecules, results in a complex series of well-characterized molecular events, culminating in lymphocyte activation, transformation, mitosis, and finally apoptosis *(1–3)*. These events are associated with early changes in membrane potential, coupled with an Na^+ influx, and with changes in pH, followed by the influx and internal release of Ca^{2+} ions. The processes linking early and late intracellular events in the course of cell activation involve conformational changes of cytosolic enzymes and/or their regulatory proteins, as well as their intracellular matrix reorganization *(4–6)*. The monitoring of these early structural changes can be performed by measuring the fluorescence polarization (FP) of intracellular fluorescent probes *(7–13)*. Specific fluorescence probes such as diphenyl hexatriene (DPH) and fluorescein diacetate (FDA) have been used to measure membrane fluidity *(14,15)* and changes in the cytoplasmic microviscosity *(7)*, respectively.

A relatively high degree of intrinsic intracellular fluorescein FP is found in many cells at their G_o-G_1 resting state *(16)*. A decrease in FP has been observed after cell stimulation *(10,12,17,18)* as well as while the cells are subjected to changes in the osmolality of the medium *(13)*. Other factors that may cause an alteration of FP include physiological changes induced by stimulation *(8,10,11)*; progression through cell cycle phases *(16)*, and the influence of stimulation inhibitors *(19)*, cytokines *(17)*, and viral infection *(20)*. In addition, FP has been used to monitor pre-lytic events in conjugated effector and target cells *(21)*.

From: *Methods in Molecular Biology, Vol. 134: T Cell Protocols: Development and Activation*
Edited by: K. P. Kearse © Humana Press Inc., Totowa, NJ

In **Subheading 1.1.** we briefly review fluorescence, fluorescence lifetime, and FP. This is followed by a discussion of a few applications of FP for monitoring T lymphocyte activation using intracellular fluorescent probes for FP measurements.

1.1. Fluorescence Transitions

Fluorescence and phosphorescence are events concerned with light emission from excited molecules after their relaxation to the lowest energy state. Excitation is a change of state resulting from the rapid absorption of energy. The sources for this energy are numerous and may be chemical, radioactive, or a light source (laser, incandescent lamps, and so forth). The laws of quantum mechanics dictate that discrete energy states and energy are expressed in the form of electronic, vibrational, rotational, translational electron spin orientation, and nuclear spin orientation. Fluorescence is related to the electronic state and its associated set of vibrational states.

The initial state of a molecule before excitation is usually the singlet ground electronic state, S_0. In many, if not most instances, after absorption, the excitation energy is lost as heat to the surroundings. This occurs through nonradiative transitions (intersystem crossing, internal conversion), that convert molecular electronic energy into vibrational energy and allow the excited molecule to relax to its ground state level.

The transitional processes resulting in fluorescence are shown in the Jablonski diagram *(22)* (**Fig. 1**). A relaxed molecule at room temperature is normally at the (lowest) ground state, S_0. A light photon is absorbed with the appropriate energy, whereby a transition to any one of several probable vibrational states and a higher electronic state (i.e., S_1, S_2,) occurs in approx 10^{-15} s. Shortly afterwards (~10^{-12} s), the molecule in a radiationless process relaxes (loses energy) to the lowest vibrational state in S_1. This process is termed internal conversion. Within an average time of usually 10^{-7}–10^{-9} s, the molecules again relax to one of the vibrational states of S_0, while emitting a photon, in a process defined as fluorescence. The energy of the emitted photon is thus lower than that of the exciting photon, resulting in an energy shift called stock shift *(23)*. The radiationless processes also participate in the evacuation of the excited state, thereby reducing its population and decreasing the observed Fluorescence Intensity (FI). FI therefore depends on the relative rates of the other competing processes. If fluorescence is the only means of depopulating the excited state, then this is kinetically a first-order process, in which the fluorescence relaxation time, τ_F, refers to a bulk property, measuring how long the molecules exist in a particular state. **Fig. 1** summarizes some of the pathways and typical values of their transition life times.

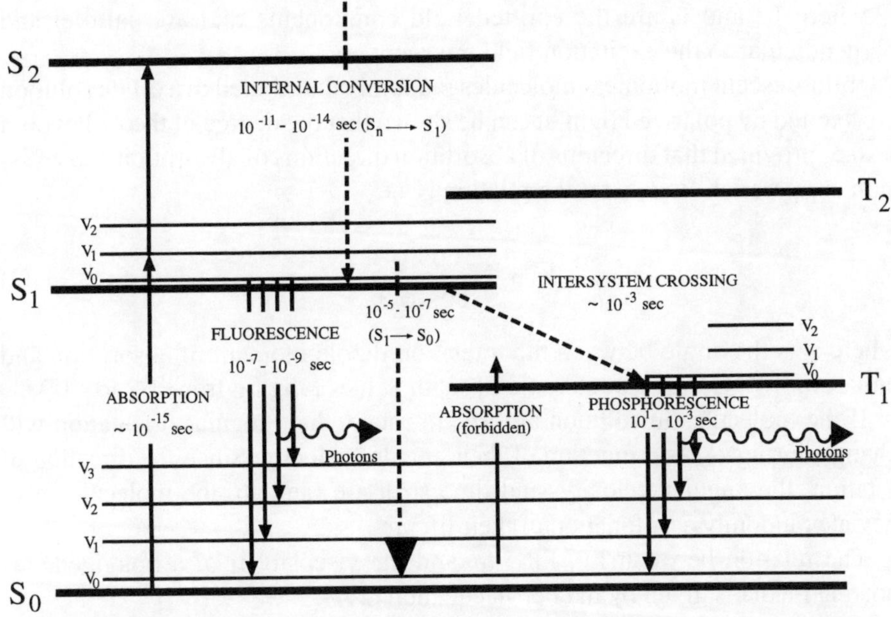

Fig. 1. Jablonsky schematic energy level diagram: S and T are electronic levels. V is the vibronic level. S_0 is the ground electronic state. Broken lines symbolize radiationless transitions and the wavy line the photon emission.

1.2. Fluorescence Polarization

Light is an electromagnetic wave whose vibrating electric and magnetic field vectors are perpendicular to one another and to the direction of the wave propagation. An emitting molecule acts as a dipole antenna transmitting electromagnetic waves. The direction of the vector of the emitted vibrating electronic field is defined as its polarization. Let us consider such a transmitting molecular antenna in the center of a sphere, its axes pointing N-S (North South). Its field would be symmetrical with respect to the antenna axes, its strength maximal at the equatorial, and 0 at the N-S direction. The same applies for the absorption of polarized radiation, where the absorbing probability distribution is not uniform. This distribution is termed photoselection, since it is directly related to the angle between the exciting field and the antenna, as $\cos^2\theta$.

The degree of the emission polarization is defined as

$$FP = \frac{(I_\parallel - I_\perp)}{(I_\parallel + I_\perp)} ,$$

(1)

where $I_{||}$ and $I_{\perp}$ are the emitted field components that are parallel and perpendicular to the excitation field, respectively.

If fluorescent motionless molecules randomly distributed in a dilute solution are excited by polarized light, it can be shown that the degree of their FP would be 0.5, provided that directons of absorbtion directions of absorption and emission are parallel. In general the relation is

$$FP_0 = \frac{3\cos^2\phi - 1}{\cos^2\phi + 3} \, ,\tag{2}$$

where ϕ is the angle between the transition dipole moment of absorption and emission. FP_0 is the characteristic FP with values ranging from $1/2$ to $-1/3$.

If the molecules in solution are free to rotate, their angular orientation will change during τ_F, as a function of their angular velocity. Since the direction of rotation, the angular velocity, and time span are random, the molecules also deviate randomly as a function of their lifetime.

The relation between FP, FP_0, τ_F, and the viscosity η of a homogeneous hosting media is given by the Perrin equation *(24)*

$$\frac{1}{FP} - \frac{1}{3} = \left(\frac{1}{FP_0} - \frac{1}{3}\right)\left(1 + \frac{RT}{\eta V}\, t_F\right),\tag{3}$$

where V is the molar volume of a spherical probe, R is the gas constant, and T the absolute temperature.

$$\left(\frac{RT}{\eta V}\right)^{-1}\tag{4}$$

is defined as τ_R, the rotational correlation time of the probe. The latter is the most dominant and variable reflecting environmental changes such as temperature, viscosity, mobility, and probe-binding as monitored by FP. Clearly, when $T/\eta \to 0$, $FP \to FP_0$.

Fluorescence and FP are powerful techniques that are used in biology and biochemistry for measuring molecular interactions, conformational changes, and chemical reactions. Specifically, the sensitivity of this technique stems from both the stock shift (*see above*), which enables the easy discrimination between the excitation and emitted fluorescence signals, and from the fact that many of these reactions and processes that affect the fluorescence and FP take place on the same time scale as the fluorescence lifetimes.

2. Materials

2.1. Cell Separation

A lymphocyte-rich fraction is isolated from heparinized or citrated peripheral blood lymphocytes (PBL) by ficoll density-gradient centrifugation. Separation procedures based on membrane antigens (receptors) such as the use of antibody-coated magnetic beads or other adhesive surfaces are not recommended (*see* **Note 1**).

2.2. Fluorescent Probes

Most of the FP measurements are carried out with fluorescein derivatives (carboxyfluorescein [CF], carboxymethyl fluorescein [CMF], 2',7'-bis-[carboxyethyl]-5-[6']-(carboxyfluorescein [BCECF]), since they all have a high fluorescent quantum yield in physiological media as well as emission spectra that can be conveniently detected.

2.3. Staining Solutions

Staining solutions prepared by dissolving nonfluorescent esters of the fluorescein derivatives mentioned above (*see* **Note 2**) (e.g., FDA, carboxyfluorescein diacetate [CFDA], carboxymethyl fluorescein diacetate [CMFDA], and 2',7'-bis-[carboxyethyl]-5-(6')-carboxy-fluorescein acetoxymethylester [BCECF/AM], *see* **Note 3**) in acetic acid or in dimethyl sulfoxide (DMSO) and only then diluted in phosphate-buffered saline (PBS) to yield a staining solution of about 0.6 μM (*see* **Note 4**). If acetic acid is used as the solvent, correction of the pH is done with either $Na_2HPO_4.12H_2O$ or NaOH.

2.4. FI and FP Standards

Three main sources are used as FI and FP standards:

1. Fluorescent beads (*see* **Note 5**).
2. Viscous fluorescent glycerol-water solutions (40, 50, 60, 65, 70, 75, 80, and 85%) (*see* **Note 6**).
3. Long-life absolute intensity standard (*see* **Note 7**).

3. Methods

3.1. Principal Methods of FP Measurements

Intracellular FP measurements can be usually carried out in three ways:

1. On cell suspension in a cuvet using spectrofluorimeters with FP accessories,
2. On single-cells using a flow-through system (flow cytometers), and
3. On individual cells using a static cytometer such as the CellScan, described in **Subheading 3.2.**

In both the cuvet and flow-through modes, the FP is measured at a 90° angle to the propagation of the excitation beam, minimizing the scattered light signal. However, in the CellScan, FI is measured at 180° using an epi-fluorescence microscope.

3.2. FI and FP Measurement by the CellScan Apparatus

1. The CellScan apparatus: The CellScan apparatus was developed with the objective of enabling repetitive FP measurements on individual cells, such as lymphocytes *(25)*. Since most of the examples presented here were analyzed by the CellScan, some of its essential features are described in detail. The apparatus has three principal components:

   a. A cell carrier, consisting of a grid of precisely dimensioned and contoured microscopic holes on a flat surface, which captures cells of a desired size and holds them in place for repeated analyses. The carrier, used for lymphocytes, has holes approx 8 µm in diameter, spaced 20 µm apart; a 2-mm squared grid can hold 10,000 cells, each located in a separate trap (**Fig. 2**).

   b. A motor-driven, microscope stage that holds and moves the cell carrier.

   c. A micro-photometer comprised of a blue laser light source, microscopic optics for illuminating the sample and collecting fluorescent light, and four photomultiplier tubes and associated optical and electronic equipment for measuring FP at two emission wavelengths.

2. General check-up: Essential requirements to ensure proper performance of the CellScan include:

   a. Check of polarizer alignment, carried out both by the reference polarizer and the standardized viscous fluorescent solutions;

   b. Alignment of cell carrier axes to define the initial coordinate points and the movement scale factor;

   c. Background measurements including dark current, autofluorescence, and fluorescence background of the working solutions;

   d. Determination of the optical system depolarization factor, to correct for distortions of FP because of the numerical aperture of the microscope objective, and asymmetric optical pass;

   e. Persistence and reproducibility tests (*see* **Note 8**); and

   f. Sensitivity tests (*see* **Note 9**).

3. Standardization: Standardization of the CellScan operation involves a few steps, some of which are performed before each run, whereas others are done daily or only as a part of maintenance. The standardization procedure incorporated in the software notifies the user of the need to perform a certain procedure and guides him through it. This includes real-time measurements, presentation of results, and comparison with internal standards incorporated in the machine.

4. FI and FP measurements: In the CellScan, FI measurements are made by the photon-counting technique. Instead of measuring all cells at fixed time intervals (preset time, as used in cuvet and flow-through systems), and determining FI from the output levels of the detectors, each cell is monitored for the time required to detect a preset number of photoelectrons at each detector. Thus, the FI is readily calculated, which is inversely proportional to the monitoring time. Because the number of photoelectrons counted is preset, the precision of the measurements is the same for all cells; coefficients of variation (CVs) are typically <2%, allowing small changes in polarization to be readily detected (*see* **Note 10**). A PC, with

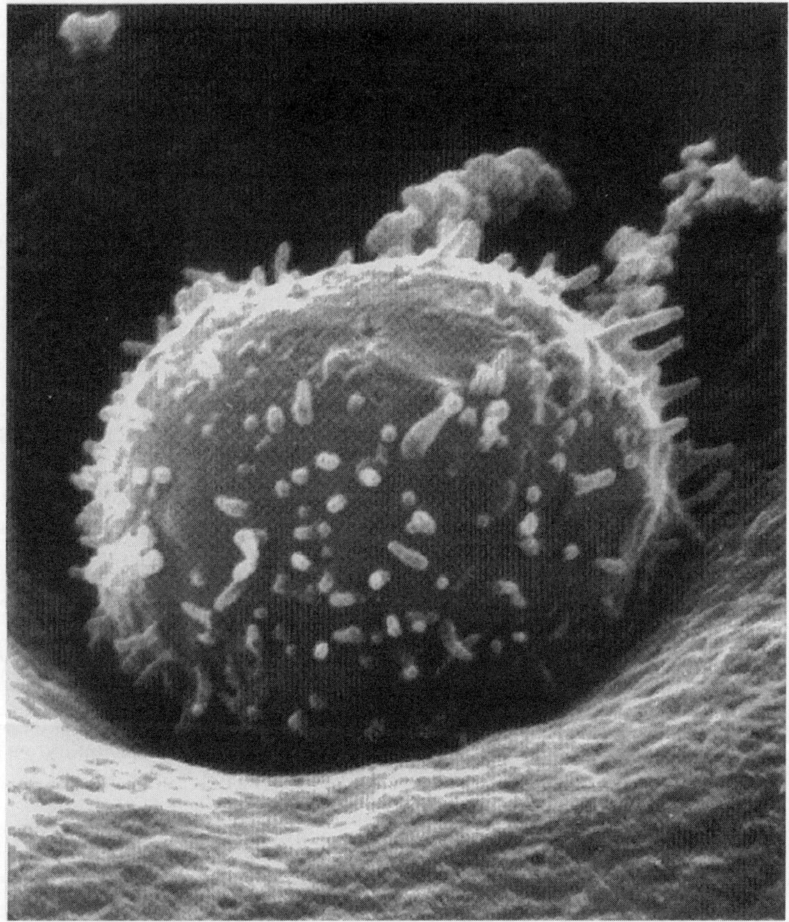

Fig. 2. A lymphocyte after settling in the cell carrier.

associated electronics, controls the motion of the microscopic stage and the steps in the measurement, and is also used for data collection, analysis, and display.

5. Data analyses: Acquired data is displayed on-line, as well as graphically and numerically. The software determines all test limits, before, during, and after the scan. All on-line statistics are displayed during the tests, as well as numerous numerical and graphic screens, e.g., histograms and scatter diagrams.

Three parameters are considered in measuring fluorescence emission from cells: fluorescence intensity (I), polarization (P), and measurement time (t). Classification of subgroups of cells may be based on any one of these parameters. The CS-*S* software provides tools that use visual analysis for cell classification. Once a cluster has been identified, it can be bounded by one or more methods:

   a. *Box mode*, whereby the position of the data is bound by cursors on the x- and y- axes;

   b. *Polygon mode*, which creates a data region bound by up to 10 vertices.

   c. The *point mode*, in which by pointing and marking a single-cell, the operator may include or exclude any of the measured cells depicted on the screen.

6. Kinetic analyses: Kinetic parameters are derived by applying both linear and nonlinear modeling. The linear model, $y(t) = at + b$, looks for the parameters a and b of the linear equation, where $y(t)$ is the measured quantity, t is the time, and a and b are the calculated parameters. The CS-S algorithm uses χ^2 as the criterion for the correctness-of-fit. Nonlinear modeling is done by least square fits using the Levenberg-Marquardt method. Two models are used: $y(t) = ae^{-bt}$ and $y(t) = a(1 - e^{-bt})$.

7. Mode of FI and FP measurements: For static and kinetic FI and FP measurements, specific procedures should be followed, which include sample loading on the cell carrier, cell staining, and rinsing *(25)*. Procedures for measuring the kinetic parameters of cells in the CS-S are as follows:

   a. Continuous measurements: a simple measurement sequence of the cells under study is taken and cells of the same clusters (determined by the use of nontemporal parameters) are then compared with them by their time sequence. Time-dependent parameters are derived by observing and calculating this relationship on a time scale plot of the results.

   b. Repetitive measurements: the cells under study are repeatedly measured and each measurement is accurately timed. The kinetic parameters are then directly determined for each individual cell. Cells can be classified by grouping according to kinetic parameters. This measurement method enables a statistically valid, short-time kinetic analysis of a cell population, along with analyzing the kinetics of individual cells in that population.

For some relevant measurements of lymphocyte activation by FI and FP performed on the CellScan, the reader is referred to Notes 11–13.

3.3. Monitoring FP of a Cell Suspension in a Cuvet

3.3.1. Spectrofluorimeters for FP Measurement on Cell Suspension in a Cuvet

FP measurements of cell suspension in a cuvet is usually carried out on spectrofluorimeters having either an L- or T-shaped optical arrangement. In both modes, detection is performed perpendicularly to the propagation of the exciting beam. In the L-shaped configuration, only one detector is used. Thus $I_{||}$ and $I_{\perp}$ are commonly measured consecutively by rotating the emission polarizer. Using the T shape, $I_{||}$ and $I_{\perp}$ can be recorded simultaneously. A schematic diagram of the two set-ups and their characteristic charts is given in **Fig. 3**.

3.3.2. Instrument Standardization

Standardization includes:

1. Polarizer alignment that ensures a perpendicular and parallel alignment between excitation and emission polarizers;

2. Grating-factor (G) determination for unequal transmission of the two polarization components;
3. Scattered light check-up (*see* **Note 4**); and
4. Determination of the fluorescence background of the staining solution, a problem stemming from the spontaneous hydrolysis of the acetic groups of the fluorescein derivatives.

3.3.3. Principal Measurement Procedures
of the FI and FP of Cell Suspensions in a Cuvet

Cuvet FP measurements of cells is carried out as follows (please refer to **Fig. 3**): after setting the excitation wavelength to 470 ± 20 nm and the emission to 510 ± 5 nm, 4 mL glass cuvets are placed into the thermostated holder in the measuring compartment (*see* **Note 15**) and filled with 3.5 mL of staining solution. When the temperature of the solution reaches 22°C, 0.2 mL of cell suspension (s) (6×10^6 cells/mL), incubated with and without (control) stimulant, is gently injected into the cuvet and the FI $I_\parallel^s\,(t)$ and $I_\perp^s\,(t)$ are recorded for about 5 min, or until $I_\perp^s\,(t)$ reaches approx 80% of the full scale used. To correct for extracellular fluorescein fluorescence due to leakage during measurements,
1. The cells must be quickly filtered away from the suspension on millipore paper (2 μm pore size) via suction by applying no more than 40 mm of Hg vacuum and collecting the filtrate;
2. The filtrate (F) background FP components, $I_\perp(F)$ and $I_\parallel(F)$ are measured using the same meticulously washed cuvet (*see* **Note 16**).

To calculate the cellular FP, the whole cell suspension (s) intensities, $I_\parallel^s\,(t)$ and $I_\perp^s\,(t)$ are first extrapolated to the half time of the filtration duration ($t_{1/2}$) and is calculated as follows:

$$FP = \frac{[\,I_\parallel^s\,(t_{1/2}) - I_\parallel\,(F)\,] - G\,[\,I_\perp^s\,(t_{1/2}) - I_\perp\,(F)]}{[\,I_\parallel^s\,(t_{1/2}) - I_\parallel\,(F)\,] + G\,[\,I_\perp^s\,(t_{1/2}) - I_\perp\,(F)]} \tag{5}$$

and the percentage of depolarization following stimulation equals

$$\frac{FP_{(control)} - FP_{(stimulant)}}{FP_{(control)}} \tag{6}$$

For examples of monitoring mitogenic activation of lymphocytes and their cell cycle, the reader is referred to **Notes 17** and **18**.

4. Notes

1. The use of antibody-coated magnetic beads as other adhesive surfaces are not recommended since they might induce undesired stimulation which will be detected by FP measurements.

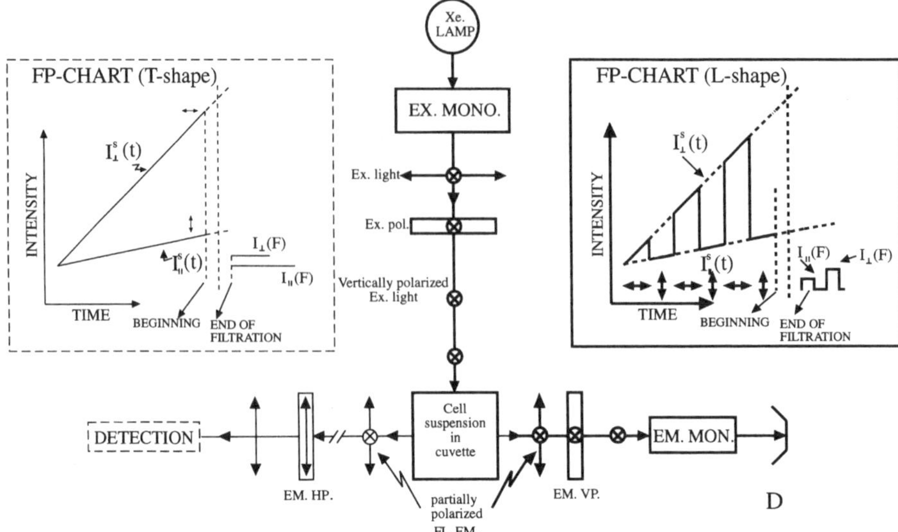

Fig. 3. Schematic upper view of L and T optical arrangement for cuvet FP measurements. L-shaped system constructed as the "L" part of the figure, illustrated in bold lines. The FI $I_\parallel^s(t)$ and $I_\perp^s(t)$ was measured consecutively by rotating the emission polarizer. A representative chart of this arrangement is given in the upper-right frame in the figure where the emission polarizer orientation is indicated by the small arrows under the chart lines. In the T-shaped system the left part (thin lines) of the optical arrangement is included. This allows simultaneous measurement of I‖(t) and I⊥(t), as representatively shown in the upper-left frame. Nomenclature: EX.MONO and EM.MON stand for excitation and emission monochromator, respectively. Ex.pol. for excitation polarizer, FL.EM. for fluorescence emission, EM.VP. and EM.HP. for vertical and horizontal emission polarizer, respectively, and D for Detector.

2. Since fluorescein is strongly fluorescent in water, its presence in the medium causes a prohibitively high fluorescent background, thus rendering the measurement of FP in cells impossible. To minimize this difficulty, nonfluorescent fluorescein esters are used.

3. The nonfluorescent fluorescein esters diffuse easily into cells, where they are converted enzymatically into fluorescent fluorescein derivatives. The extent of leakage differs for each of these derivatives. For example, BCECF leaks slowly compared to fluorescein, since under physiological conditions it holds 4–5 extra negative charges compared to one in fluorescein. The penetration, conversion, and accumulation of such dyes is called fluorochromasia *(26)*.

4. The acetic derivatives of fluorescein (as well as other fluorophores) are only slightly soluble in water. Therefore, they must be first dissolved in acetic acid or in DMSO at the concentration range of few m*M*, and only then diluted in PBS.

5. In choosing fluorescent beads as FI and FP standards, the following features should be noted:
   a. Beads with broad-band emission spectra to allow detection by all channels, as well as narrow band emission for testing separate channels;
   b. A homogeneous scattering characteristic having a round shape and accurate size, with minimal adsorbance of the bead material;
   c. Good stability and easy storage over time;
   d. Scattering and FI similar to those of living lymphocytes.
6. The FI of such solutions should be in the range emanating from stained lymphocytes.
7. As a long-life absolute intensity standard, the use of a ^{3}H-fluorescent ('beta light') tube is recommended.
8. To ensure proper performance, it is recommended to periodically run persistence and reproducibility tests, which should yield an average FP per bead or cell not exceeding 2.5 and 3%, respectively. An example of such a persistence and reproducibility test is given in **Fig. 4**. It shows the results of 25 routine scans of a field of 10×10 traps of fluorescent beads and 10 scans of FDA-stained lymphocytes. For each bead or cell, the persistence on the carrier, FP values, and CV are presented in panels I, II, and III, respectively. Note that although the particles have been rinsed throughout the scans, no beads have been lost (reflected by the length of the persistence lines, **Fig. 4A, I**) and the majority of the cells have survived the ten measurements (**Fig. 4B, I**).
9. The sensitivity of the CellScan in detecting minute changes of FP is tested by monitoring the changes in FP resulting from alterations in microviscosity induced by varying osmolarity. Varying medium osmolarity brings about changes in the water content of the cells and consequently in intracellular viscosity. An example is illustrated with a sample cell in **Fig. 5**. FP increases when the cell is rinsed (R) with a buffer of 0.350 osmol/Kg and decreases at 0.250 osmol/Kg.
10. The flexible sampling time in the CellScan enables the use of very low excitation intensities and low dye concentrations. In addition, the cells are held gently in traps (**Fig. 2**), minimizing problems in FI and FP measurements related to shear forces.
11. Mitogenic stimulation of lymphocytes results in changes in their intracellular microviscosity; the degree of change is quantifiable and can be calculated by single-cell or population analyses. Changes of FP were observed after phytohemagglutinin (PHA) (and ConA) stimulation. Lymphocytes isolated from peripheral blood were stimulated with PHA, and analyzed by the CellScan. **Fig. 6** shows a three-dimensional histogram of FP vs FI before and after PHA stimulation. A substantial decrease in FP and an increase in FI accompanied lymphocyte activation with PHA.

Using the CS-*S*, the characteristic kinetic behavior of FDA hydrolysis was observed after lymphocyte activivation by mitogen (**Fig. 7**). The kinetic pattern of the unstimulated cells resembled an exponential decay function, whereas the stimulated cells typically exhibited a linear pattern. From the slope, intercepts, and overall pattern of the plots, the cell kinetics before and after lymphocyte stimulation can be clearly distinguished.

 Deutsch et al.

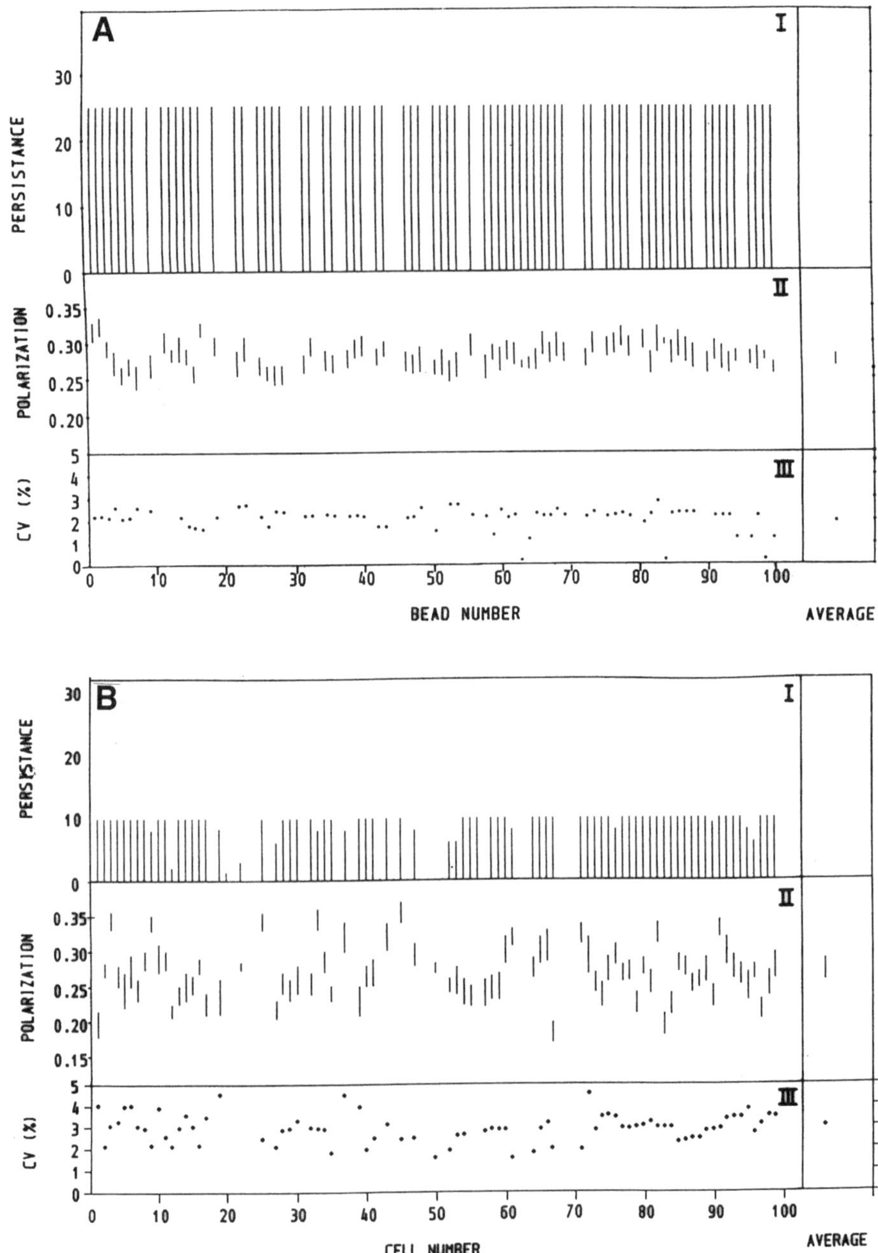

Fig. 4. Reproducibility of CellScan Performances (I) Persistence of particles; (II) Spread of polarization; (III) CV of polarization. **(A)** 25 consecutive scans of beads, **(B)** 10 consecutive scans of cells. The vacancies between lines indicate empty traps.

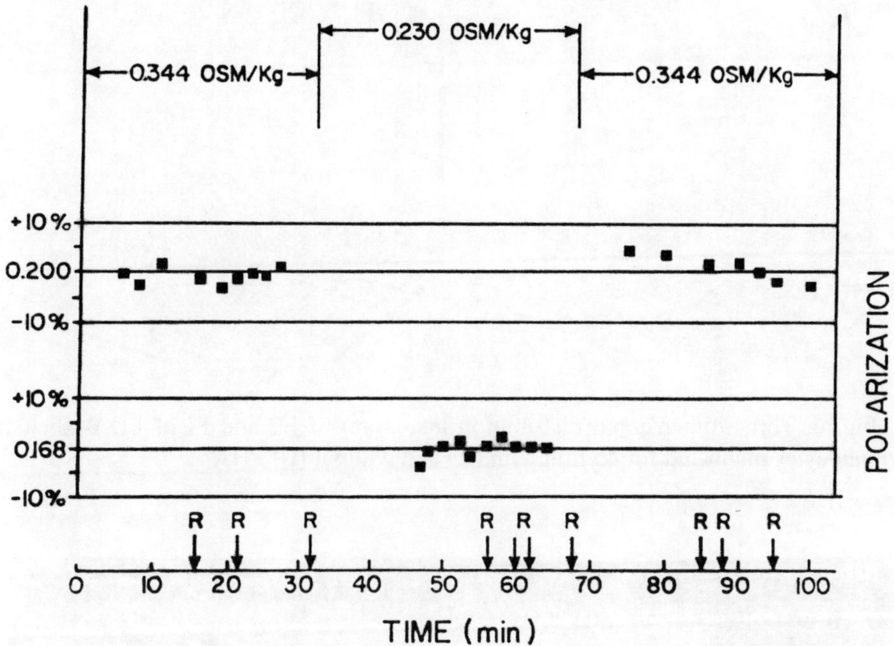

Fig. 5. Modulation of intracellular FP (microviscosity) effected by different osmolality. R-Rinsing.

12. Antigenic stimulation of lymphocyte subpopulations: **Fig. 8** depicts a typical distribution of FI vs FP for populations of untreated PBL. Using the CS-*S* cluster analysis, two subpopulations were apparent, characterized by their FI. The mean FI of the high-intensity subpopulation was three times higher than that of the lower population (99.8 ± 25 and 29.3 ± 15, respectively). The mean FP value of unstimulated, high-intensity lymphocyte subpopulations loaded on an individual cell carrier was 0.209 ± 0.019 (CV of about 10%). A very low variation from this mean value was found among various cell populations derived from all blood donors tested (CV of the average mean value between 60 individuals was approx 9.5 %).

The FI and FP of PBL from patients with advanced atherosclerosis and from control subjects stimulated by oxidized-LDL (oxLDL) in vitro were determined. After exposure to oxLDL, changes in FI, as well as in FP were evident (**Fig. 9**). In patients with advanced atherosclerosis, a specific and dose-dependent reduction of FP within the high-intensity cell population accompanying higher FI, were apparent upon exposure to low doses of oxLDL (up to 25 μg/mL); higher concentrations of oxLDL (200 μg/mL) induced an increase in FP concurrently with a marked decrease in FI. The maximum decrease in FP values upon triggering with oxLDL was found to be at antigen concentrations of 2 μg/mL. This dual effect of oxLDL, namely, depolarization at a low dose and hyperpolarization at a

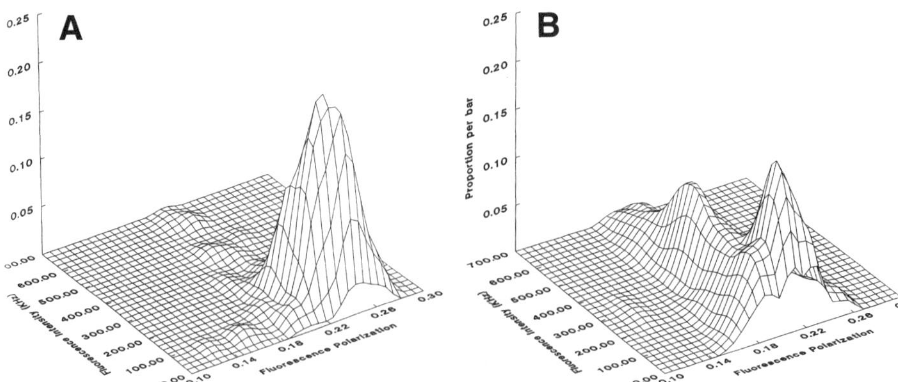

Fig. 6. Three-dimensional distribution histogram of FP and FI of FDA-labeled lymphocytes incubated for 45 min with (**A**) and without (**B**) PHA.

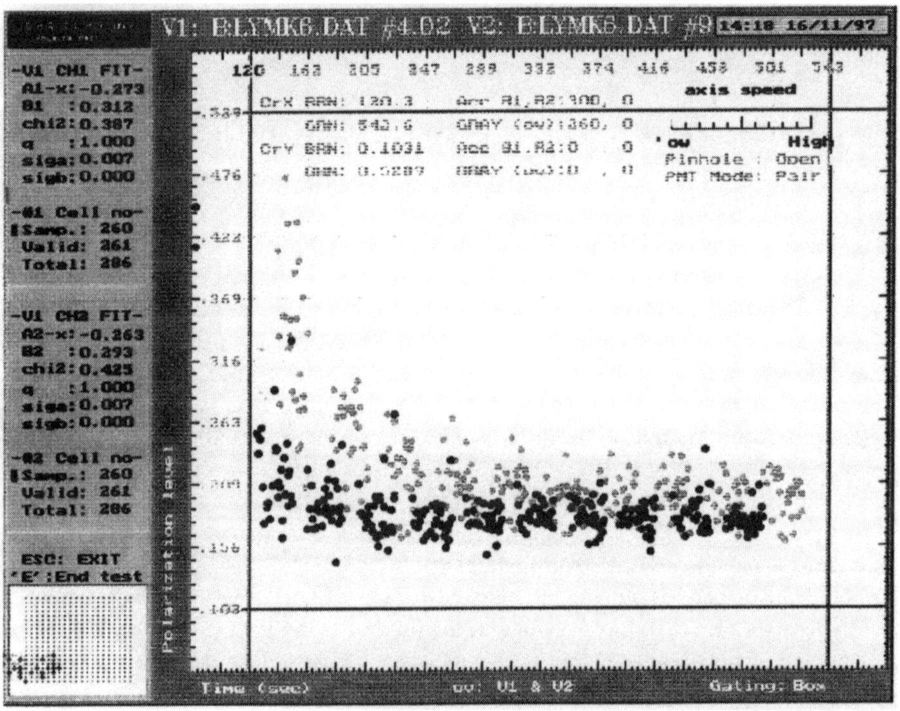

Fig. 7. CS-*S* scatter diagram of FP (ordinate) vs time (abscissa). Lymphocytes were incubated for 40 min with (dark dots) and without (light dots) PHA, loaded on the cell carrier and stained with FDA. Repetitive measurements of selected cells were performed by the CellScan at 30-second intervals.

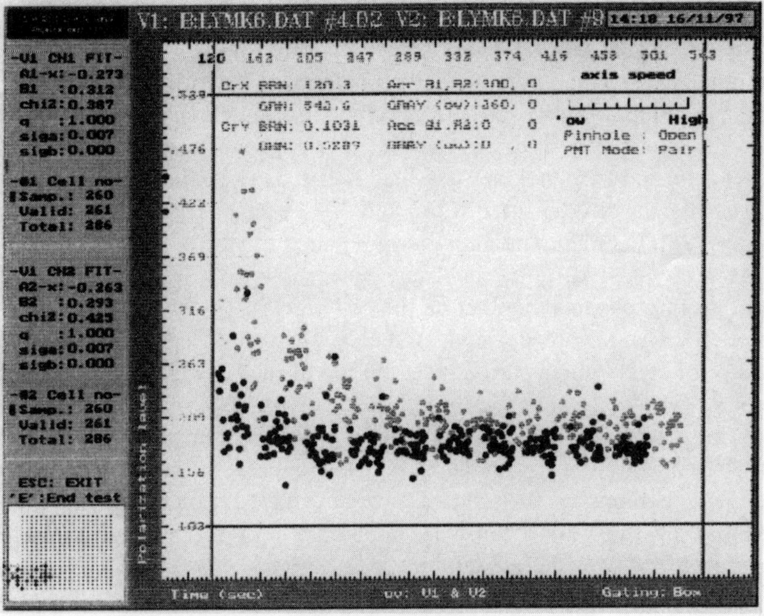

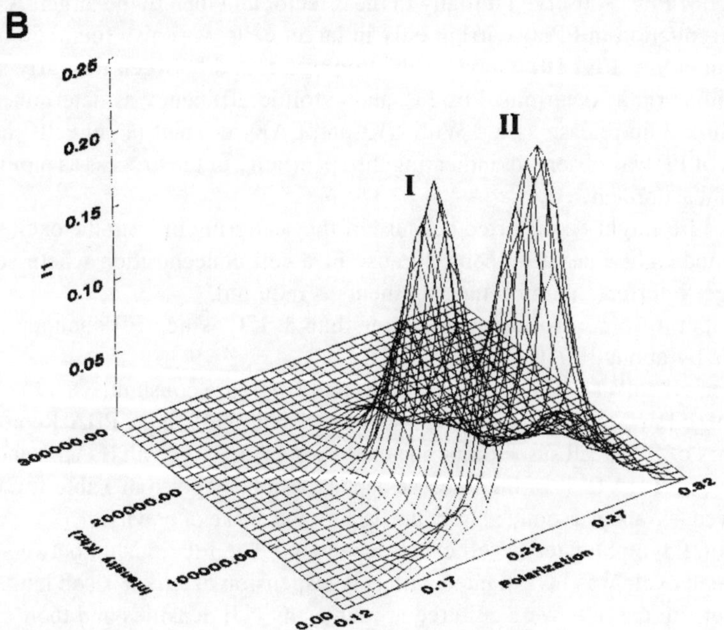

Fig. 8. Identification of clusters by the CS-*S*. Two lymphocyte cluster populations, I and II, are evident in **(A)** FI (abscissa) vs FP (ordinate) scatter diagram as well as in **(B)** a three-dimensional distribution histogram of the same data.

high dose, was seen in patients with active ischemic heart disease but not in the control group *(27)*.

13. Monitoring effector and target cell stimulation during killer-target conjugation: The aim of this study was to detect prelytic intracellular changes induced in both effector and target cells during their interaction (conjugation). Both natural killer (NK) cells and Lymphokine Activated Killer (LAK) cells were used as effector cells, whereas NK-sensitive K562 and NK-resistant Daudi cells were used as targets *(28)*. In order to monitor the stimulation of an effector cell induced by the bound (conjugated) target cell, and vice versa ($FP_{(stimulant)}$), both cells were brought into physical contact on the cell carrier. The stained cells occupying the cell carrier were defined as the 'first group'. The unstained, 'second group' of cells, which were loaded on top of the 'first group', could either be another type of cells or the same type of cells. FP control and post-conjugation measurements were carried out as follows: Immediately after the initial measurement of $FP_{(control)}$ of the 'first group' of cells, 50 µL of cell suspension, of the second group, 4×10^6 cells/mL, were overlayed upon the 'first group'. Upon settling of the cell, occurring approx 3 min after loading, $FP_{(stimulant)}$ measurements were carried out.

    FP measurements were carried out on the same individual cells for a period of approx 4 h. Within minutes after effector/target conjugation, a transient reduction of FP was observed initially in the effector and then in the target. A continuous reduction in FP, occurring only in target cells, was also found 50 min after conjugation (**Fig. 10**). Good correlation was found between the early stages of conjugation as determined by FP, and cytolitic efficiency as determined by the ^{53}Chromium release assay. With NK- and LAK-resistant target cells, no reduction of FP was observed, indicating the specificity of the process as monitored by FP measurements.

14. Since FP might be distorted because of the scattering of both the excitation and emitted light caused by cells; the use of a cell concentration where scatter no longer interferes with FP measurements is required.

15. Temperature control must be better than $\pm\ 1°C$, since FP changes in living cells by about 3%/°C.

16. When all cells are filtered away, $I_{\perp}(F)$ and $I_{||}(F)$ are constant.

17. FP of cell suspensions, incubated for 45' in 37°C with and without PHA. Representative values of FP of cell suspensions, incubated for 45' in 37°C with (FP_{PHA}) and without ($FP_{control}$) PHA of % of fluorescence depolarization are given in **Table 1**. CV did not exceed 4% and was omitted from the data for the   sake of brevity.

18. FP of T lymphocytes is cell cycle-dependent: The relationship between FP and the cell cycle was investigated with cell suspension of Jurkat T cell leukemia in a cuvet. Jurkat cells were cultured at increasing cell densities and their cell cycle progression was monitored by FP.

    Jurkat cells were maintained in complete medium, RPMI 1640 supplemented with 10% (v/v) fetal calf serum (FCS), 2 m*M* L-glutamine, 1 m*M* Na pyruvate, 50 U/mL penicillin, and 50 µg/mL streptomycin, in a humidified

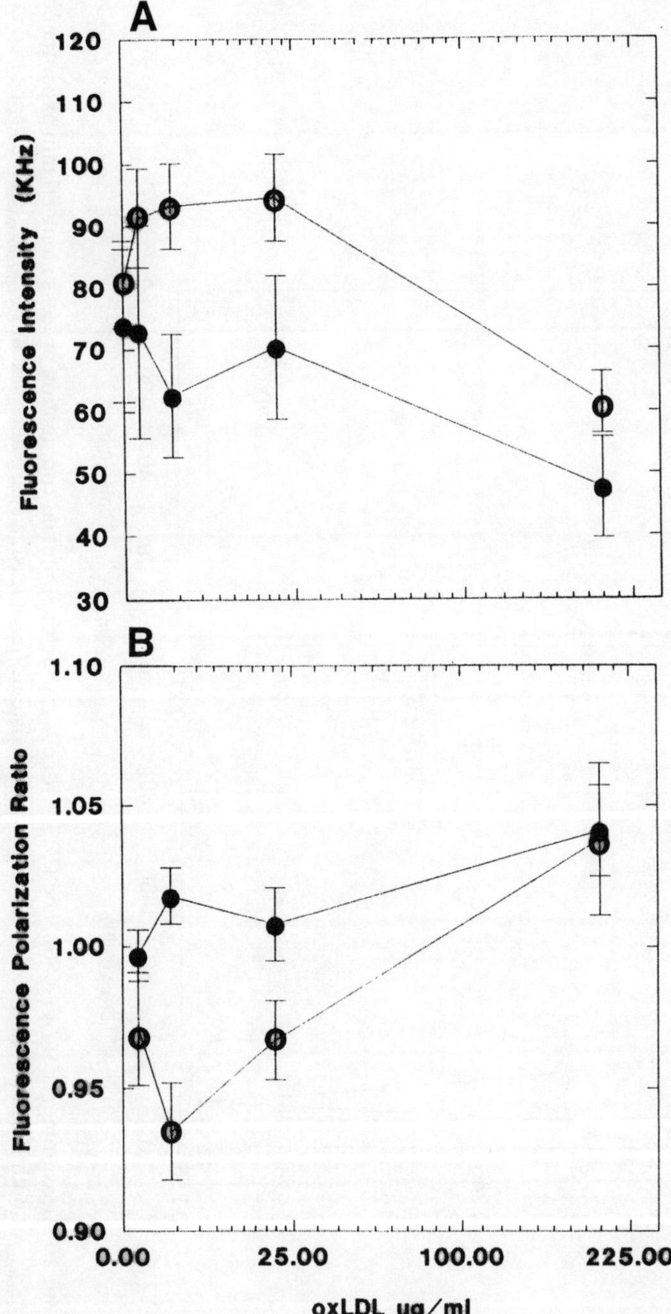

Fig. 9. Activation of lymphocytes by oxLDL. Titration curves of oxLDL concentration vs. FI (**A**) and of FP ratio (**B**). Each dot represents the mean value of lymphocyte subpopulations obtained from 17 control subjects (●), and 21 atherosclerosis patients (◐).

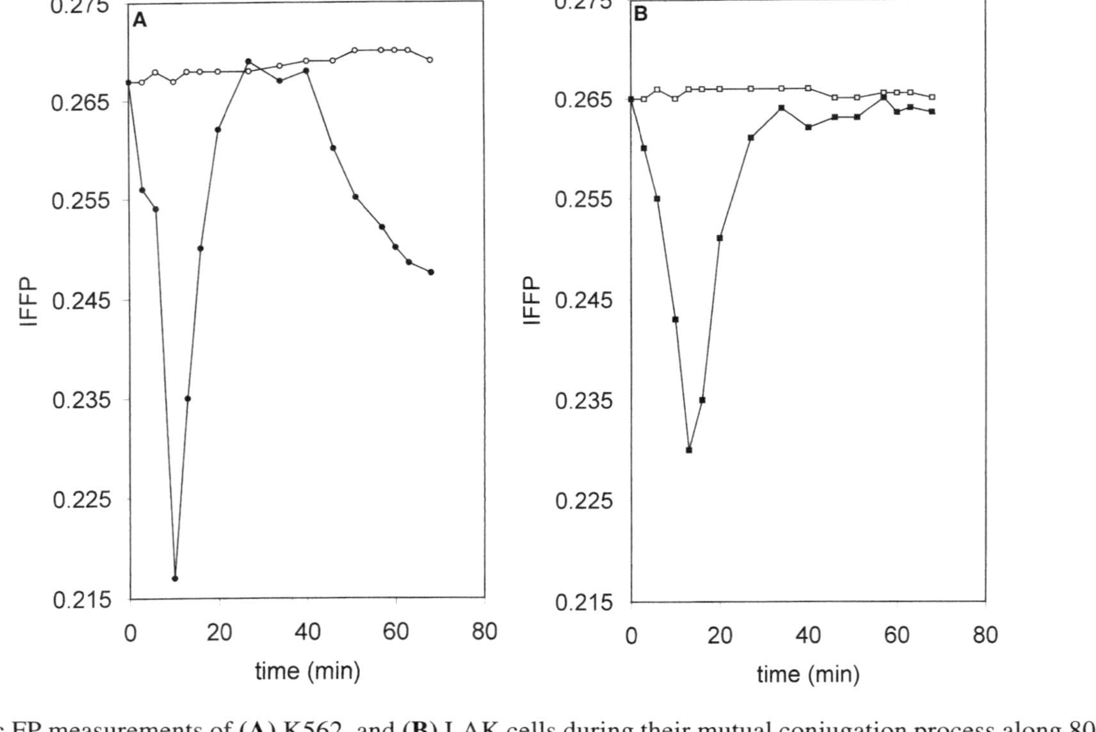

Fig. 10. Kinetic FP measurements of (**A**) K562, and (**B**) LAK cells during their mutual conjugation process along 80 min experiment period. The FP$_{(control)}$ of both K562 (O) and LAK (□) cells was consistent. In contrast, a sharp decrease in FP$_{(stimulant)}$ values appeared at 10 and 12 min after conjugation when K562 (●) and LAK (■) cells correspondingly were used as a 'first' group. Approximately 10 min later, FP$_{(stimulant)}$ levels increased and reached the corresponding FP$_{(control)}$ values. About 50 min post conjugation, the FP$_{(stimulant)}$ of target cells alone (not of effector cells), again decreased, but moderately with time. Each mark represents the results of at least five measurements. In order to simplify the figures, the SD (average ± 0.005) bars were omitted from the data presented.

Table 1
Lymphocyte Activation by Fluorescence Depolarization

FP$_{(control)}$	FP$_{(PHA)}$	Depolarization (%)
0.196	0.174	11
0.187	0.165	12
0.195	0.156	20
0.198	0.182	8
0.185	0.157	15
0.192	0.169	12
0.201	0.167	17
0.190	0.177	7
0.188	0.164	13
0.191	0.168	12

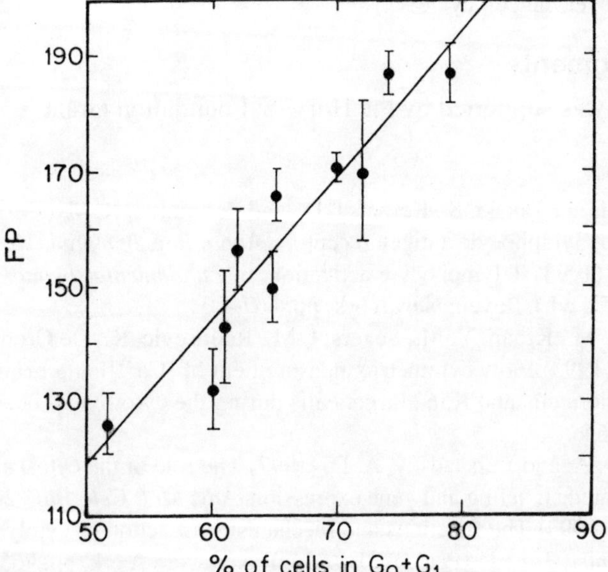

Fig. 11. Mean FP of Jurkat T cells as a function of the percentage of cells in the G$_0$/G$_1$ phases. In each experiment the measurements were performed in triplicate.

atmosphere containing 5% CO_2. Cells were cultured at 5 cell densities (1, 2, 4, 5, 7 × 10^6/mL) for 24 h, then washed three times with Dulbecco PBS, and incubated in the same buffer for 1 h before cell cycle and FP measurements.

For phase-arrest, Jurkat cells were cultured in complete medium containing 1 μM hydroxyurea or 1 μM nocodazole for 24 h. After incubation, cells were washed 3 times with Dulbecco PBS, and incubated in the same buffer for 1 h before cell cycle and FP measurements. Cell staining, FP measurement and stimulation were as mentioned in **Subheading 3.3.**

At the highest cell density, cells at the resting phases (G_0/G_1) predominated, and the mean FP was 0.186 ± 0.015. At the lowest density, with a diminished proportion of cells in the G_1/G_2 stages, the mean FP decreased to 0.126 ± 0.01 (**Fig. 11**). Treatment of the Jurkat T-cell line with phase-arresting agents, $1~\mu M$ hydroxyurea, or $1~\mu M$ nocodazole, arrested the cells in the S and G_2/M phases, respectively. The treated cells exhibited substantially lower FP values, and a mean FP value of 0.140, compared to 0.171 ± 0.009 in control cells. Preincubation of Jurkat cells in buffer resulted in the accumulation of the cells in the G_0/G_1 phases as well as a parallel increase in FP. A characteristic decrease in FP was demonstrated upon triggering the cells with PHA. A high correlation (Pearson correlation $=0.942$) was found between the percentage of cells in the G_0/G_1 phases and the mean FP of the measured cell population (**Fig. 11**). These results suggested that the intracellular microviscosity of Jurkat T cells, as measured by FP, changed over the cell cycle.

Acknowledgments

This work was supported by the Horwitz Foundation Grant.

References

1. Alberola-Ila, J., Takaki, S., Kerner, J. D., and Perlmutter, R. M. (1997) Differential signaling by lymphocyte antigen receptors. *Annu. Rev. Immunol.* **15,** 125–154.
2. Weiss, A. (1993) T lymphocyte activation, in *Fundamental Immunology*, 3rd ed. (Paul, W. E., ed.), Raven, New York, pp. 467–504.
3. Van Graft, M., Kraan, Y. M., Segers, I. M., Radosevic, K., De Grooth, B. G., and Greve, J. (1993) Flow cytometric measurement of [Ca^{2+}]I and pH$_i$ in conjugated natural killer cells and K562 target cells during the cytotoxic process. *Cytometry* **14,** 257–264.
4. Ben-Ze'ev, A. and Bershadsky, A. D. (1997) The role of the cytoskeleton in adhesion-mediated signaling and gene expression. *Adv. Mol. Cell. Biol.* **24,** 125–163.
5. Berke, G. (1993) The functions and mechanisms of action of cytolymphocytes, in *Fund. Immun.*, 3rd ed., (Paul, W. E., ed.), Raven, New York, pp. 965–1014.
6. Geiger, B., Rosen, D., and Berke, G. (1982) Spatial relationships of MTOC and the contact area of Cytotoxic T lymphocytes. *J. Cell. Biol.* **95,** 137–143.
7. Cercek, L. and Cercek, B. (1977) Application of the phenomenon of changes in the structuredness of cytoplasmic matrix (SCM) in the diagnosis of malignant disorders: A review. *Europ J. Cancer* **13,** 903–915.
8. Deutsch, M. and Weinreb, A. (1983) Validation of the SCM-tst for the diagnosis of Cancer. *Eur J. Cancer Clin Oncol.* **19,** 187–193.
9. Chaitchik, S., Deutsch, M., Asher, O., Krauss, G., Lebovich, P., Michlin, H., and Weinreb, A. (1988) An evaluation of the SCM test for the diagnosis of cancer of the breast. *Eur. J. Cancer Clin. Oncol.* **25,** 861–866.

10. Ron, I. G., Deutsch, M., Tirosh, R., Weinreb, A., Eisenthal, A., and Chaitchik, S. (1995) Fluorescence polarization changes in lymphocyte cytoplasm as a diagnostic test for breast carcinoma. *Eur. J. Cancer* **31A,** 917–920.
11. Deutsch, M., Ron, I., Weinreb, A., Tirosh, R., and Chaitchik, S. (1996) Lymphocyte fluorescence polarization measurements with the CellScan system: Application to the SCM cancer test. *Cytometry* **23,** 159–165.
12. Eisenthal, A., Marder, O., Dotan, D., Baron, S., Lifschitz-Mercer, B., Chaitchik, S., Tirosh, R., Weinreb, A., and Deutsch, M. (1996) Decrease of intracellular fluorescein fluorescence polarization (IFFP) in human peripheral blood lymphocytes undergoing stimulation with phytohaemagglutinin (PHA), concanavalin A (ConA), pokeweed mitogen (PWM) and anti-CD3 antibody. *Biol. Cell* **86,** 145–150.
13. Deutsch, M. and Weinreb, A. (1994) Apparatus for high precision repetitive sequential measurements of living cells. *Cytometry* **16,** 214–226.
14. Duportail, G. and Weinreb, A. (1983) Photochemical changes of fluorescent probes in membranes and their effect on the observed fluorescence anisotropy values. *Biochim. Biophys. Acta* **736,** 171–177.
15. Lenz, B. R. (1989) Membrane 'fluidity' as detected by diphenyl hexatriene probes. *Chem. Phys. Lipids* **50,** 171–179.
16. Zurgil, N., Deutsch, M., Tirosh, R., and Brodie, C. (1996) Indication that intracellular fluorescence polarization of T lymphocytes is cell cycle dependent. *Cell Struct. Funct.* **21,** 1–6.
17. Marder, O., Shoval, S., Eisenthal, A., Fireman, E., Skornick, Y., Lifschitz-Mercer, B., Tirosh, R., Weinreb, A., and Deutsch, M. (1996) Effect of interleukin-1α, interleukin-1β and tumor necrosis factor-α on the intracellular fluorescein fluorescence polarization of human lung fibroblasts. *Pathobiology* **64,** 123–130.
18. Eisenthal, A., Marder, O., Lifschitz-Mercer, B., Skornick, Y., Tirosh, R., Weinreb, A., and Deutsch, M. (1996) Inhibition of mitogen-induced changes in intracellular fluorescence polarization of human peripheral blood lymphocytes by colchicine, vinblastine and cytochalasin B. *Cell Struct. Funct.* **21,** 159–166.
19. Kaplan, M., Trebnyikov, E., and Berke, G. (1997) Fluorescence depolarization as an early measure of T lymphocyte stimulation. *J. Immunol. Methods* **201,** 15–24.
20. Eisenthal, A., Marder, O., Lifschitz-Mercer, B., Skornick, I., Tirosh, R., Irlin, Y., and Deutsch, M. (1997) Infection of K562 cells with influenza A virus increases their susceptibility to NK lysis. *Pathobiology* **65,** 331–340.
21. Fixler, D., Tirosh, R., Eisenthal, A., Lalchuk, S., Marder, O., Irlin, Y., and Deutsch, M. (1998) Prelytic stimulation of target and effector cells following conjugation as measured by intracellular fluorescein fluorescence polarization. *J. Biomed. Optics* **3,** 312–325.
22. Jablonsky, A. (1935) Uber den mechanismus des photoluminescenz von farbstoff- phosphoren. *Z. Phys.* **94,** 38–46.
23. Stokes, G. G. (1852) On the change of refrangibility of light. *Philos. Trans.* **143,** 385.
24. Perrin, F. (1929) La fluorscence des solutions. *Ann. Phys. (Paris)* **12,** 169–275.
25. Deutsch, M. and Weinreb, A. (1994) Apparatus for high-precision repetitive sequential optical measurement of living cells. *Cytometry* **16,** 214–226.

26. Rotman, B. and Papermaster, B. W. (1966) Membrane properties of living mammalian cells studied by enzymatic hydrolysis of fluorogenic esters. *Proc. Natl. Acad. Sci. USA* **55,** 134–141.
27. Zurgil, N., Levy, Y., Deutsch, M., Gilburd, B., George, J., Haratz, D., Kaufman, M., and Shoenfeld, Y. (1998) Reactivity of peripheral blood lymphocytes (PBL) to oxLDL: A novel system to estimate atherosclerosis employing the CellScan. *Clin. Cardiol.* **22,** in press.
28. Fixler, D., Tirosh, R., Eisenthal, A., Marder, O., Irlin, Y., Lalchuk, S., and Deutsch, M. (1997) Monitoring of effector and target cell stimulation during conjugation by fluorescence polarization. *Biol. Cell.* **89,** 443–452.

19

Measurement of Lymphoproliferation at the Single-Cell Level by Flow Cytometry

Hans Gaines and Gunnel Biberfeld

1. Introduction

The recognition phase of the cell-mediated immune response is studied in vitro by monitoring responses of CD4[+] T cells, cultured in the presence of specific antigen. Conventional cultures include mononuclear cells separated from peripheral blood by a complex and time-consuming procedure. Several investigators *(1–7)* have suggested the use of whole-blood cultures which is easier to perform and involve less manipulations, thus reducing the risk of contamination, preactivation, or selective depletion or enrichment of cell subsets. The cell-mediated immune response involves a broad spectrum of measurable mechanisms. Multiparameter flow cytometry analysis permits the simultaneous detection of cell surface and intracellular molecules, as well as light-scatter characteristics of individual cells. In this chapter, a method is described for the measurement of proliferative responses in whole-blood cultures, using flow cytometric detection of lymphoblast development. The method is simple and reproducible, and can be combined with immunostaining for the detection of cytokine production, cell-surface expression of costimulatory molecules, and DNA synthesis.

2. Materials

1. Test samples: specimens of peripheral blood drawn into evacuated tubes containing heparin.
2. Culture media: RPMI 1640 (Gibco-BRL Ltd, Middlesex, UK) supplemented with 2 mM L-glutamine (Gibco-BRL Ltd), 10,000 IU/mL penicillin (Gibco-BRL Ltd) and 10,000 µg/mL streptomycin (Gibco-BRL Ltd).
3. Test tubes: 12 × 75 mm polystyrene round-bottom tubes with caps (Falcon 2054, Becton Dickinson Labware, Franklin Lakes, NJ).

From: *Methods in Molecular Biology, Vol. 134: T Cell Protocols: Development and Activation*
Edited by: K. P. Kearse © Humana Press Inc., Totowa, NJ

4. Activators: mitogens, e.g., phytohemagglutinin (Sigma Chemical Co. St. Louis, MO), concanavalin A (Pharmacia-LKB, Uppsala, Sweden), poke-weed mitogen (PWM; Wellcome Reagents Ltd, Beckenham, UK), CD3 MAb (OKT3, Ortho Diagnostics, Stockholm, Sweden); and antigens, e.g., PPD (SBL Vaccin AB, Stockholm, Sweden), or TT (SBL Vaccin AB).
5. Washing buffer: phosphate-buffered saline (PBS).
6. Lysing solution: Ortho-mune Lysing Reagent (Ortho Diagnostics). Bring vial to room temperature (15–30°C). Prepare the lysing solution by adding the vial contents to 100 mL of distilled water. Store the solution at room temperature in a tightly stoppered container with minimal air space. Discard solution after 1 wk. Do not refrigerate or freeze.
7. Fixing solution: CellFIX 10X concentrate (Becton Dickinson). Store at room temperature (20–25°C). For use, dilute CellFIX 1:10 with distilled and deionized water. Store in a glass container at room temperature (20–25°C) for up to 1 mo.

3. Methods

3.1. Whole-Blood Culture

1. Collect peripheral blood specimens by venipuncture into evacuated tubes containing heparin. Mix the blood well with the anticoagulant to prevent clotting. Specimens should be maintained at 18–22°C during transportation and storage, and should be processed within 24 h after collection (*see* **Notes 1** and **2**).
2. Dilute samples 1/10 in culture media (*see* **Note 3**).
3. Distribute the blood suspensions in 900 µL aliquots in test tubes. Add activators or culture medium in aliquots of 100 µL to each tube (*see* **Notes 4–6**).
4. Keep cultures in a humidified environment at 37°C with 5% CO_2 in the air for the required period of time, usually 5 d (*see* **Note 7**).
5. Centrifuge tubes for 5 min at 300*g* at room temperature. Remove supernatants.
6. Add 1 mL lysing solution to each tube and vortex sample tubes immediately. Incubate for 10 min at 15–25°C to lyse remaining erythrocytes (*see* **Note 8**).
7. Repeat **step 5**.
8. Add 1 mL phosphate-buffered saline to each tube. Vortex sample tubes.
9. Repeat **step 5**.
10. Add 0.5 mL fixing solution. Vortex sample tubes. Store in the dark at 4°C for up to 24 h (*see* **Note 9**).

3.2. Flow Cytometric Analysis

1. Select flow cytometer instrument settings, used for acquisition of whole-blood specimens. Acquire a few hundred events from various sample tubes to control and, if necessary, optimize instrument settings, e.g., negative controls to set threshold on forward scatter below the left margin of resting lymphocytes, and positive controls to ensure that all cells, including lymphoblasts, are on scale. The expected scatter profiles for different leukocyte populations in the absence or presence of activator are shown in **Fig. 1** (*see* **Note 10**).

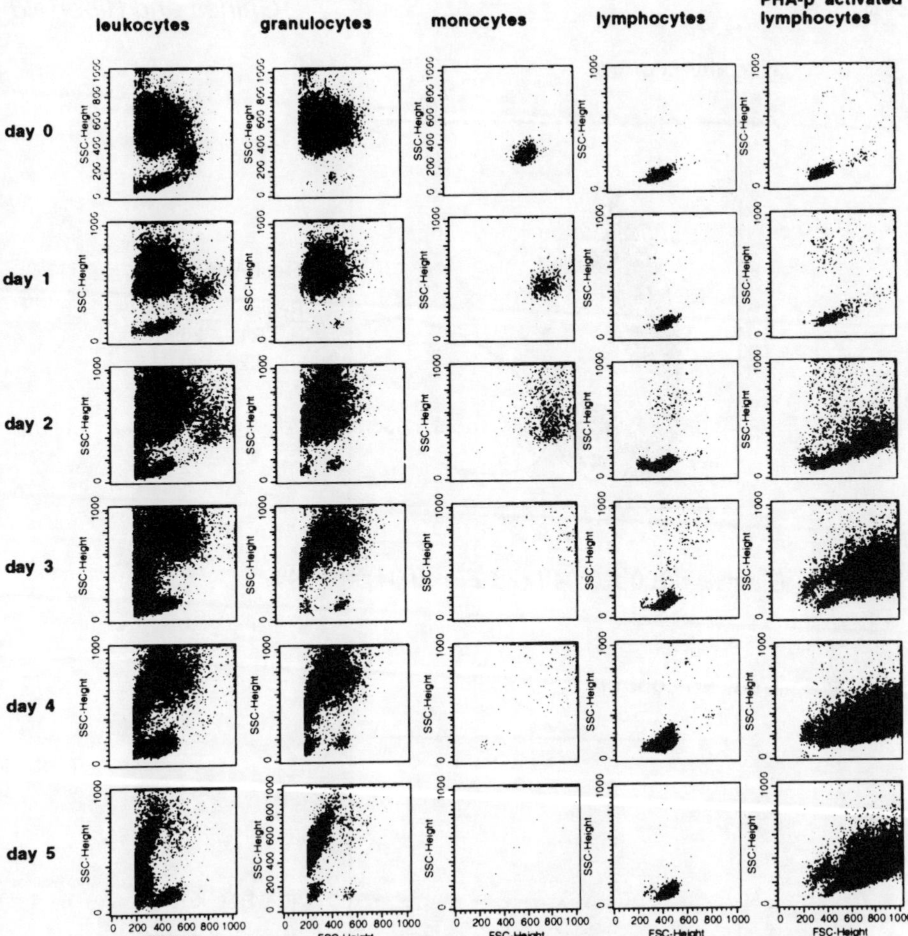

Fig. 1. Flow cytometric dot plots illustrating the scatter profiles of different leukocyte populations in whole-blood cultured in medium only, or with phytohemagglutinin-protein 5 µg/mL (PHA-p) 0–5 d. Plots show all leukocytes, or populations gated by their expression of surface markers: granulocytes (CD45$^\pm$, CD14$^-$); monocytes (CD45$^+$, CD14$^+$); and lymphocytes (CD45$^+$, CD14$^-$).

2. Acquire the required number of events, e.g., 10,000 events, from each tube and save results electronically in list mode data format. Visualize the collected events on a forward scatter × side scatter dot plot continuously during acquisition, to ensure that representative data are collected from each sample (*see* **Note 11**).

3. Analyze light scatter (forward scatter × side scatter) dot plots for negative and positive controls (**Fig. 2**). Draw a region (**R1**) around the cluster of resting lymphocytes identified in the negative control sample. Copy R1 to the positive control sample and draw another region (**R2**) around the cluster of lymphoblasts identified in the positive control sample.

Negative control

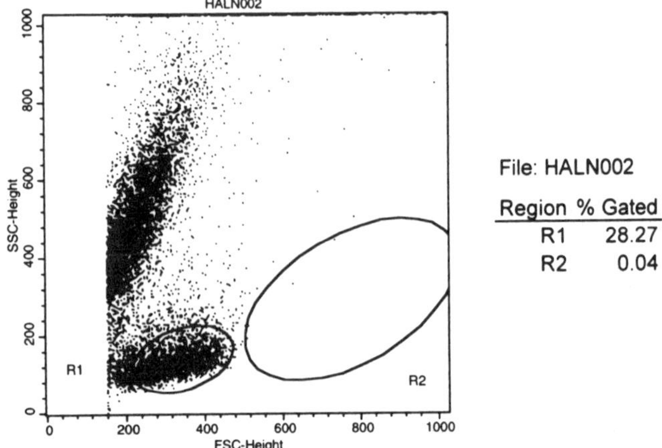

Blast% = 100 x 0.04 / (28.27 + 0.04) = 0.14%

Positive control

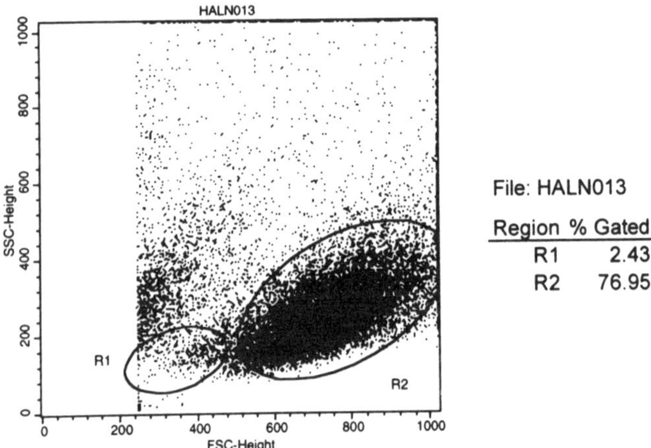

Blast% = 100 x 76.95 / (2.43 + 76.95) = 96.94%

Fig. 2. Flow cytometric analysis of negative control (medium only) and positive control (phytohemagglutinin 5 µg/mL) samples of whole-blood cultured 5 d.

Dot plots show light scatter profiles with one region (**R1**) around the cluster of resting lymphocytes, identified in the negative control sample, and another region (**R2**) around the cluster of lymphoblasts, identified in the positive control sample. Percentage of lymphocytes that are lymphoblasts are calculated for both samples.

4. Determine the number of cells in R1 and R2 for each sample tube.
5. Express the results for each tube as "blast%"; percentage of lymphocytes that are lymphoblasts [$100 \times R2 / (R1 + R2)$].
6. Validate the test using the blast% for negative and positive control, which usually should be around 0.1–0.6% and 30–100%, respectively.
7. Express results as stimulation-index; blast%$_{test\ sample}$/blast%$_{negative\ control\ sample}$ (*see* **Notes 12–15; Figs. 3–6**).

4. Notes

4.1. Whole-Blood Culture

1. Specimens that should be used for whole-blood cultures cannot be collected into tubes containing tripotassium ethylenediamine tetra-acetate (K_3EDTA), since K_3EDTA, present in whole-blood cultures, binds calcium and inhibits specific immune reactions.
2. Cultures of whole-blood are more influenced than cultures of isolated peripheral blood mononuclear cells (PBMC) by mishandling during collection and maintenance of specimen affecting specimen integrity. Hemolysis or partial clotting may:
   a. Induce preactivation of cells, thus increasing the background stimulation and decreasing the resolution power of the test;
   b. Cause lysis and damage to cells, increasing the rate of accumulation of toxic substances, thus decreasing the duration of time that the culture can be maintained; and
   c. Cause selective loss of subpopulations or soluble factors, thus affecting results. Such problems are rare, however, when recommended procedures for collection and maintenance of specimen are followed.
3. A dilution of whole-blood 1/10 in culture media is usually optimal when measuring specific immune responses. Other dilutions may be used for other purposes. The rate of accumulation of toxic substances because of the lysis of erythrocytes and granulocytes will increase in cultures using less diluted whole-blood, which will decrease the duration of time that the culture can be maintained: usually cultures of 1/2 diluted whole-blood cannot be maintained for more than 48 h, whereas cultures of 1/10 diluted whole-blood are usually stable for 120–168 h.
4. Whole-blood cultures may also be set up in round-bottom microtiter plates (immune responses to specific antigens will not develop in flat-bottom microtiter plates). Wells containing cultures in volumes of 200 µL can be used for measurement of immune responses to mitogens, but may be less valuable when testing for specific immune responses: such cultures will usually include only 20,000–40,000 lymphocytes and a sufficient number of T cells specific for the antigen tested may, in some cases, not be present among that number of lymphocytes.
5. The amounts of mitogens or antigens that should be added to whole-blood cultures have to be determined for each purpose. Generally, the final concentrations are identical to those used for PBMC cultures; e.g., phytohe-

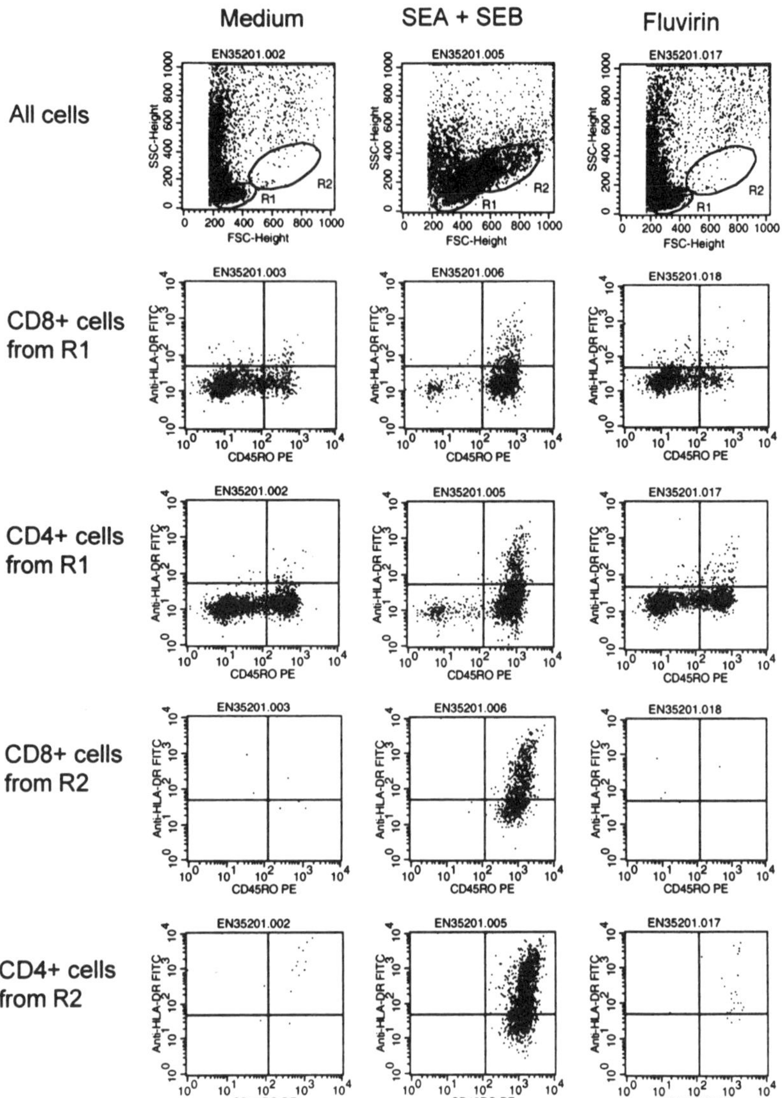

Day 1 after onset of influenza infection

Fig. 3. Flow cytometric analysis demonstrating development of a cell-mediated immune response against influenza antigens following an onset of influenza infection. Whole-blood, taken from a patient with acute influenza infection 1 and 6 d, respectively, after onset of symptoms, was cultured 6 d in medium only, or in the presence of either a superantigen mixture (staphylococcal enterotoxin A 10 ng/mL; SEA, and staphylococcal enterotoxin B 5 ng/mL; SEB, Sigma-Aldrich Co., Stockholm, Sweden), or influenza virus surface antigens (Fluvirin® 1/80, SBL Vaccin AB); and therafter immunostained with FITC-conjugated anti-

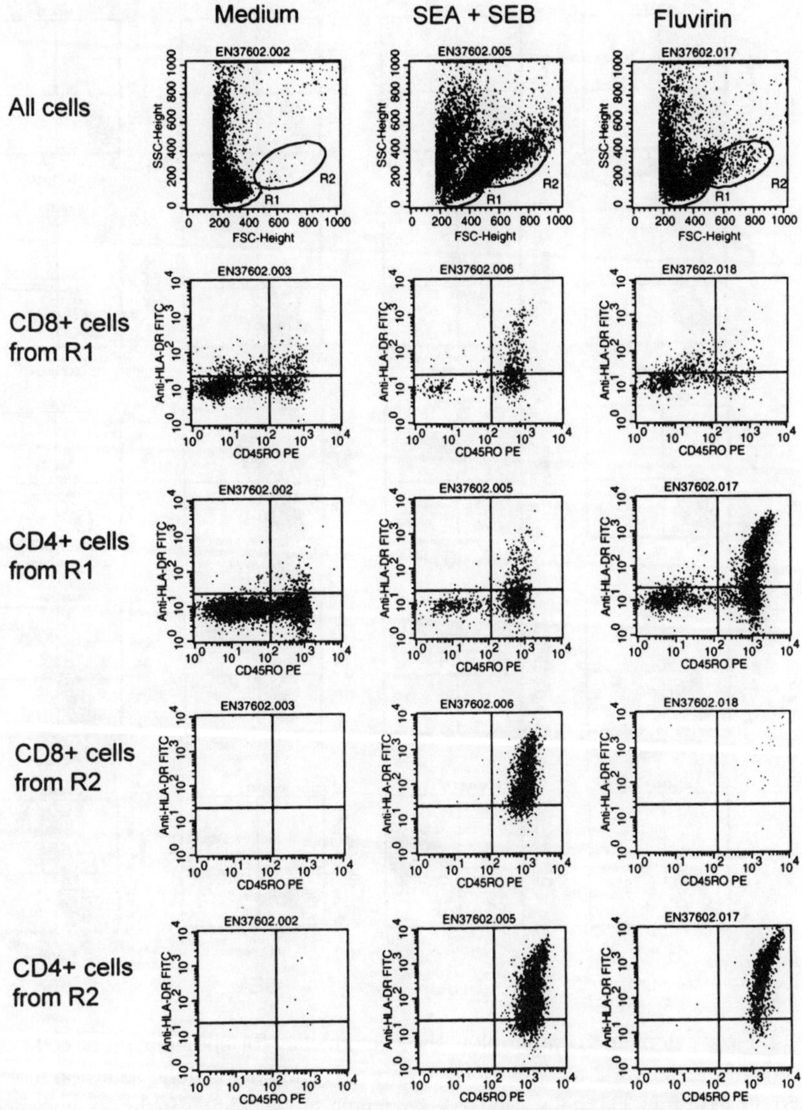

Day 6 after onset of influenza infection

HLA-Dr antibody, PE-conjugated CD45RO antibody, and PerCP-conjugated antibody against either CD8 or CD4 (all antibodies from Becton Dickinson, Franklin Lakes, NJ). The first obtained sample displayed no significant reactivity to influenza antigen. In the sample obtained 6 d after onset of influenza infection, activated (HLA-Dr$^+$) memory (CD45RO$^+$) CD4$^+$ cells to influenza had appeared. These cells were detected within R1 as well as within R2, and all cells with a lymphoblast scatter profile (R2), developed following activation with influenza antigens, were activated memory CD4$^+$ cells.

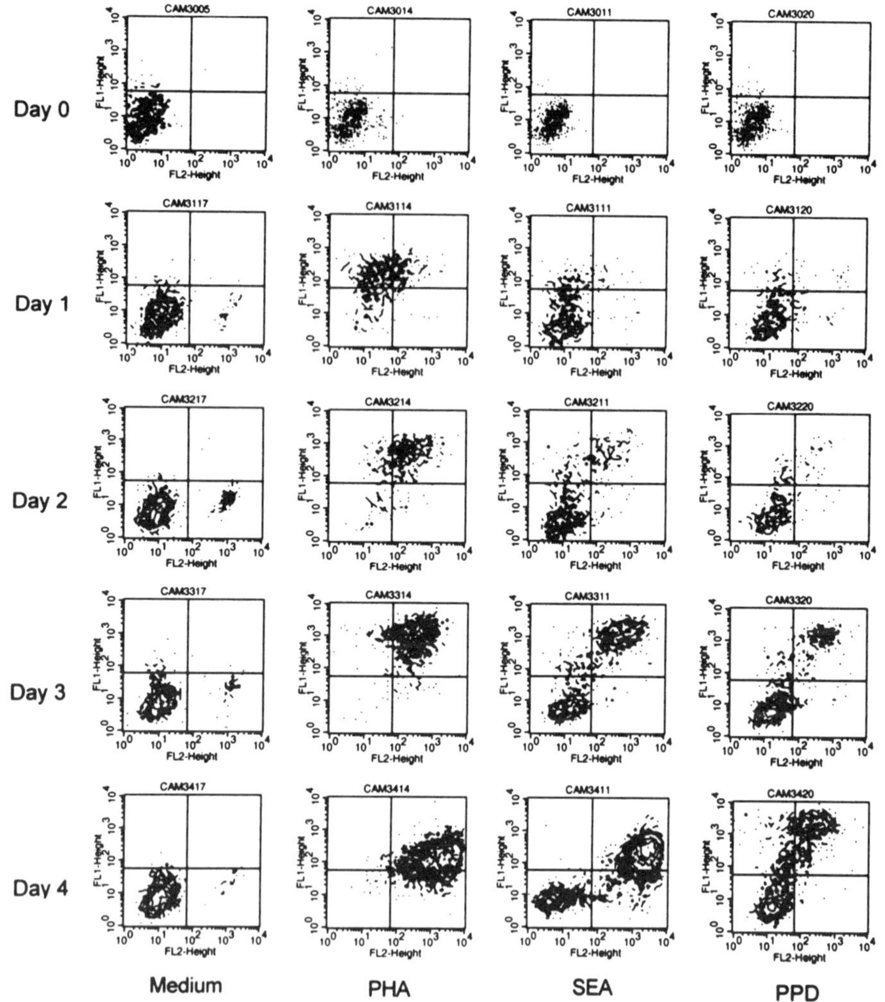

Fig. 4. Flow cytometric contour plots showing kinetics for upregulation of cell surface expression of interleukin-2 receptor (CD25) on *y*-axis and inter cellular adhesion molecule (CD54) on *x*-axis, for CD4+ cells gated d 0–4 of whole-blood cultures in the presence of only medium, mitogen (phytohemagglutinin 5 µg/mL; PHA), superantigen (staphylococcal enterotoxin A 10 ng/mL; SEA), or antigen (tuberculin purified protein derivate 5 µg/mL; PPD).

     magglutinin 5 µg/mL, concanavalin A 5 µg/mL, poke-weed mitogen 10 µg/mL, CD3 MAb OKT3 0.1 µg/mL, PPD 1.2 µg/mL, TT 5 µg/mL.

6. Conventional cultures, using PBMC are generally run in triplicates since adverse results occur at varying frequencies. Whole-blood cultures can be run in duplicates, or even as single tests, as it is technically easier to perform, less manipulations are involved, increasing the reproducability of the test.

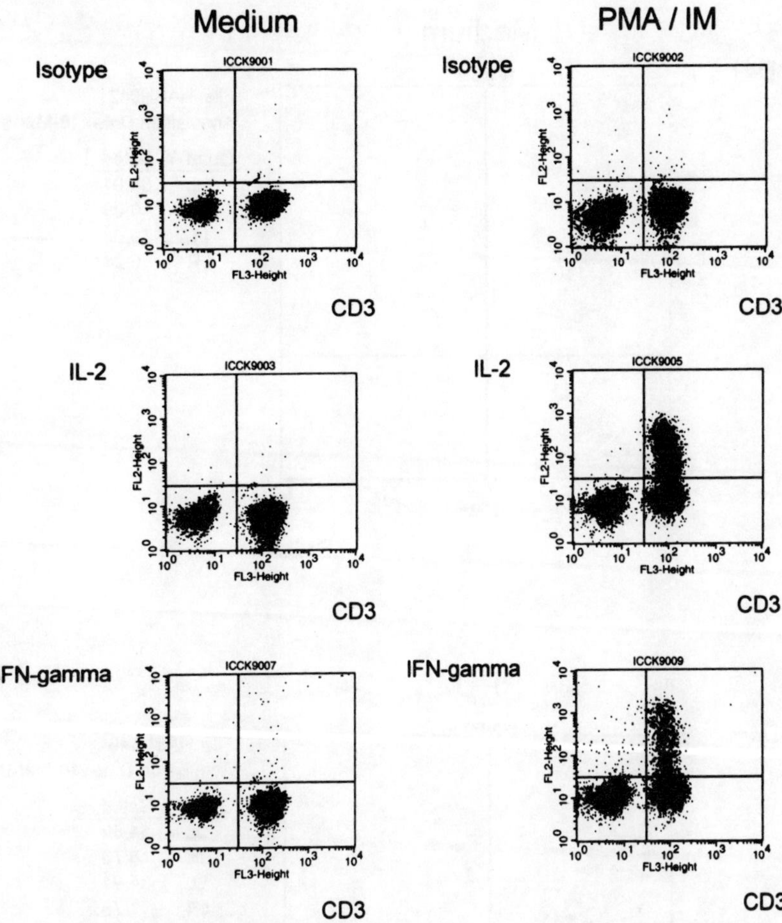

Fig. 5. Flow cytometric detection of intracellular IL-2 and IFN-gamma in T cells. Whole-blood was cultured over night in the abscence or presence of phorbol 12 — myristate 13 — acetate (PMA, Sigma-Aldrich) 25 ng/mL and ionomycin (IM, Sigma-Aldrich) 1 µg/mL and following permeabilization with saponin immunostained with PerCP-conjugated anti-CD3 antibody and PE-conjugated antibody to either IL-2, IFN-gamma, or irrelevant isotype-matched control antibody (all anitbodies from Becton Dickinson).

7. The duration of time that is needed for culturing is dependent on the immune response being lmeasured. Very strong activators, e.g., PMA and ionomycin, can induce responses within 24–48 h; conventional activators like phytohemaggluti-nin (PHA), concanavalin A, poke-weed mitogen, anti-CD3 MAbs, or strong anti-gens can induce responses within 72–120 h; whereas weak antigens may require 120–168 h to induce measurable responses. Conventional proliferative cultures measuring incorporation of tritiated thymidine should optimally be harvested at

Medium

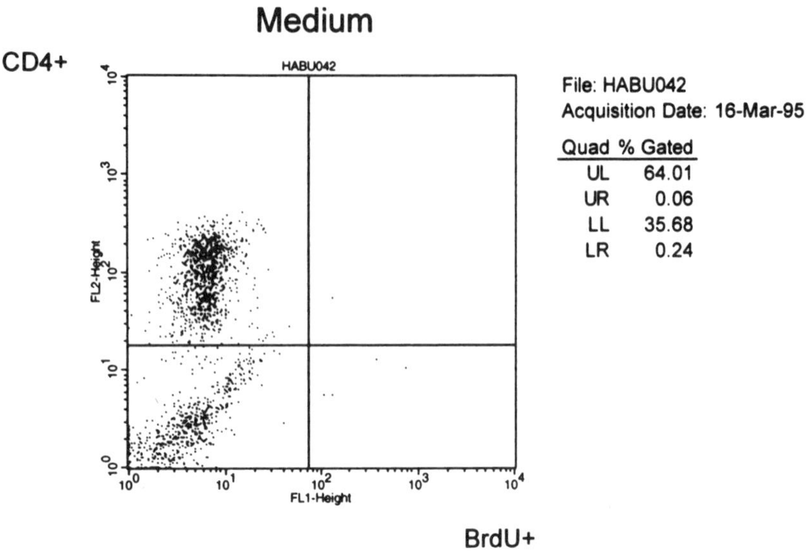

PPD

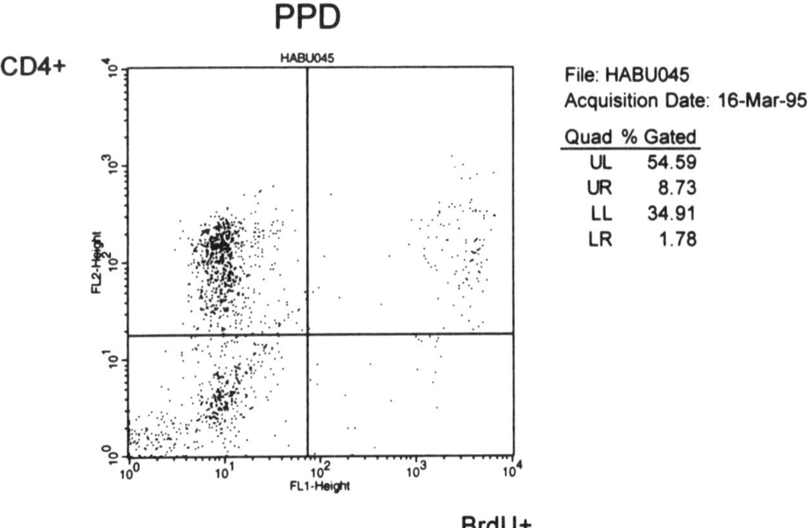

Fig. 6. Flow cytometric dotplots showing DNA replication in a subset of CD4+ T cells following activation by tuberculin purified protein derivate (PPD) 5 µg/mL in whole-blood cultures. Cells were cultured 4 d in the absence or presence of PPD, and 5-bromo-2-deoxyuridine (BrdU) — a thymidine analogue — was added to the cultures during the last 7 h. Uptake of BrdU indicating DNA synthesis was detected by intracellular staining with a FITC-conjugated anti-BrdU antibody.

two time-points since the maximal DNA-synthesis occurs at different periods of time for strong and weak activators; e.g., 3 d for PHA and 5 d for specific antigen. Split harvesting is usually not needed when proliferative responses are monitored as development of lymphoblasts since these cells accumulate during time; e.g., 5 d for both PHA and specific antigen.

8. The lysing procedure should be repeated if the cell pellets are red, indicating the presence of unlysed erythrocytes, following the removal of the supernatants after the lysing procedure. Add 0.5 mL of lysing solution to tubes containing red cell pellets, vortex immediately, and incubate for 5 min. Then, add 0.5 mL phosphate-buffered saline to each tube, vortex, and continue according to the procedure at **step 9**. Another possibility is to use 2.0 mL instead of 1.0 mL of lysing solution, at **step 6**, to achieve a more efficient lysation.

9. For fixation of samples, other fixing reagents like 1% paraformaldehyde may also be used. Alternatively, samples may be resuspended in phosphate-buffered saline, and stored unfixed in the dark at 4°C, but not for more than 4 h before acquisition.

4.2. Flow Cytometric Analysis

10. The performance of the flow cytometer is very stable if standardized procedures are employed for calibration and setting of the instrument. The regions drawn for gating of resting lymphocytes and lymphoblasts, respectively, during one experiment, can usually be employed for analysis of data collected during succeeding experiments.

11. Conventional procedures for maintenance of the flow cytometer can generally be employed at analysis of cultured whole-blood. However, if the samples contain high concentrations of cells, cleaning of the flow system between samples or dilution of samples should be done to avoid precipitation of cells and debris and clogging of the instrument's tubes.

4.3. Variations/Alternative Techniques

12. The methods described in this chapter measures the proliferative responses in whole-blood cultures using flow cytometric identification of lymphoblasts by their light scatter profile. The method can be combined with immunostaining procedures and multiparameter flow cytometer analysis of different mechanisms of cell-mediated immune responses. The cultured specimens can be immunostained to study the expression of cell-surface molecules on the lymphoblasts; to identify the phenotypes of the lymphocytes responding to a given mitogen or antigen, or to study the kinetics of expression of costimulatory molecules, cell-adhesion molecules, and cytokine receptors. The staining procedure is very easy to add to the preparation outlined in **Subheading 3.1.** Following removal of supernatants in **step 5**, the cell pellets are incubated with fluorochrome-conjugated monoclonal antiobodies for 15 min at room temperature, followed by **step 6**. Multiparameter analysis following immunostaining is demonstrated in **Figs. 3** and **4**.

13. Flow Cytometry monitors development of lymphoblasts expressed as proportion of lymphocytes, but absolute number of blasts can also be used; either by examining the samples with a flow cytometer especially suited for determination of cell concentrations *(8)*, or by adding a known number of beads that can be detected by the cytometer (TruCounts; Becton Dickinson Ltd).

14. Antigen-specific immune responses are also induced and regulated through the production and secretion of soluble mediators e.g., cytokines which can be detected and measured in the supernatants of whole-blood cultures by specific ELISAs. Cytokines can also be detected at the intracellular level in whole-blood cultures by flow cytometric analysis following fixation, permeabilization, and staining with cytokine-specific MAb *(9)*. The advantage of this method over the measurement of soluble cytokines in culture supernatants is that it enables the identification of the phenotype of cytokine-producing cells, and permits the simultaneous detection of several cytokines in individual cells. Flow cytometric detection of cytokines in cells following whole-blood culture is demonstrated in **Fig. 5**.

15. Flow cytometric measurement of lymphoproliferation can also be used for cultures of peripheral blood mononuclear cells *(8)*. DNA synthesis can be measured in whole-blood cultures using the conventional method of detecting the uptake of tritiated thymidine *(5)*. DNA-replicating lymphoblasts can also be detected in whole-blood cultures by flow cytometry *(7)*, following addition to cultures of 5-bromo-2-deoxyuridine (BrdU, Sigma-Aldrich) — a thymidine analogue, fixation, permeabilization, and staining with BrdU-antibody (Becton Dickinson), as illustrated in **Fig. 6**.

References

1. Junge, U., Hoekstra, J., Wolfe, L., and Deinhardt, F. (1970) Microtechnique for quantitative evaluation of in vitro lymphocyte transformation. *Clin. Exp. Immunol.* **7(3),** 431–437.

2. Luquetti, A. and Janossy, G. (1976) Lymphocyte activation VIII. The application of a whole blood test to the quantitative analysis of PHA responsive T cells. *J. Immunol. Methods* **10(1),** 7–25.

3. Leroux, M., Schindler, L., Braun, R., Doerr, H. W., Geissen, H. P., and Kirchner, H. (1985) A whole blood lymphoproliferation assay for measuring cellular immunity against herpes viruses. *J. Immunol. Methods* **79(2),** 251–262.

4. Frankenburg, S. (1988) A simplified microtechnique for measuring human lymphocyte proliferation after stimulation with mitogen and specific antigen. *J. Immunol. Methods* **112(2),** 177–182.

5. Bloemena, E., Roos, M. T. L., Van Heijst, J. L. A. M., Vossen, J. M. J. J., and Schellekens, P. T. A. (1989) Whole-blood lymphocyte cultures. *J. Immunol. Methods* **122(2),** 161–167.

6. Weir, R. E., Morgan, A. R., Britton, W. J., Butlin, C. R., and Dockrell, H. M. (1994) Development of a whole blood assay to measure T cell responses to

leprosy: a new tool for immuno-epidemiological field studies of leprosy immunity *J. Immunol. Methods* **176(1),** 93–101.
7. Gaines, H., Andersson, L., and Biberfeld, G. (1996) A new method for measuring lymphoproliferation at the single-cell level in whole blood cultures by flow cytometry. *J Immunol Methods* **195(1–2),** 63–72.
8. Medina, E., Borthwick, N., Johnson, M. A., Miller, S., and Bofill, M. (1994) Flow cytometric analysis of the stimulatory response of T cell subsets from normal and HIV-1+ individuals to various mitogenic stimuli in vitro. *Clin. Exp. Immunol.* **97(2),** 266–272.
9. Yssel, H. and Cottrez, F. (1998) Measuring human cytokine responses, in *Methods in Microbiology volume 25: Immunology of Infection* (Kaufman, S. H. E. and Kabelitz, D., eds.), Academic Press, San Diego, CA, pp. 621–649.

20

Digital Image Analysis
of Lymphocyte Activation

Bradley W. McIntyre, T. Kent Teague,
Darren G. Woodside, and David K. Wooten

1. Introduction

The size and shape of an individual T lymphocyte can reflect activation or functional status. Therefore, information from a visual assessment of morphology can provide important criteria for determining extrinsic factors that regulate the physiological responses of lymphocytes. The combination of video microscopy and digital imaging can detect and quantify differences in cellular morphology, and therefore, it has been exploited and developed into a reproducible, sensitive method for the direct study of lymphocyte behavior. We have used this method to quantitate human T-lymphocyte coactivation, leading to cellular blastogenesis and proliferation *(1)*, the induction and kinetics of lymphocyte aggregation *(2)*, and lymphocyte adhesion and the formation of pseudopodia *(3)*.

Upon activation, small resting lymphocytes transform into larger blasts and proliferate. We have developed a method to quantitate this blastogenesis and use these values as indicators of lymphocyte proliferation *(1)*. Conventional methods widely used for determining proliferation are the [^{3}H]-thymidine incorporation, MTT (3-[4,5-dimethylthiazol-2-yl]-2,5-diphenyltetrazolium bromide) assays, and flow cytometry *(4–9)*. The video microscopy and digital imaging assay for determining lymphocyte activation and proliferation has many characteristics that offer advantages over these conventional methods. It does not produce radioactive waste, does not require cell harvesting nor sample manipulations; allows for continuous monitoring of single-cell events; has the potential to analyze subpopulations; and allows direct scoring of cellular activation, DNA synthesis, and proliferation. Although flow cytometry also has

From: *Methods in Molecular Biology, Vol. 134: T Cell Protocols: Development and Activation*
Edited by: K. P. Kearse © Humana Press Inc., Totowa, NJ

some of these advantages, sample manipulations and harvesting are still required, and it is not possible to continuously monitor cells with this method. The MTT assay produces no radioactive waste, and sample harvesting is not required, but MTT possesses none of the other aforementioned advantages of the video microscopy and digital imaging assay, whereas the [3H]-thymidine incorporation method is limited solely to direct measurements of DNA synthesis.

Since video microscopy and digital imaging can detect subtle differences in cell shape and size, we have also used this technology to develop assays for studying the morphological changes that occur when lymphocytes adhere and activate to spread, extend pseudopodia, or become motile *(3)*. Once the subjectivity of the experimenter is removed from the analysis of cell morphology, along with the increased accuracy and sensitivity, the digital image analysis of cells can be exploited to detect and characterize the multiple biochemical signaling pathways that regulate the different aspects of lymphocyte behavior. With this new dimension, the combination of the microscope, video camera, and computer should become a mainstay in immunology laboratories in the future.

2. Materials

2.1. Cells

1. Human T-cell lines used include HPB-ALL, Jurkat, Molt-4, and PEER.
2. Human peripheral blood T lymphocytes are freshly isolated from normal donors.

2.2. Monoclonal Antibodies

1. Monoclonal antibodies used for these studies should be purified.

2.3. Microscopy, Image Acquisition, and Image Analysis (Fig. 1)

1. Nikon DIAPHOT-TMD inverted microscope with 37°C incubator ×10, ×20, and ×40 objectives.
2. VI-470 CCD video camera with camera processor (Optronics Engineering, Goleta, CA).
3. Sony Trinitron monitor.
4. Macintosh IIVX computer with minimum of 20 MB RAM.
5. QuickCapture frame grabber board (Data Translation, Inc., Marlboro, MA).
6. Read/write magneto-optical disk drive.
7. National Institutes of Health public domain Image software (ftp://codon.nih.gov/pub/nih-image/nih-image161_fat.hqx).

3. Methods

3.1. Immobilization of Activating Proteins to Plastic

Monoclonal antibodies, extracellular matrix components, such as fibronectin, or recombinant proteins, such as VCAM-Ig, are used to activate the lymphocytes.

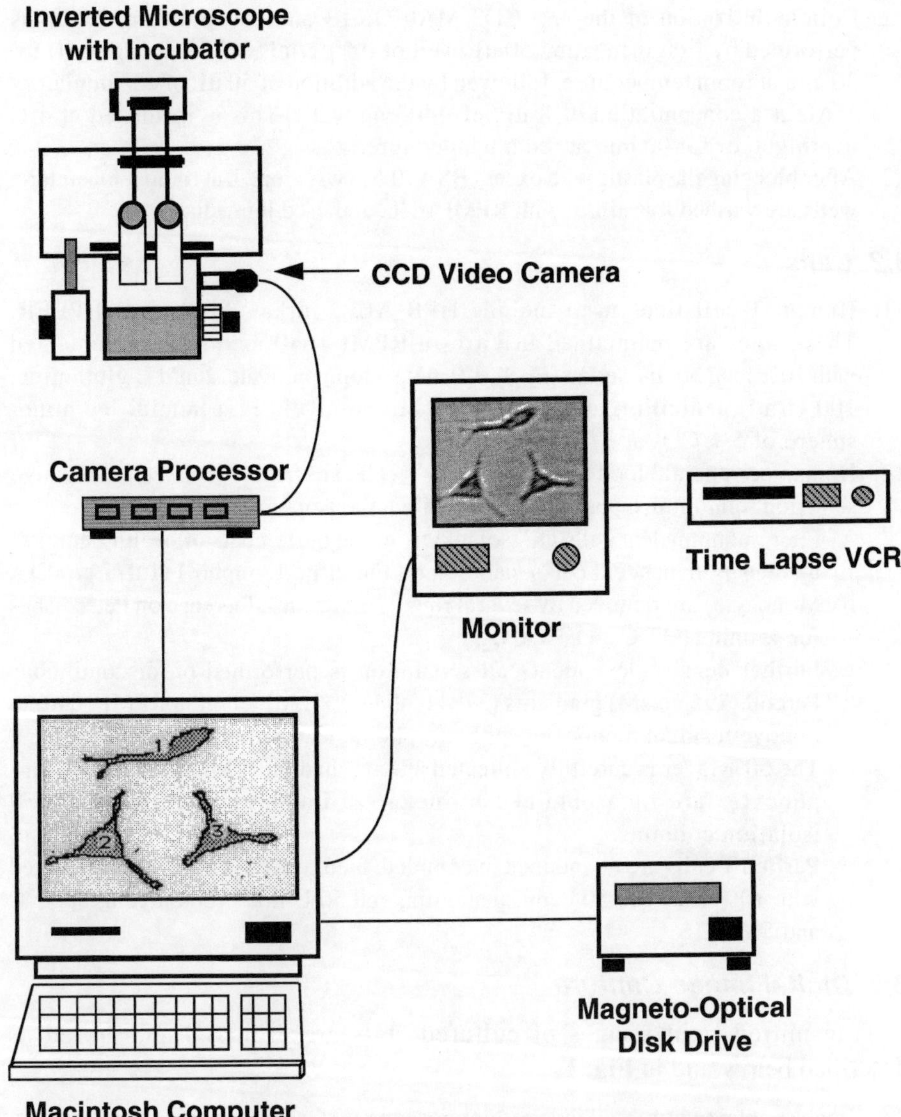

Fig. 1. The image acquisition setup. The video signal passes from the CCD video camera attached to the inverted microscope to either the computer or to the time-lapse VCR. Images can be stored on either VCR tape or on magneto-optical disks, allowing analog or digital recording of experiments.

1. Purified proteins are diluted in PBS to the desired concentrations and then immobilized in 96-well Covalink plates at room temperature for 2 h or overnight at 4°C.

2. Coimmobilization of the anti-CD3 MAb OKT3 and costimulatory MAbs is performed by first incubating 50 µL/well of 0.5 µg/mL OKT3 (25 ng/well) for 30 min at room temperature, followed by the addition of 50 µL of costimulatory MAb at a concentration of 8 µg/mL (400 ng/well). This is incubated at 4°C overnight, or for 90 min at room temperature.
3. After blocking the plastic with excess BSA (0.5% w/v) for 2 h at room temperature, wells are washed four times with RPMI 1640, and used immediately.

3.2. Cells

1. Human T-cell lines used include HPB-ALL, Jurkat, Molt-4, and PEER. These lines are maintained in vitro in RPMI 1640 medium supplemented with 10% fetal bovine serum (FBS), 1.0 mM sodium pyruvate, 2 mM L-glutamine, 100 U/mL penicillin, and 100 µg/mL streptomycin in a humidified atmosphere of 5% CO_2 at 37°C.
2. Human peripheral blood T cells. Human T cells are freshly isolated by negative selection to minimize possible activation via the isolation protocol.
   a. First, mononuclear cells are isolated from the buffy coats of healthy donors by density-dependent cell separation on Fico/Lite-LymphoH (1.077 g/mL).
   b. Monocytes are removed by several rounds of plastic adherence on Petri dishes for 45 min at 37°C and 5% CO_2.
   c. Further density-dependent cell separation is performed on discontinuous Percoll (295 mosM) gradients (37, 44, and 60% v/v Percoll in RPMI 1640) to remove residual monocytes, polymorphonuclear leukocytes, and RBC.
   d. The 60% layer is carefully collected and washed in RPMI 1640, and T lymphocytes are then obtained by negative immunoselection on T-cell isolation columns.
   e. Purfied T cells are maintained in complete media (RPMI 1640, supplemented with 10% v/v FBS, 50 U/mL penicillin, and 50 U/mL streptomycin) at 37°C and 5% CO_2.

3.3. Digital Image Capture

Transmitted light images of cultured cells are digitized and stored as described below and in **Fig. 1**.

1. Images obtained with an inverted microscope and a CCD video camera system are observed on a monitor.
2. To obtain the highest contrast between cells and background, the phase contrast ring is removed, the condenser aperture diaphragm is stopped to a minimum setting, and the focus is set slightly above the midplane of the cells. This arrangement in conjunction with the phase contrast objective produces strong contrast between the cells and background, with the cells appearing as dark spots on a bright field.
3. The camera passes the video signal to the Macintosh computer.
4. A frame grabber board digitizes the images, that are stored on a magneto-optical disk cartridge.

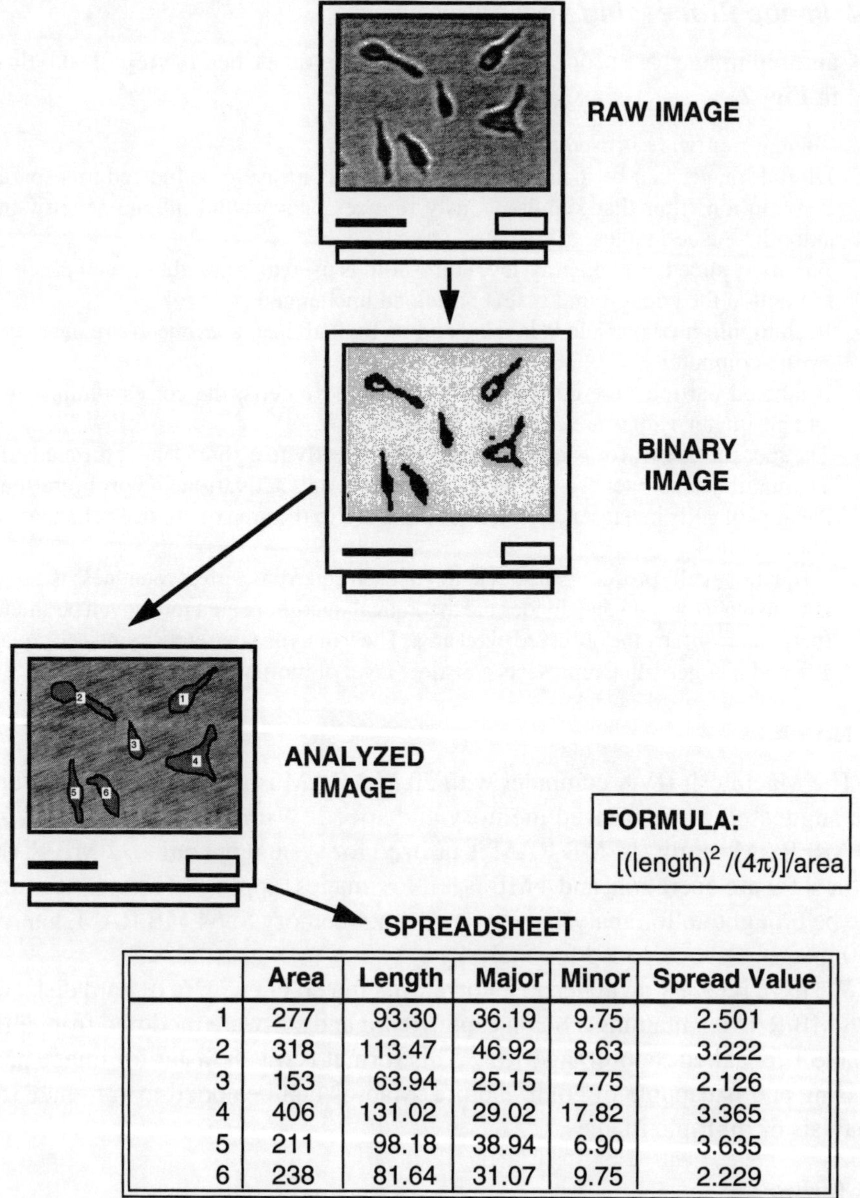

	Area	Length	Major	Minor	Spread Value
1	277	93.30	36.19	9.75	2.501
2	318	113.47	46.92	8.63	3.222
3	153	63.94	25.15	7.75	2.126
4	406	131.02	29.02	17.82	3.365
5	211	98.18	38.94	6.90	3.635
6	238	81.64	31.07	9.75	2.229

Fig. 2. Image processing. Raw digitized images are subjected to threshold segmentation to produce a binary image. The binary images are processed by the computer and analyzed using the Image software to measure a variety of parameters such as area, length (perimeter), and major and minor axis. The measurements for each cell can be automatically exported to a spreadsheet for calculations and analysis.

3.4. Image Processing and Analysis

Captured images are processed and analyzed as described in **steps 1–8** below and in **Fig. 2**.

1. "Image" software is used to analyze the images.
2. Digital images can be manipulated to enhance contrast, or subjected to a spatial convolution filter that simultaneously reduces background inhomogeneity and smooths the cell edges.
3. A density slice based on gray-level threshold is used to highlight the cell pixels in red, while the background pixels remained unchanged.
4. Each highlighted particle is labeled and its total area and perimeter are measured by the computer.
5. If labeled particles are composed of two or more cells, the corresponding area and perimeter values are excluded manually.
6. The measurements for each image are sent directly to a spreadsheet for analysis.
7. To quantify blastogenesis (as an indicator of T-cell activation and proliferation), the area of cells in a test activation is compared to the area of control cells that are not activated.
8. To quantify cell spreading, the deviation of each cell from perfect roundness is calculated using a formula that divides the theoretical maximum area for a given perimeter (perimeter^2/4π) by the observed pixel area. The value for a perfectly round cell equals 1.0, and a larger value represents a distinct level of morphologic change.

4. Notes

The Macintosh IIVX computer with 20 MB RAM is sufficient, but upgrades are suggested for increased memory and speed. With the Macintosh IIVX/ 20 MB RAM set-up, 14 MB RAM is utilized for system operation, 2 MB RAM is for software operation, and 4 MB is left for images (approx 12 images at a time can be brought up for analysis). By increasing memory to 64 MB RAM, approx 150 images can be opened for analysis.

We have recently switched to a Power Macintosh G3 with 6GB hard disk and 128 MB RAM containing a Scion capture card and software modified from NIH Image 1.62 called ScionImage 1.62. This format is much faster for image processing and is capable of color capture. Macros can be added to automate the analysis of multiple images.

References

1. Teague, T. K., Munn L., Zygourakis, K., and McIntyre, B. W. (1993) Analysis of lymphocyte activation and proliferation by video microscopy and digital imaging. *Cytometry* **14,** 772–782.
2. Munn, L. L., Glacken, M. W., McIntyre, B. W., and Zygourakis, K. (1993) Analysis of lymphocyte aggregation using digital image analysis. *J. Immunol. Methods* **166,** 11–25.

3. Szabo, M. C., Teague, T. K., and McIntyre, B. W. (1995) Regulation of lymphocyte pseudopodia formation by triggering the integrin $\alpha4\beta1$. *J. Immunol.* **154,** 2112–2124.
4. Miller, O. J. (1970) Autoradiography in human genetics. *Adv. Hum. Genet.* **1,** 35–130.
5. Taylor, J. H., Woods, P. S., and Hughes, W. L. (1957) The organization and duplication of chromosomes as revealed by autoradiographic studies using tritium-labeled thymidine. *Proc. Natl. Acad. Sci. USA* **43,** 122–127.
6. Mossman, T. (1983) Rapid colorimetic assay for cellular growth and survival: Application to proliferation and cytotoxicity assays. *J. Immunol. Methods* **65,** 55–63.
7. Hulett, H. R., Bonner W. A., Barrett, J., and Herzenberg, L. A. (1969) Cell sorting: Automated separation of mammalian cells as a function of intracellular fluorescence. *Science* **166,** 745–749.
8. Braylan, R. C., Benson, N. A., Nourse, V., and Kruth, H. S. (1982) Correlated analysis of cellular DNA, membrane antigens and light scatter of human lymphoid cells. *Cytometry* **2,** 337–343.
9. Dolbcare, F., Gratzner, H., Pallavicini, M. G., and Gray, J. W. (1983) Flow cytometric measurement of total DNA content and incorporated bromodeoxyuridine. *Proc. Natl. Acad. Sci. USA* **80,** 5573–5577.

21

Induction of T-Cell Signaling
by Immobilized Integrin Ligands

Jean Maguire van Seventer and Gijs A. van Seventer

1. Introduction

The integrin supergene family of adhesion molecules are cell surface $\alpha\beta$ heterodimers (reviewed in **ref. 1**). Although most integrins are involved in the binding of cells to extracellular matrix (ECM) components, many T-cell integrins can also bind to cell surface ligands. CD4$^+$ T helper (Th) cells can express several integrins, of which the best studied are the leukocyte function-associated antigen-1 (LFA-1), $\alpha_L\beta_2$ (CD11a/CD18), and the very late activation antigen-4 (VLA-4), $\alpha_4\beta_1$ (CD49d/CD29). The highest affinity ligand for LFA-1 is the intercellular adhesion molecule-1 (ICAM-1) (CD54), which is a member of the immunoglobulin (Ig) supergene family. Other ligands for LFA-1 are the Ig supergene family members ICAM-2 (CD102) and ICAM-3 (CD50). VLA-4, the second functionally important integrin expressed on Th cells, can bind to both the ECM protein fibronectin and the cell surface expressed Ig supergene family member vascular adhesion molecule-1 (VCAM-1) (CD106).

The T-cell integrins LFA-1 and VLA-4 are adhesion molecules that have been shown to play an important role both in the adhesion of T cells to inflamed endothelium and their subsequent migration into tissues, and in the binding of T cells to antigen presenting cells (APC) (reviewed in **refs. 1–3**). T-cell integrins are distinct from integrins expressed on adherent cell types in that they are in a low ligand-binding state on resting T cells, and require activation through "inside-out" signaling to revert to a high ligand-binding state (**4**). This high ligand-binding state can be achieved either by increasing the affinity of the integrin for its ligand through a conformational change in the integrin's extracellular binding domains, or by increasing the avidity of integrin:integrin

From: *Methods in Molecular Biology, Vol. 134: T Cell Protocols: Development and Activation*
Edited by: K. P. Kearse © Humana Press Inc., Totowa, NJ

ligand binding, as by the clustering or patching of integrins on the T-cell surface *(5)*. Examples of physiological signals that upregulate integrin binding activity are chemokines *(6)* and antigen-specific recognition by the T cell receptor (TCR)/CD3 complex *(4,7)*. While much research has been devoted to the "inside-out" signaling that regulates integrin binding to ligand, details of such research will not be discussed in this chapter.

In recent years, it has become clear that T-cell integrins, including LFA-1 and VLA-4, can function not only as adhesion molecules, but also as signal-transducing molecules capable of providing T-cell stimulatory, or "outside-in" signals *(8)*. This chapter will focus on the methodology used to induce "outside-in" integrin signals by crosslinking of T-cell integrins with immobilized integrin natural ligands.

Crosslinking of T-cell integrins by integrin ligands induces the generation of signals that, along with TCR/CD3-derived signals, can costimulate T cells. The first direct evidence that T-cell integrin ligands could induce T-cell costimulatory signals came from studies demonstrating that resting Th cell proliferation could be achieved by stimulation with coimmobilized anti-CD3 MAb and purified ICAM-1 *(9)*. Subsequently, the other LFA-1 ligands, ICAM-2 *(10)* and ICAM-3 *(11)*, and the VLA-4 ligands VCAM-1 *(12)* and fibronectin *(13)*, were also shown to provide costimulation for Th cells in similar model systems.

Naive Th cell differentiation leading to functionally distinct Th cell subsets, as defined by cytokine secretion profiles, is critically regulated by the cytokine milieu present at the time of TCR/CD3 ligation, and by the costimulatory signals provided by the antigen presenting cell (APC). The cytokines IL-4 and IL-12 are well known inducers of Th2-like and Th1-like cells, respectively (reviewed in **ref. *14***). Naive Th cell stimulation with coimmobilized anti-CD3 MAb and ICAM-1 or VCAM-1 induces differentiation into Th cells that secrete the Th1 cytokines IFN-γ and TNF-α, but not the Th2 cytokines IL-4 or IL-5 *(15)*. Th1-like cells that are generated in this way have, however, low viability and do not show significant expansion after the second stimulation in vitro (R. T. Semnani and G. A. van Seventer unpublished). Damle et al. has shown that integrin-mediated costimulation of naive Th cells in these model systems leads to cell death through apoptosis, and can be prevented by CD28-mediated signals *(16)*. Recently, we found that addition of exogenous rIL-12 to coimmobilized anti-CD3 MAb and ICAM-1 not only significantly increases the levels of secreted IFN-γ, but also allows for repeated stimulations with good cell viability and high cell expansion rates. In contrast, addition of exogenous rIL-4 does not rescue integrin-stimulated naive Th cells from cell death (E. M. Palmer and G. A. van Seventer, manuscript in preparation). These results indicate that integrin-mediated costimulation can provide the necessary T-cell costimulatory signals required for cell proliferation, but not for clonal expansion and cell viability. In addition, they demonstrate that when integrin-mediated costimulatory signals are combined with signals provided by IL-12, clonal expansion can be induced, with the subsequent generation of Th1 cells. Interestingly, these results imply that the generation of Th1 cells can be CD28-independent, in contrast to the generation of Th2 cells which is CD28-dependent.

Although in vitro models of T-cell costimulation clearly show that T-cell integrins can mediate T-cell costimulatory signals, the signaling pathways that transduce these T-cell integrin-derived costimulatory ("outside-in") signals are still not well defined. Biochemical data on the specific intracellular signals transduced by T-cell integrins is mainly descriptive, and there is little, if any, direct evidence indicating which signals are involved in the induction of T-cell proliferation. Crosslinking of LFA-1 on T cells is reported to activate phospholipase C-γ1 (PLC-γ$_1$) and its downstream effector molecules *(17,18)*. In contrast, many more signaling molecules are known to be affected by β$_1$ integrin signaling. T cell binding to immobilized fibronectin, VCAM-1, or anti-β$_1$ integrin MAb is reported to induce tyrosine phosphorylation of not only PLC-γ$_1$, but also pp59^{FYN}, pp56^{LCK}, pp125^{FAK}, MAP kinase *(19)*, Pyk2 *(20)*, pp105^{CAS-L} *(21)*, and paxillin *(22)*, as well as induction of the DNA-binding protein AP-1 *(23)* A role for focal adhesion kinase family members in β$_1$-integrin-mediated T-cell costimulation has been implied by experiments showing that signals generated by the binding of T cells to immobilized VCAM-1 and anti-CD3 MAb can synergize to induce tyrosine phosphorylation of both pp125^{FAK} and Pyk2 *(20,24)*. Interestingly, CD28-mediated T-cell costimulation does not upregulate tyrosine phosphorylation of pp125^{FAK} and Pyk2 *(20)*.

This chapter outlines a protocol for the activation of T cells by crosslinking of integrin receptors with immobilized integrin ligands, in the presence or absence of TCR crosslinking with immobilized anti-CD3 MAb (*see* **Note 1**). Although the protocol specifically describes details for the activation of primary resting human CD4$^+$ T cells and Jurkat T leukemia cells, it may be modified for the study of other primary T cells and T-cell lines.

2. Materials

2.1. Cells to Be Analyzed

1. CD4$^+$ T cells (*see* **Note 2**): *See* Chapter 28, for details on materials needed for negative immunomagnetic isolation of resting CD4$^+$ T cells from peripheral blood mononuclear cells (PBMC).
2. Jurkat T cells (*see* **Note 3**): The Jurkat T leukemia cell line is available from the ATTC. Culture in RPMI 1640 supplemented with 10% FCS, L-glutamine, and antibiotics, at densities not exceeding 1×10^6 cells/mL of culture medium.

2.2. Integrin Ligands and MAbs

1. Integrin ligands (*see* **Note 4**): Extracellular matrix integrin ligands, such as fibronectin and laminin, can be purchased from various commercial sources (e.g., Gibco-BRL, Grand Island, NY). Cell surface integrin ligands are commonly used as Ig-fusion proteins (e.g., ICAM-1-Ig or VCAM-1-Ig).
2. Anti-integrin MAbs (*see* **Note 5**): Many antibodies against the extracellular domains of integrin receptors are commercially available as purified MAb, or can be obtained as hybridomas from the ATTC.
3. Anti-CD3 MAb OKT3: OKT3 is available as a hybridoma from the ATTC.
4. Polyclonal antisera (*see* **Note 6**): Anti-human IgG and anti-mouse IgG polyclonal sera are available from commercial sources, such as NCI/Cappel (Durham, NC).

2.3. Biochemical Analysis of Integrin-Mediated Signaling in Human T Cells

1. Labware and equipment: Tissue culture treated 6-well plates (*see* **Note 7**), 15- and 50-mL polyprolylene centrifuge tubes, and Eppendorf tubes. Refrigerated table top centrifuge with holders for tissue culture plates, and refrigerated microcentrifuge.
2. Assay media (*see* **Note 8**): X-Vivo 20 serum-free media (BioWhittaker, Walkersville, MD) supplemented with HEPES (10 mM) and antibiotics.
3. Phosphate-buffered saline (PBS): PBS with Ca^{2+}/Mg^{2+} for washing cells prior to stimulation, and PBS without Ca^{2+}/Mg^{2+} for harvesting cells. For studies of protein tyrosine phosphorylation, the PBS for harvesting cells should be Ca^{2+}/Mg^{2+} free, and contain EDTA (2 mM final) and sodium orthovanadate (1 mM final) to inhibit tyrosine phosphatase activity.
4. Lysis buffer (*see* **Note 9**):

Solution	Amount for 10 mL buffer	Final concentration
1 M Tris-HCl (pH 7.4)	0.5 mL	50 mM
5 M NaCl	0.6 mL	300 mM
20% Triton X-100	0.5 mL	1.0%
0.5 M EDTA (pH 8.0)	40 µL	2 mM
10 mg/mL aprotinin	10 µL	10 µg/µL
5 mg/mL leupeptin	10 µL	5 µg/µL
100 mM Pefabloc®SC	100 µL	1 mM
0.5 M NaF	200 µL	10 mM
dH$_2$O to 10 mL		

For experiments studying protein tyrosine phosphorylation events, the lysis buffer should also include 1 mM sodium orthovanadate (100 µL of 100 mM) (Sigma), a tyrosine phosphatase inhibitor. A stock solution (100 mM) of sodium orthovanvadate should be prepared immediately before use, and be kept chilled on ice.

Protease inhibitors (aprotinin, leupeptin, and Pefabloc®SC) may be purchased as lyophilisates from Boehringer Mannheim (Indianapolis, IN) and other commercial sources. They should be reconstituted according to the manufacturers' suggestions, and stock solutions should be stored in aliquots, at –20°C to avoid repeat thawing. Aprotinin and leupeptin are stable for at least 6 mo at –20°C. Pefabloc®SC is stable for at least 2 mo at –20°C. A stock solution of 0.5 M NaF in H_2O may be stored at room temperature.

3. Methods

3.1. Cells to Be Analyzed

1. CD4[+] T cells: The isolation procedure (Chapter 28) can be initiated a day in advance and the cells can be kept at 4°C overnight.
2. Jurkat T cells: Cells should be split the day before the experiment, so that they are growing in log phase the day of the experiment.

3.2. Integrin Ligands and MAbs: Preparation of Plates for Stimulation

1. Day 1: Coat tissue culture treated 6-well plates overnight at 4°C with 5–10 µg/mL polyclonal antihuman IgG (for immobilization of chimeric integrin:human Ig fusion proteins) and/or antimouse IgG (for immobilization of mouse MAb), diluted in PBS containing Ca^{2+} and Mg^{2+}. Add 2 mL/well of each antibody dilution. All wells should be coated with the same polyclonal antibodies. If only one type of polyclonal antibody is required for an experiment, bring the final volume of wells to 4 mL with PBS.
2. Day 2: Wash wells 3× with sterile PBS containing Ca^{2+} and Mg^{2+}. After the last wash, add 2 mL/well of the ligand and/or MAb to be used for stimulation, diluted in PBS with Ca^{2+} and Mg^{2+}. The concentration of ligands and MAbs will vary according to the signaling event being studied. Suggested starting points for ligand/ MAb dilutions are: integrin ligands as purified extracellular matrix proteins: 1 µg/ mL; integrin ligands as fusion proteins: 0.3 µg/mL; anti-integrin MAbs: 0.1–0.3 µg/mL; and anti-CD3 MAb OKT3: 0.1 µg/mL. For control, nonstimulating conditions cells should be incubated in wells that are coated with only human- and/or mouse-specific polyclonal antisera. Bring the final volume of all wells to 4 mL with PBS. Reagents may contain azide, because the wells will be extensively washed before cells are added. This second step in the coating process can be done overnight at 4°C or, alternatively, for 2–3 h at room temperature. The number of wells required per stimulating condition will depend upon the proteins being studied and assays to be performed on final lysates.
3. Day 3: Wash wells 3× with PBS, and add 1 mL of assay media/well after the last wash. Incubate plates at 37°C before adding cells for stimulation.

3.3. Biochemical Analysis of Integrin-Mediated Signals in Human T Cells

3.3.1. Preparation of Reagents and Solutions

1. Warm serum free media to 37°C.
2. Prepare lysis buffer and chill on ice.

3. Fill 15 or 50 mL polypropylene centrifuge tubes with chilled PBS without Ca^{2+}/Mg^{2+}, containing tyrosine phosphatase inhibitors (2 mM EDTA, 1 mM sodium orthovanadate) if required. Add enough of the PBS solution to dilute harvested media containing nonadherent cells by at least half. Keep filled tubes chilled at 4°C.

3.3.2. Preparation of Cells

1. Wash Jurkat T cells or CD4+ T cells once in PBS (with Ca^{2+}/Mg^{2+}) before resuspending in assay media at 2×10^6/mL for Jurkat T cells, and $5–10 \times 10^6$ cells/mL for CD4+ T cells.
2. Warm cells to 37°C before adding to the wells to initiate experiment. If the stimulation is not carried out immediately, it is advisable to keep the cells in a flask, on its side, in the incubator. This will minimize T-cell:T-cell interactions, which otherwise may be of some significance in cells settling to the bottom of a centrifuge tube.

3.3.3. Preparation of Plates

See **Subheading 3.2.**, Day 3.

3.3.4. Initiation of Experiment

1. Add 1 mL of cells in assay media to each well of the 6-well plates, already containing 1 mL of media (final volume is 2 mL/well).
2. Immediately spin plate at 180g for 30 s in room temperature centrifuge, to allow for immediate contact between cells and antibodies/ligands. The combined time for the centrifuge to come up to speed, spin for 30 s, and then brake completely should be ~1.5 min.
3. Remove plates and incubate at 37°C for as long as the assay further requires. For many early integrin-mediated signaling events 10 min (or less) incubations are sufficient. *Note*: Cells are stimulated at low densities to prevent the induction of integrin signaling pathways (e.g., LFA-1:ICAM-1, VLA-4:VLA-4) as a result of T-cell:T-cell interactions.

3.3.5. Harvest

1. Place tissue culture plate at a slight angle and transfer media, containing nonadherent cells, from wells of the same stimulating condition to either a 15 or 50 mL polypropylene v-bottom centrifuge tube. Centrifuge tubes should be prefilled with cold Ca^{2+}/Mg^{2+}-free PBS, as described in **Subheading 3.3.1.**
2. Perform *in situ* lysis of adherent cells remaining in wells by adding 150–200 μL lysis buffer to each well. Spread lysis buffer evenly over the well by gently rocking the plate. Incubate plates at 4°C for at least 15 min.
3. While plates are incubating, spin down nonadherent cells in a 4°C centrifuge. Resuspend the cell pellet in 1 mL of cold Ca^{2+}/Mg^{2+}-free PBS, and transfer to an Eppendorf tube. Spin down pellet cells again in a 4°C microcentrifuge by giving a quick (~30 s) spin. Remove supernatant.

4. Remove plates, containing adherent cell homogenate, from 4°C. Loosen homogenates by tapping the plates briskly, while being careful to avoid loss of homogenate by spilling. Transfer homogenates to Eppendorf tubes containing nonadherent cells from the same wells. Vortex to thoroughly resuspend pellet of nonadherent cells.

5. Continue lysis on ice for an additional 15 min, vortexing every few minutes.

6. Pellet cell membranes by microcentrifugation at 4°C for 15 min.

7. Transfer lysate containing supernatant to a fresh Eppendorf tube. Each tube will contain lysate from an equivalent number of cells.

4. Notes

1. Jurkat cells adhere spontaneously to VCAM-1, and it has been shown that on certain Jurkat cell lines a majority of the $\alpha_4\beta_1$ integrin receptors are in a high ligand-binding state and capable of binding soluble VCAM-1-Ig *(25)*. Resting primary T cells, however, do not significantly bind to integrin ligands because of the low binding state of their cell surface expressed integrin receptors. Thus, integrin signaling studies with resting primary T cells and natural integrin ligands are, in general, not very informative. Certain anti-integrin MAbs, such as the anti-CD29 MAb TS2/16 (available from the ATTC), can induce integrins to become high-affinity ligand binding receptors. Alternatively, induction of high-affinity integrins can be achieved by altering the presence of certain divalent cations in the media. For example, chelating Ca^{2+} in the media with EGTA in the presence of sufficient Mg^{2+} will increase β_2 integrin binding, while addition of Mn^{2+} increases β_1 integrin binding *(26)*. Another approach that can be used to induce the binding of primary T cells to integrin ligands is to activate the T cells through anti-CD3 MAb crosslinking *(4)*. One should keep in mind, however, that when T cells are stimulated by the combination of anti-CD3 crosslinking and binding of integrin receptors to their natural ligands, the activation of a given downstream signal transduction pathway may be the result of integrin receptor-dependent signaling, TCR/CD3-dependent signaling, or synergistic integrin receptor- and TCR/CD3-dependent signaling.

2. Take necessary precautions when working with human blood products. Assume that all blood-derived products are hazardous. This includes cell lysates, culture supernatants, and any other reagents that come in contact with human blood products. For isolation of $CD4^+$ T cells from PBMC modify the protocols described in Chapter 28 by omitting in the antibody cocktail the anti-CD45RO MAb. The expected yield of PBMC from a 25–50 mL buffy coat ranges from 0.3 to 1×10^9 cells. The yield of resting $CD4^+$ T cells is usually between 15 and 25% of that of the PBMC.

3. The Jurkat T leukemia cell line is one of, if not the most, commonly used T-cell line for signaling studies, which is why we describe its use in this chapter. However, other T-cell lines (e.g., H9) exist, which may be more appropriate for a given investigator's studies. Be aware that there are many different clones of the Jurkat cell line, and that these clones differ slightly in their functional and pheno-

typic properties. For example, not all Jurkat T-cell clones will readily secrete detectable levels of IL-2 following appropriate surface receptor crosslinking. It may be necessary to obtain a subclonal population of Jurkat cells, through limiting dilution, that satisfactorily expresses the cell surface molecules of interest (e.g., high expression of CD3, CD28, CD11a [α_L chain] and CD49d [α_4 chain]).

4. Cell surface expressed integrin ligands, such as ICAM-1 and VCAM-1, are often used as recombinant chimeric molecules in the form of fusion proteins between the extracellular domains of the integrin ligand and the Fc-domain of human IgG$_1$. (For details on the generation of such fusion proteins *see* **refs.** *25,27.*)

5. Anti-integrin MAbs may be used to mimic the integrin aggregation induced by natural integrin ligands in many T-cell costimulation and signaling systems. However, it should be noted that studies in fibroblasts indicate that the integrin-mediated signals resulting from integrin aggregation alone (as induced by nonblocking, anti-integrin MAbs) differ from those resulting from integrin aggregation plus integrin receptor occupancy (as induced by natural integrin ligands and certain ligand blocking, anti-integrin MAbs) *(28)*.

6. Optimal TCR/CD3 and integrin signaling requires the formation of clusters of receptors on the T-cell surface, and can be achieved by immobilizing integrin ligands and MAbs on the plastic of tissue-treated culture wells. Indirect binding to plastic of integrin natural ligands, in the form of Ig fusion proteins, and of anti-integrin MAb through polyclonal "capture" antibodies, allows for the use of much less of these stimulatory reagents than is required for direct binding to plastic. In the indirect binding approach, plates are first coated with a polyclonal anti-immunoglobulin sera (e.g., sheep-antihuman IgG and goat-antimouse IgG). Subsequently, integrin ligand fusion proteins (e.g., ICAM-1-Ig) or anti-integrin MAbs are added, with or without anti-CD3 MAb. The concentration of T-cell stimulatory reagents required with the "indirect" immobilization technique is in the order of 0.1–0.3 µg/mL, while the less efficient "direct" immobilization frequently requires concentrations in the order of 1–3 µg/mL.

7. The method outlined may be modified so as to be performed in 96- or 24-well plates, or in individual tissue culture plates. Simply increase or decrease the amount of antibody solution used to coat each well/plate, and the number of cells stimulated in each well/plate, according to the change in surface area from that of a well of a 6-well plate (i.e., 9.6 cm^2).

8. Serum-free media is used as assay media so as to prevent the stimulation of T cells by soluble ECM integrin ligands present in serum (e.g., plasma fibronectin). It should be noted, however, that for optimal expression of T-cell effector functions (e.g., IL-2 secretion), following incubation periods that are usually significantly longer that those required for most biochemical studies, serum containing media is often required.

9. Depending on the type of analysis to be performed, Triton X-100 can be substituted with other detergents of choice. It should be noted, however, that coprecipitation studies to analyze integrin-associated proteins are likely to fail in this stimulation protocol with immobilized integrin-ligands, as

integrin ligand:integrin complexes may remain attached to plastic after cell lysis. Thus, integrin-associated proteins may be best studied by stimulating cells with soluble integrin-ligands/anti-integrin MAbs, crosslinked with secondary, polyclonal antibodies.

References

1. Springer, T. A. (1994) Traffic signals for lymphocyte recirculation and leukocyte emigration: The multistep paradigm. *Cell* **76,** 301–314.
2. Spits, H., Van Schooten, W., Keizer, H., Van Seventer, G., Van de Rijn, M., Terhorst, C., and De Vries, J. E. (1986) Alloantigen recognition is preceded by nonspecific adhesion of cytotoxic T cells and target cells. *Science* **232,** 403–405.
3. Shaw, S., Luce, G. E. G., Quinones, R., Gress, R. E., Springer, T. A., and Sanders, M. E. (1986) Two antigen-independent adhesion pathways used by human cytotoxic T cell clones. *Nature* **323,** 262–264.
4. Dustin, M. L. and Springer, T. A. (1989) T-cell receptor cross-linking transiently stimulates adhesiveness through LFA-1. *Nature* **341,** 619–624.
5. Kucik, D. F., Dustin, M. L., Miller, J. M., and Browm, E. J. (1996) Adhesion-activation phorbol ester increases the mobility of leukocyte integrin LFA-1 in cultured lymphocytes. *J. Clin. Invest.* **97,** 2139–2144.
6. Weber, C., Katayama, J., and Springer, T. A. (1996) Differential regulation of beta 1 and beta 2 integrin avidity by chemoattractants in eosinophils. *PNAS USA* **93,** 10,939–10,944.
7. Shimizu, Y., van Seventer, G. A., Horgan, K. J., and Shaw, S. (1990) Regulated expression and function of three VLA (β1) integrin receptors on T cells. *Nature* **345,** 250–253.
8. van Seventer, G. A., Shimizu, Y., and Shaw, S. (1991) Roles of multiple accessory molecules in T-cell activation. *Curr. Opin. Immunol.* **3,** 294–303.
9. van Seventer, G. A., Shimizu, Y., Horgan, K. J., and Shaw, S. (1990) The LFA-1 ligand ICAM-1 provides an important costimulatory signal for T cell receptor-mediated activation of resting T cells. *J. Immunol.* **144,** 4579–4586.
10. Damle, N. K., Klussman, K., and Aruffo, A. (1991) Intercellular adhesion molecule-2, a second counter-receptor for CD11a/CD18 (leukocyte function-associated antigen-1), provides a costimulatory signal for T-cell receptor-initiated activation of human T cells. *J. Immunol.* **148,** 665–671.
11. Hernandez-Caselles, T., Rubio, G., Campanero, M. R., Del Pozo, M. A., Muro, M., Sanchez-Madrid, F., and Aparicio, P. (1993) ICAM-3, the third LFA-1 counterreceptor, is a co-stimulatory molecule for both resting and activated T lymphocytes. *Eur. J. Immunol.* **23,** 2799–2806.
12. van Seventer, G. A., Newman, W., Shimizu, Y., Nutman, T. B., Tanaka, Y., Horgan, K. J., Gopal, T. V., Ennis, E., O'Sullivan, D., Grey, H., and Shaw, S. (1991) Analysis of T-cell stimulation by superantigen plus major histocompatibility complex class II molecules or by CD3 monoclonal antibody: costimulation by purified adhesion ligands VCAM-1, ICAM-1 but not ELAM-1. *J. Exp. Med.* **174,** 901–913.

13. Shimizu, Y., van Seventer, G. A., Horgan, K. J., and Shaw, S. (1990) Costimulation of proliferative responses of resting CD4[+] T cells by the interaction of VLA-4 and VLA-5 with fibronectin or VLA-6 with laminin. *J. Immunol.* **145,** 59–67.

14. Paul, W. E. and Seder, R. A. (1994) Lymphocyte responses and cytokines. *Cell* **76,** 241–251.

15. Semnani, R. T., Nutman, T. B., Hochman, P., Shaw, S., and van Seventer, G. A. (1994) Costimulation by purified intercellular adhesion molecule 1 and lymphocyte function-associated antigen 3 induces distinct proliferation, cytokine and cell surface antigen profiles in human "naive" and "memory" CD4 T cells. *J. Exp. Med.* **180,** 2125–2135.

16. Damle, N. K., Klussman, K., Leytze, G., Aruffo, A., Linsley, P. S., and Ledbetter, J. A. (1993) Costimulation with integrin ligands intercellular adhesion molecule-1 and vascular cell adhesion molecule-1 augments activation-induced death of antigen-specific CD4[+] T lymphocytes. *J. Immunol.* **151,** 2368–2379.

17. Kanner, S. B., Grosmaire, L. S., Ledbetter, J. A., and Damle, N. K. (1993) Beta2-integrin LFA-1 signaling through phospholipase C-gamma-1 activation. *Proc. Natl. Acad. Sci. USA* **90,** 7099–7103.

18. van Seventer, G. A., Bonvini, E., Yamada, H., Conti, A., Stringfellow, S., June, C. H., and Shaw, S. (1992) Costimulation of TCR/CD3-mediated activation of resting human CD4[+] T-cells by LFA-1 ligand ICAM-1 involves prolonged inositol phospholipid hydrolysis and sustained increase of intracellular Ca++ levels. *J. Immunol.* **149,** 3872–3880.

19. Sato, T., Tachibana, K., Nojima, Y., D'Aviro, N., and Morimoto, C. (1995) Role of the VLA-4 molecule in T cell costimulation. Identification of the tyrosine phosphorylation pattern induced by the ligation of VLA-4. *J. Immunol.* **155,** 2938–2947.

20. van Seventer, G. A., Mullen, M. M., and van Seventer, J. M. (1998) Pyk2 is differentially regulated by β_1 integrin- and CD28-mediated costimulation in human CD4[+] T lymphocytes. *Eur. J. Immunol.* **28,** 3867–3877.

21. Milnegishi, M., Tachibana, K., Sato, T., Iwata, S., Nojima, Y., and Morimoto, C. (1996) Structure and function of Cas-L, a 105-kD Crk-associated substrate-related protein that is involved in beta-1 integrin-mediated signaling in lymphocytes. *J. Exp. Med.* **184,** 1365–1375.

22. Tachibana, K., Sato, T., D'Aviro, N., and Morimoto, C. (1995) Direct association of pp125FAK with paxillin, the focal adhesion targeting mechanism of pp125FAK. *J. Exp. Med.* **182,** 1089–1099.

23. Yamada, A., Nikaido, T., Nojima, Y., Schlossman, S. F., and Morimoto, C. (1991) Activation of human CD4 T lymphocytes. Interaction of fibronectin with VLA-5 receptor on CD4 cells induces the AP-1 transcription factor. *J. Immunol.* **146,** 53–56.

24. Maguire, J. E., Danahey, K., Burkly, L., and van Seventer, G. A. (1995) A T cell receptor-mediated signal synergizes with Beta-1 integrin-dependent tyrosine phosphorylation of focal adhesion kinase in human T cells. *J. Exp. Med.* **182,** 2079–2090.

25. Jakubowski, A., Rosa, M. D., Bixler, S., Lobb, R., and Burkly, L. C. (1995) Vascular Cell Adhesion Molecule (VCAM)-Ig fusion protein defines distinct affinity states of the Very Late Antigen (VLA-4) receptor. *Cell Adhes. Communication* **3,** 131–142.
26. Shimizu, Y. and Mobley, J. L. (1993) Distinct divalent cation requirements for integrin-mediated CD4$^+$ T lymphocyte adhesion to ICAM-1, fibronectin, VCAM- 1, and invasin. *J. Immunol.* **151,** 4106–4115.
27. Fawcett, J., Holness, C. L. L., Needham, L. A., Turley, H., Gatter, K. C., Mason, D. Y., and Simmons, D. L. (1992) Molecular cloning of ICAM-3, a third ligand for LFA-1, constitutively expressed on resting leukocytes. *Nature* **360,** 481–484.
28. Miayamoto, S., Akiyama, S. K., and Yamada, K. M. (1995) Synergistic roles for receptor occupancy and aggregation in integrin transmembrane function. *Science* **267,** 883–885.

22

Cytotoxic T-Cell Adherence Assay (CAA)

Graham R. Leggatt and Jay A. Berzofsky

1. Introduction

Cytotoxic T lymphocytes (CTL) play an important role in the control of intracellular pathogens through their capacity to lyse infected target cells or secrete immunostimulatory cytokines, such as IFN-γ or TNF-α *(1–3)*. These features of cytotoxic T cells are termed "effector" mechanisms and have been measured extensively in the past using assays, such as cytokine ELISAs, or radioactive chromium release from target cells *(4,5)*. However, several other important changes occur within CTL in conjunction with these effector mechanisms. Triggering of the T-cell receptor (TCR) by cognate peptide/major histocompatability complex (MHC) class I complexes leads to a cascade of intracellular signaling events which, among other outcomes, results in increased cell surface adhesion to extracellular matrix and surrounding cells *(6,7)*. Increased surface adhesion may be caused by the provision of new cell surface adhesion receptors from the intracellular pool or conformational changes in existing cell surface receptors following antigen-specific TCR triggering *(8)*. Several studies have now demonstrated the specific binding of activated CTL to plate-bound MHC class I molecules and fibronectin using an assay system that involves wash steps to remove unbound cells *(9–11)*. In the current chapter, the increased adhesiveness of CTL, following specific peptide/MHC class I recognition, forms the basis of a simple, peptide-specific assay, the cytotoxic T-cell adherence assay (CAA) *(12)*, which correlates well with more traditional effector assays, such as ^{51}Cr release, and does not involve washing steps. This technique has the advantage of being inexpensive and rapid, and not requiring radioactive nuclides.

From: *Methods in Molecular Biology, Vol. 134: T Cell Protocols: Development and Activation*
Edited by: K. P. Kearse © Humana Press Inc., Totowa, NJ

2. Materials

1. Murine CTL line or clone (prepared according to standard methods; *see* **ref. *12***).
2. Growth medium: A 1:1 mixture of RPMI-1640 liquid and Eagle-Hank's amino acids (EHAA; Life Technologies, Gaithersburg, MD) liquid supplemented with 2 m*M* L-glutamine, 100 U/mL penicillin, 100 µg/mL streptomycin, 5×10^{-5} *M* 2-mercaptoethanol and 10% fetal calf serum (FCS) (Sigma, St. Louis, MO).
3. Lympholyte M ficoll (Accurate Chemical and Scientific Corporation, Westbury, NY).
4. 96-well round-bottom plates (Corning [Costar plates], Acton, MA).
5. 15 mL tubes.
6. Trypan blue (Sigma, St. Louis, MO).
7. Peptide — minimal CTL epitope.

3. Methods

1. Harvest the CTL line or clone from the bottom of a 24-well plate by vigorous pipeting. The CTL culture should be at least 7 d poststimulation with antigen at the time of harvesting.
2. Place the harvested cells in 10 mL tubes with 5 mL of cells for every 2 mL of Lympholyte M. Lympholyte M is carefully layered beneath the cells using a pipet such that an interface exists between the ficoll and the culture. Centrifuge the cells at 400*g* for 15 min (*see* **Note 1**).
3. At the completion of the centrifugation, carefully remove cells from the interface and transfer to a new tube. Add fresh growth media and wash the cells by centrifugation at 250*g* for 5 min.
4. Resuspend cells in 1 mL of growth medium and count live cells by trypan blue exclusion.
5. Add ficolled cells to each well of a 96-well round-bottom plate at 100,000 viable cells per well in a 100 µL volume.
6. As a negative control, 100 µL of growth medium (no peptide) is added to duplicate wells containing the CTL (*see* **Note 2**). The positive control consists of 100 µL of the cognate peptide (if known) in growth medium.
7. Prepare titrated concentrations of the test peptides and add to duplicate wells, containing the CTL, in a 100 µL volume.
8. Place the 96-well plates in an incubator and monitor visually by inspection through the plate bottom for the presence of a cell pellet in the negative control and evidence of a dispersed pellet in the peptide-treated wells (*see* **Fig. 1**) (*12*). The assay is complete when the negative control forms a pellet which is clearly distinguishable from the positive control. Pellets may form within 5 h but are mostly clearly seen after overnight incubation (*see* **Note 3**). A CAA titer is given as the lowest concentration of peptide which results in a dispersed pattern of CTL visibly different from the negative control pellet.

4. Notes

1. Ficolling of the CTL line or clone is important in removing cell debris produced by dying, irradiated, antigen presenting cells. The CAA has been shown to require

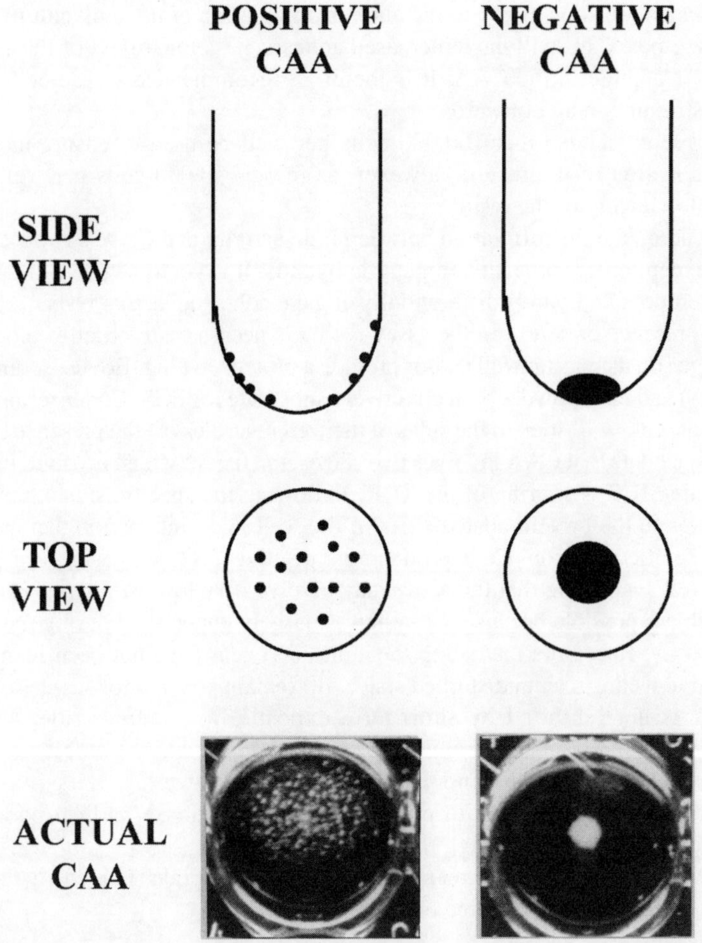

Fig. 1. The appearance of positive and negative CAA results as illustrated by the side and top view of a single well from a 96-well round bottom plate. A photograph of an actual positive and negative CAA is included as a reference.

    live cells. Additionally, the presence of large numbers of nonantigen specific CTL, such as would be the case for CAA performed on spleen cells freshly isolated from an immunized mouse, is incompatible with the CAA. Dead or nonantigen specific CTL will contribute to the pellet thus making the experimental well more like the no peptide control well.

2. Negative control wells with CTL but without peptide are critical to the visible interpretation of the experiment because all other wells with added peptide will be compared with this control. If the negative control does not form a pellet then the experiment cannot be interpreted. This situation can arise if the CTL are

harvested too soon after routine antigen stimulation of the bulk culture. At these early times, CTL will have increased adhesiveness regardless of the addition of further peptide in the CAA. It is therefore recommended to use cells from d 7 poststimulation and onwards.

3. It is recommended that 100,000 cells per well be used to ensure macroscopic visualization of the result. However, as few as 50,000 cells per well will still enable viewing of the result.

4. In general, a tight correlation between lytic activity and CAA was observed with the exception of some altered peptide ligands. It is yet to be determined whether altered peptide ligands differentially engage adhesion versus lysis.

5. The presence of serum in the assay media is necessary in order to block surface charges on the plastic well and/or provide a protein coating. Bovine serum albumin (BSA) and milk powder both effectively substitute for FCS. Under serum free conditions, cells will stick to the sides of the well regardless of the presence of peptide.

6. We speculate that CAA involves two stages, the first of which involves the cognate peptide/MHC triggering of the TCR. Following the specific signal, the cell then adheres to the protein-coated sides of the well in an interaction that can involve nonspecific adhesion. Cells producing a positive CAA are easily resuspended in the well suggesting that the assay may involve very low affinity adhesion events which are possible because the system is largely unpertubed during the course of the assay. Receptors mediating the adhesion event have not been identified and positive wells, in an undisturbed state, will remain positive for several days.

7. CAA is not inhibited by short-term exposure to sodium azide, colchicine, cytochalasin B, cyclohexamide, or actinomycin, which inhibit metabolism, cytoskeleton, protein and RNA synthesis. However, it is inhibited by wortmannin, an inhibitor of phosphoinositide-3-kinase, indicating a need for signal transduction through the TCR or integrins.

8. CAA is ideally suited to screening minimal sized peptides to identify the cognate peptide for a given CTL line or clone.

References

1. Berke, G. (1993) The functions and mechanisms of action of cytolytic lymphocytes, in *Fundamental Immunology* (Paul, W. E., ed.), vol. 3, Raven, New York, pp. 965–1014.

2. Kägi, D., Vignaux, F., Ledermann, B., Bürki, K., Depraetere, V., Nagata, S., Hengartner, H., and Golstein, P. (1994) Fas and perforin pathways as major mechanisms of T cell-mediated cytotoxicity. *Science* **265,** 528–530.

3. Takeshita, T., Kozlowski, S., England, R. D., Brower, R., Schneck, J., Takahashi, H., DeLisi, C., Margulies, D. H., and Berzofsky, J. A. (1993) Role of conserved regions of class I MHC molecules in the activation of CD8+ CTL by peptide and purified cell-free class I molecules. *Int. Immunol.* **5,** 1129–1138.

4. Li, Y., Stefura, W. P., Simons, F. E., Jay, F. T., and HayGlass, K. T. (1994) Limiting dilution analysis of antigen stimulated IL-4 and IFN-gamma production in human mononuclear cell populations. *J. Immunol. Methods* **175,** 169–179.

5. Brunner, K. T., Mauel, J., Cerrotini, M. C., and Chapius, B. (1968) Quantitative assay of the lytic action of immune lymphoid cells on 51 Cr-labeled allogeneic target cells in vitro: inhibition by isoantibody and by drugs. *Immunology* **14**, 180–181.

6. Dustin, M. L. and Springer, T. A. (1991) Role of lymphocyte adhesion receptors in transient interactions and cell locomotion. *Ann. Rev. Immunol.* **9,** 27–66.

7. O'Rourke, A. M. and Mescher, M. F. (1992) Cytotoxic T-lymphocyte activation involves a cascade of signaling and adhesion events. *Nature* **358,** 253–255.

8. Lub, M., Van Kooyk, Y., and Figdor, C. G. (1995) Ins and outs of LFA-1. *Immunol. Today* **16,** 479–483.

9. O'Rourke, A. M. and Mescher, M. F. (1993) The roles of CD8 in cytotoxic T lymphocyte function. *Immunol. Today* **14,** 183–188.

10. O'Rourke, A. M., Rogers, J., and Mescher, M. F. (1990) Activated CD8 binding to class I protein mediated by the T-cell receptor results in signalling. *Nature* **346,** 187–189.

11. Kane, K. P. and Mescher, M. F. (1993) Activation of CD8-dependent cytotoxic T lymphocyte adhesion and degranulation by peptide class I antigen complexes. *J. Immunol.* **150,** 4788–4797.

12. Leggatt, G. R., Alexander-Miller, M. A., Kumar, A., Hoffman, S. L., and Berzofsky, J. A. (1997) Cytotoxic T lymphocyte (CTL) adherence assay (CAA): a non-radioactive assay for murine CTL recognition of peptide-MHC class I complexes. *J. Immunol. Methods* **201,** 1–10.

23

Detecting Ubiquitinated T-Cell Antigen Receptor Subunits by Immunoblotting

Allan M. Weissman

1. Introduction

An increasing number of transmembrane proteins are being identified as substrates for ubiquitination. Ubiquitin is a highly conserved 76 amino acid polypeptide that is covalently added to proteins as monomers or chains as a consequence of the formation of an isopeptide linkage between the carboxyl terminus of ubiquitin and the ε-amino groups of lysine side chains of target proteins (reviewed in **ref. 1**). Classically, modification by ubiquitin results in a change in migration on SDS-PAGE such that modified proteins take on a ladder-like appearance with a periodicity of ~8 kDa. Alternatively, ubiquitinated species can appear as a high molecular weight smear. Our current understanding is that, for transmembrane proteins, this modification may occur while in the endoplasmic reticulum (ER) or at the plasma membrane. In both cases ubiquitination occurs on the cytosolic (intracellular) domain. Thus, this modification should not affect recognition by antibodies directed against luminal (or extracellular) domains.

Ubiquitination of transmembrane proteins located in the ER is generally associated with targeting for proteasomal degradation (reviewed in **ref. 2**). For a number of mammalian cell surface receptors, ubiquitination occurs as a consequence of early signaling events, particularly the activation of protein tyrosine kinases, however in most cases ubiquitination of cell surface receptors has not been linked to degradation by 26S proteasomes. Interestingly, in yeast, there are now several well-studied examples where ubiquitination of transmembrane proteins at the plasma membrane actually functions as a targeting signal for endocytosis and subsequent degradation in lysosomes (reviewed in **ref. 2**).

From: *Methods in Molecular Biology, Vol. 134: T Cell Protocols: Development and Activation*
Edited by: K. P. Kearse © Humana Press Inc., Totowa, NJ

The T cell antigen receptor (TCR) has been studied both as a model for assembly of a multi-subunit transmembrane complex and as a cell surface signaling molecule. TCRs undergo ubiquitination, presumably at the cell surface, in response to receptor engagement *(3,4)*. Unassembled TCR subunits undergo ubiquitination in the ER, in this case as part of a process leading to destruction in 26S proteasomes *(5)*.

Ubiquitinated TCR subunits can be demonstrated by immunoblotting using antibodies that recognize ubiquitin (as described below). Alternatively, higher molecular weight forms indicative of ubiquitination may be visualized by immunoblotting using antibodies directed against individual TCR components. The relative sensitivity of these two approaches is influenced both by the number of ubiquitinated TCR subunits and by the number of ubiquitins attached. Additionally, a role for proteasomes (and therefore likely ubiquitin) in the turnover of the TCR subunits and other proteins may be discerned by use of proteasome inhibitors in combination with either metabolic labeling or immunoblotting (*see* **ref. 5** for examples). It is our experience that treatment of cells with proteasome inhibitors does not alter detection of ubiquitinated forms of the TCR that are generated in response to receptor ligation. However, such treatment is essential to visualize ubiquitinated forms of CD3-δ and TCR-α bound for degradation from the endoplasmic reticulum (*see* **Notes 7** and **8**).

2. Materials

1. Lysis buffer: 50 m*M* Tris-HCl (pH 7.6) and 300 m*M* NaCl. The detergent that forms the basis for these lysis buffers is usually either 0.5% Triton -X-100 (v/v) or 1% digitonin (w/v).
2. Wash buffer: Same as lysis buffer, except that the detergent concentrations are reduced to one fifth that of lysis buffer, i.e., 0.1% Triton -X-100 or 0.2% digitonin.
3. Protease inhibitors: Protease Inhibitors are added fresh to lysis and wash buffers. The final concentrations are: 1 m*M* phenylmethylsulphonyl fluoride (PMSF), 10 μg/mL aprotinin, 10 μg/mL leupeptin, 10 m*M* iodoacetamide. We generally omit iodoacetamide from the wash buffer. PMSF is made as a 100 m*M* stock in ethanol, aprotinin, and leupeptin are from 10 mg/mL stocks in water, and iodoacetamide is weighed out fresh for each use (*see* **Note 3**).
4. Phosphatase inhibitors: In cases where it is desirable to detect phosphory-lated species either by changes in migration or by immunoblotting with antiphosphotyrosine reagents, phosphatase inhibitors are added to the PBS used for harvesting the cells, and most importantly to the lysis and wash buffers. This cocktail of phosphatase inhibitors is generally prepared as a 10-fold concentrated stock, with its pH adjusted to 7.4. This can be stored for 1–2 wk at 4°C. The stock includes: 4 m*M* NaVO$_4$, 4 m*M* EDTA, 100 m*M* NaF, and 100 m*M* sodium pyrophosphate.

5. Antibody-bound beads: Antibodies are pre-bound to protein A or G beads (available from a number of sources) for at least one hour prior to addition of postnuclear supernatant.
6. SDS/PAGE gels: For detection of TCR subunits, we generally use 12.5% gels (*see* **Note 4**).
7. Membranes, washing, fixing, and blocking: Samples that have been resolved on SDS-PAGE are transferred to Immobilon-P membranes. BSA used in blocking is fraction V (ICN) that is dissolved in Tris-buffered saline (TBS) (100 m*M* Tris, pH 7.4, 300 m*M* NaCl) and filtered (0.45 µ) before use.
8. 0.1 *M* potassium phosphate buffer pH 7.0 containing 0.5% (v/v) glutaraldehyde.

3. Methods

1. Cells (typically $1–2 \times 10^7$ cell equivalents) are manipulated as appropriate, rapidly cooled to 4°C by addition of cold PBS, with phosphatase inhibitors added if necessary, and harvested by centrifugation. It is important that for all subsequent steps until gel electrophoresis that material be maintained at 4°C "on ice."
2. Cell membranes are solubilized using either 800 µL Triton -X-100- or digitonin-containing lysis buffer supplemented with protease inhibitors and, in some cases, phosphatase inhibitors.
3. After 30–60 min with intermittent vortexing, nuclei and insoluble material are pelleted at 15,000*g* for 15 min.
4. The soluble "postnuclear" supernatant is transferred to a microcentrifuge tube containing 50 µL protein A or protein G beads prebound with the desired antibody. Samples are tumbled in the cold for at least 1 h.
5. Beads are washed at least 3 times with 1 mL volumes of detergent-based "wash buffer. " Samples should be mixed at each wash.
6. Material is resuspended in SDS-PAGE sample buffer and subject to gel electrophoresis using standard protocols.
7. Using standard western blotting protocols samples are transferred to Immobilon P membranes (Millipore), (*see* **Note 5**).
8. After transfer, filters are rinsed in several changes of PBS for 20 min prior to a 20 min incubation in 0.1 *M* potassium phosphate buffer, pH 7.0, containing 0.5% (v/v) glutaraldehyde. Membranes are again rinsed in several changes of PBS for 20 min. They are then blocked in 5% BSA in TBS for at least 1 h at room temperature prior to immunoblotting.
9. There are several commercial sources of anti-ubiquitin reagents and several labs have generated their own. Immunoblotting with these reagents is generally carried out using standard washing and development protocols (*see* **Note 6**) and concentration of antibody suggested by the supplier.

4. Notes

1. Triton -X-100 is a more effective and by far less costly reagent than digitonin. However, the human ζ subunit does not co-immunoprecipitate consistently with

other TCR subunits after lysis in Triton -X-100. This is generally not a problem for mouse TCR, nor is it a problem if ζ is to be directly immunoprecipitated.

2. Digitonin is available from sources including Sigma (check availability) and Wako (Kyoto, Japan). Digitonin should be prepared as a 2% stock in water. Solubility can be a problem, which can be overcome by boiling. After cooling, the 2% solution should be filtered. Digitonin stock solutions are generally made fresh every 7 d.

3. It is crucial that an alkylating agent (iodoacetamide or *N*-ethyl maleimide) be included in the lysis buffer. There are a number of active deubiquitinating enzymes, these contain active sulfhydryls.

4. When resolving TCR subunits by SDS-PAGE we generally use 12.5% gels to retain non-modified ζ (16 kDa reduced). If this is not an issue, lower percentage gels, which will help resolve ubiquitinated species may be used.

5. Immobilon-P is used as the transfer membrane when glutaraldehyde fixation is carried out. It is important that the membrane not be exposed to BSA prior to washing and glutaraldehyde fixation. Some labs use nitrocellulose instead of Immobilon and autoclave the membranes rather than fix in glutaraldehyde.

6. There are an increasing number of sources of anti-ubiquitin antibodies. These reagents vary in their ability to detect monoubiquitin relative to multiubiquitin chains. Additionally, anti ubiquitin reagents are generally of relatively low affinity, and commercial polyclonal reagents may be of low and inconsistent titer. The issue of antibody quality coupled with low steady state abundance of ubiquitinated forms frequently makes detection challenging.

7. It is becoming apparent that there are several other ubiquitin-like proteins that are capable of modifying proteins these include SUMO-1 *(6)* and a 15 kDa γ interferon-inducible protein known as UCRP *(7)*.

8. Reagents that are used to inhibit proteasome function include peptide aldehydes such as LLNL (*N*-acetyl-Leu-Leu-norleucinal) *(8)* and MG132 *(9)*. Lactacystin *(10)* is perceived to be a specific proteasome inhibitor.

References

1. Weissman, A. M. (1997) Regulating protein degradation by ubiquitination. *Immunol. Today* **18,** 189–198.
2. Bonifacino, J. S. and Weissman, A. M. (1998) Ubiquitin and the control of protein fate in the secretory and endocytic pathways. *Annu. Rev. Cell Dev. Biol.* **13,** 19–57.
3. Cenciarelli, C., Hou, D., Hsu, K.-C., Rellahan, B. L., Wiest, D. L., Smith, H. T., Fried, V. A., and Weissman, A. M. (1992) Activation-induced ubiquitination of the T cell antigen receptor. *Science* **257,** 795–797.
4. Cenciarelli, C., Wilhelm, K. J., Jr., Guo, A., and Weissman, A. M. (1996) T cell antigen receptor ubiquitination is a consequence of receptor-mediated tyrosine kinase activation. *J. Biol. Chem.* **271,** 8709–8713.
5. Yang, M., Omura, S., Bonifacino, J. S., and Weissman, A. M. (1998) Novel aspects of degradation of TCR subunits from the ER in T cells: importance of

oligosaccharide processing, ubiquitination, and proteasome-dependent removal from ER membranes. *J. Exp. Med.* **187,** 835–846.

6. Satioh, H., Pu, R. T., and Dasso, M. (1997) SUMO-1: wrestling with a new ubiquitin-related modifier. *TIBS* **22,** 374–376.

7. Narasimhan, J., Potter, J. L., and Haas, A. L. (1996) Conjugation of the 15-kDa interferon-induced ubiquitin homolog is distinct from that of ubiquitin. *J. Biol. Chem.* **271,** 324–330.

8. Rock, K. L., Gramm, C., Rothstein, L., Clark, K., Stein, R., Dick, L., Hwang, D., and Goldberg, A. L. (1994) Inhibitors of the proteasome block the degradation of most cell proteins and the generation of peptides presented on MHC class I molecules. *Cell* **78,** 761–771.

9. Chen, Z., Hagler, J., Palombella, V. J., Melandri, F., Scherer, D., Ballard D., and Maniatis, T. (1995) Signal-induced site-specific phosphorylation targets IkBa to the ubiquitin-proteasome pathway. *Genes Devel.* **9,** 1586–1597.

10. Fenteany, G., Standaert, R. F., Reichard, G. A., Corey, E. J., and Schreiber, S. L. (1994) A β-lactone related to lactacystin induces neurite outgrowth in a neuroblastoma cell line and inhibits cell cycle progression in an osteosarcoma cell line. *Proc. Natl. Acad. Sci. USA* **91,** 3358–3362.

24

Determination of CD45 Tyrosine Phosphatase Activity in T Lymphocytes

David H. W. Ng, Jackie Felberg, and Pauline Johnson

1. Introduction

CD45 is a leukocyte specific protein tyrosine phosphatase and is a major lymphocyte cell surface glycoprotein (*see* **refs.** *1–3* for reviews). CD45 has been shown to be important for the transmission of signals by the T and B cell antigen receptors during both development and antigen induced activation. The phosphatase activity of CD45 has been shown to be required for efficient signaling by the T-cell receptor complex, yet little is known of how or whether the phosphatase activity of CD45 is regulated. In this chapter, we describe a simple and sensitive method to measure the phosphatase activity of CD45 isolated directly from T cells.

1.1. CD45 Phosphatase Activity

CD45 is thought to dephosphorylate and thereby help regulate the activity of src family kinase members, particularly $p56^{lck}$ and $p59^{fyn}$ in T lymphocytes *(4–8)*. CD45 allows these kinases to effectively participate in T-cell receptor mediated signaling events. CD45 can thus modulate the signal transmitted via the T-cell antigen receptor by regulating the participation of these src family kinases. Consequently, one could envisage that changes in CD45 phosphatase activity could potentially alter the outcome of an immune response. Ideally, one would like to be able to monitor the phosphatase activity of CD45 *in situ* during T-cell activation. However, this is not presently feasible given current technical restraints. As an alternative, the assay described below permits the assessment of phosphatase activity of CD45 isolated from cells undergoing cellular activation or differentiation. Thus, comparisons of the activity of CD45 isolated from different cell types and from similar cells experiencing a variety

From: *Methods in Molecular Biology, Vol. 134: T Cell Protocols: Development and Activation*
Edited by: K. P. Kearse © Humana Press Inc., Totowa, NJ

of stimuli (such as T-cell activation) can now be performed. Using this assay as a tool, we hope to gain a better understanding of how CD45 phosphatase activity is regulated under different cellular conditions in T cells.

1.2. Malachite Green Assay

The malachite green assay has been used for several years to measure the amount of inorganic phosphate in a sample *(9)*. Over the years the sensitivity of the assay has been improved *(10)* and has been adapted to measure the release of free phosphate occurring as a result of phosphatase activity *(11)*. More recently, assay volumes have been scaled down to allow the measurement of pmol amounts of phosphate *(12)* and have been adapted for high-throughput screening procedures *(13)*. Here, we outline an adaptation of this micro-assay for the measurement of CD45 phosphatase activity isolated from as few as 1×10^4 lymphoid cells *(14)*. This is a discontinuous, colorimetric phosphatase assay performed in microtiter plate wells. Although the assay is streamlined for use in assessing CD45 phosphatase activity, the assay can be easily applied to other phosphatases where immunoprecipitating antibodies, preferably monoclonal antibodies (MAbs), are available. Likewise, by varying the choice of peptide substrate used, either serine, threonine, or tyrosine, phosphatase activity can be measured.

The malachite green phosphatase assay has several advantages over previous methods. The use of radioactive substrates is laborious, as it involves the initial generation, purification, and quantitation of radioactively labeled phosphorylated substrate, in addition to the separation of the released radioactive phosphate *(4,15)*. Furthermore, only relatively small quantities of labeled substrate are available with a limited lifetime, which restricts the type of enzymatic analysis that can be performed. Another method utilizes the differential absorption of phosphotyrosine and tyrosine at a wavelength of 282 nm during a phosphatase assay *(16,17)*, but it cannot easily be used to measure multiple samples. Phosphatases are often assayed with the nonspecific substrate, para-nitrophenyl phosphate (pNPP), which upon hydrolysis generates a colored product that can be measured continuously at 405 nm. Although this can be a useful and simple method, pNPP is not an optimal substrate for CD45 and in a direct comparison with the malachite green assay using phosphopeptide substrates, immunoprecipitated CD45 gave 50-fold lower rates with pNPP (unpublished data). CD45 immunoprecipitated from $1–2 \times 10^5$ BW5147 T cells was required to get a significant increase in absorbance at OD_{405nm} over a 30 min period. Thus, the malachite green assay is at least an order of magnitude more sensitive than the colorimetric assay using pNPP.

The assay described in this article involves immunoprecipitating CD45 from cells, performing the phosphatase assay with the immunoprecipitated material, and then stopping the reaction at specific time points with the addition of malachite green. The amount of phosphate accumulated is then determined by measuring the absorption of the reaction samples at 650 nm and comparing the value to a standard curve derived from known amounts of phosphate. With the accumulation of data from at least three time points, one can then calculate the rate of hydrolysis. An aliquot of immunoprecipitated CD45 can be electrophoresed using SDS PAGE and transferred to polyvinylidene difluoride (PVDF) membrane, where the relative amount of CD45 can be estimated by Western blot analysis.

2. Materials

2.1. CD45 Immunoprecipitation

1. Sepharose CL-4B (Amersham Pharmacia Biotech, Amersham, UK) and purified CD45 MAb conjugated to CNBr activated Sepharose CL-4B. Antibody is coupled to the Sepharose according to manufacturer's instructions at a concentration of 4 mg/mL packed beads. We routinely use a pan specific anti-mouse CD45 MAb, I3/2 *(18)*, although hybridomas are available from the American Type Culture Collection that produce other CD45 MAbs, or purified anti-CD45 MAbs are available from various companies (for e.g., PharMingen, San Diego, CA) (*see* **Note 1**). Antibody coupled beads can be kept at 4°C for several months in PBS supplemented with 0.02% azide.
2. Cell lysis buffer: 0.5% Triton X-100, 20 mM Tris-HCl, pH 7.5, 150 mM NaCl, 2 mM EDTA, 0.2 mM phenylmethylsulfonyl fluoride, 1 µg/mL pepstatin, leupeptin, and aprotinin.
3. Wash buffer: same as cell lysis buffer except with 0.2% Triton X-100. Both cell lysis buffer and wash buffer can be prepared without protease inhibitors and stored at room temperature for several weeks. Both buffers should be supplemented with protease inhibitors just prior to the experiment and kept on ice.
4. Phosphatase (PTP) buffer: 50 mM Tris-HCl, pH 7.2, 1 mM EDTA, ± 0.1% β-mercaptoethanol (14.3 mM). PTP buffer should always be prepared fresh and kept on ice (*see* **Note 2**).

2.2. Malachite Green Assay

1. Phosphotyrosine peptide. 9–15-mer phosphotyrosine peptides corresponding to either the sequence surrounding the autoregulatory or negative regulatory site of src family kinases were synthesized and purified as described *(12)*. Other peptide sequences can be used and tyrosine phosphorylated peptides can be purchased (*see* **Note 3**). Phosphopeptides can be kept in lyophilized form or solubilized in HPLC grade water or buffer at a concentration of 10–100 mM and stored at –20°C. We routinely use the following peptides to measure CD45 phosphatase activity:

fyn pY531: TATEPQpYQPGENL
src pY416: LIEDNEpYTARQGA
lck pY394: EDNEpYTARE
CD3ζ pY83: LGRREEpYDVLEKKRA

Purified phosphopeptides are quantitated by determining phosphate concentration after chemical hydrolysis *(19)*. Briefly, lyophilized peptide is dissolved in HPLC grade water, aliquoted and heated to 100°C until dry; the solid peptide is then resuspended in 30 μL of 1 part 50% sulfuric acid, 1 part 60% perchloric acid and heated to 160°C in reacti-vials (Pierce, Rockford, IL) for 4–5 h. The solutions are cooled and aliquoted into microtiter wells. Known amounts of a phosphopeptide or KH_2PO_4 are treated identically and used to generate a standard curve. 80 μL of malachite green reagent is then added to all samples and 5 μL increments of 10 *N* NaOH are added until all the samples are neutralized (indicated by a graduated color change to green in the phosphate standards). This results in a colorimetric response proportional to the amount of free phosphate present in the samples. Quantitation is determined by comparison to the standard curve.

2. Malachite green reagents. Reagent #1: 0.135% malachite green-oxalate salt in distilled, deionized water (ddH_2O); reagent #2: 4.2% ammonium molybdate in 4.0 *M* HCl. Both reagents can be stored at room temperature for several months.
3. PTP buffer: 50 m*M* Tris-HCl, pH 7.2, 1 m*M* EDTA, 0.1% β-mercaptoethanol (14.3 m*M*) (*see* **Note 4**).
4. Phosphate solution for standard curve: 1 m*M* potassium dihydrogen phosphate (KH_2PO_4) in ddH_2O.
5. Microtiter plates (half-area, tissue culture treated, flat-bottomed 96-well microtiter plates, Costar, Cambridge, MA).
6. Shaker capable of attaining a speed of 120 rpm.
7. Standard ELISA microtiter plate reader capable of obtaining absorption values at 650 nm.

2.3. Western Blot (Quick Method)

1. Standard minigel electrophoresis and transfer equipment.
2. Standard electrophoresis reagents and PVDF membrane (Immobilon P, Millipore) (*see* **Note 5**).
3. Antibody that will recognize CD45 on a Western blot. We routinely use rabbit anti-mouse CD45 antisera raised against either the extracellular domain of CD45 *(20)* or against the cytoplasmic domain of CD45 *(4,21)*. Horseradish peroxidase conjugated Protein A (Bio-Rad).
4. TTBS buffer: 20 m*M* Tris-HCl, pH 7.5, 150 m*M* NaCl, 0.1% Tween 20 (prepared fresh).
5. Skim milk powder (local supermarket).
6. Scanning densitometer.

3. Methods

3.1. CD45 Immunoprecipitation

1. $1–5 \times 10^6$ BW5147 T lymphoma cells are lysed in 200–500 µL ice-cold cell lysis buffer and incubated on ice for 10 min. Lysates are then centrifuged at 14,000g for 10 min. The supernatant is kept and precleared with 10 µL of a 50% slurry of Sepharose CL-4B beads at 4°C for 1 h (*see* **Note 6**).
2. The lysate solution is centrifuged and the supernatant transferred to a fresh Eppendorf tube where 10 µL of a 50% slurry of I3/2 coupled Sepharose CL-4B is added and allowed to incubate end over end for 2 h at 4°C (*see* **Note 7**).
3. The immunoprecipitate is subsequently washed three times in wash buffer, and washed twice in PTP buffer (without 0.1% β-mercaptoethanol) (*see* **Note 8**).
4. Beads are then resuspended in a volume of PTP buffer (with 0.1% β-mercaptoethanol) such that 10 µL aliquots provide measurable optical density (OD) readings in the malachite green assay at initial time points that fall within the linear range of the standard curve (*see* **Fig. 1**). In studies using BW5147 T lymphoma cells, we typically find that $2–5 \times 10^4$ cell equivalents per 10 µL gives suitable values within this range (*see* **Fig. 2**).

3.2. Malachite Green Assay

1. Prepare a fresh working solution of malachite green reagent: Add 1 part reagent #1, 1 part reagent #2, 2 parts ddH$_2$O and Tween 20 tp 0.01%; agitate 5 min at room temperature, place on ice for 5 min, then filter through 0.2 µm filter (*see* **Note 9**).
2. Prepare 1X and 10X PTP buffer. Dilute stock solution of phosphotyrosine peptide with 10X PTP buffer and ddH$_2$O to a final concentration of 1X PTP buffer and twice the final desired molarity of the phosphopeptide (*see* **Note 10**).
3. Aliquot reagents and peptide into a half area microtiter plate such that they are in slight excess. For example, for three time points including zero, aliquot 22–24 µL peptide solution in final well and 100 µL malachite green reagent into three successive wells in the middle of the plate.
4. Add 10 µL of 1X PTP buffer to well # 1 of the microtiter plate. This will be time 0. Then add 10 µL of immunoprecipitated CD45 bead suspension in 1X PTP buffer to well #1 and to successive wells for each time point to be tested.
5. At the same time, aliquot 10 µL of KH$_2$PO$_4$ serially diluted with 1X PTP buffer to successive wells on a separate area of the plate. Also, aliquot 100 µL malachite green working reagent to adjacent wells.
6. Place plate at 30°C for 5 min to equilibrate the temperature of the reagents.
7. Initiate reaction by adding 10 µL of peptide to wells containing CD45 (but not to time 0 well) and begin timing. During the reaction, agitate microtitre plate at 120 rpm (*see* **Note 11**).
8. Stop the reaction by adding 80 µL of malachite green working reagent to each assay after the appropriate incubation time, as well as to the time 0 min well containing 1X PTP buffer and CD45, and to the wells containing the KH$_2$PO$_4$ standards. Leave for 10 min to allow the color to develop (*see* **Note 12**).

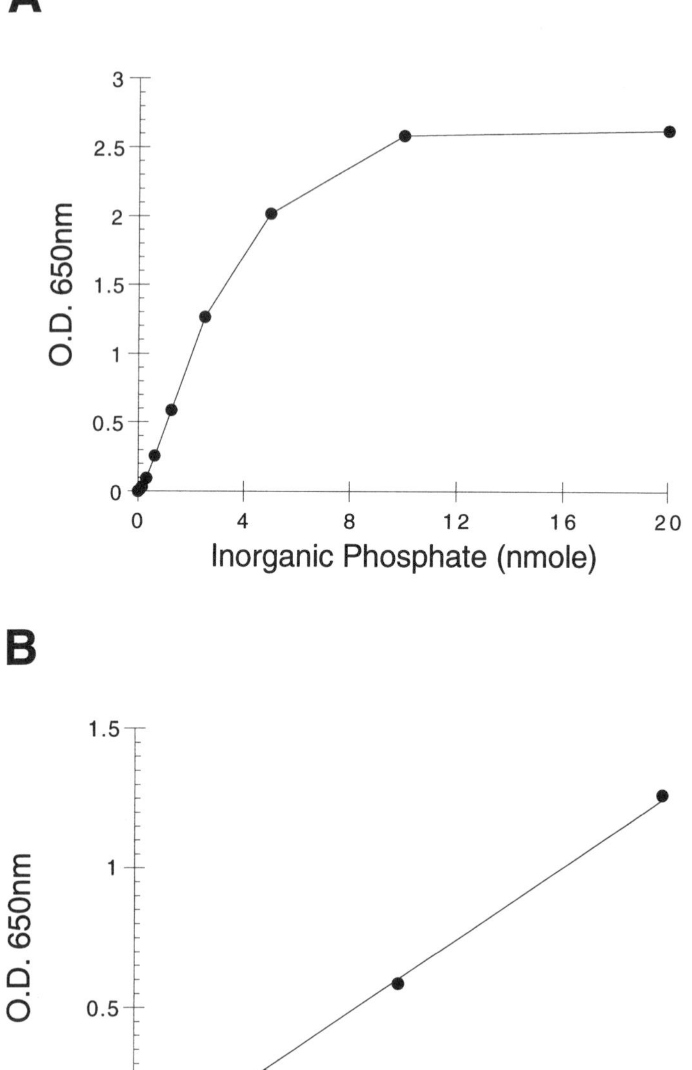

Fig. 1. (**A**) Graph of $OD_{650\,nm}$ vs amount of inorganic phosphate. (**B**) Linear part of standard curve used in determination of CD45 phosphatase activity. Absorbance at a wavelength of 650 nm (●) was measured for different concentrations of potassium dihydrogen phosphate (KH_2PO_4), after addition of the malachite green reagent.

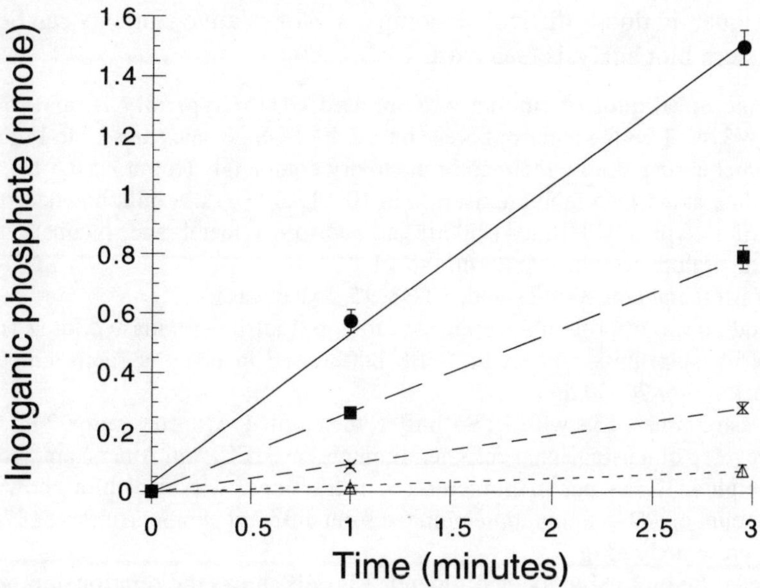

Fig. 2. PTP activity of CD45 immunoprecipitated from different numbers of BW5147 T lymphoma cells: (●) 1×10^5, (■) 5×10^4, (×) 2×10^4, (△) 1×10^4, using 3.4 m*M* src pY416 as the substrate. Assay readings were taken at 0 min, 1 min and 2 min 55 s. Optimal activity falling within the range of the standard curve (*see* **Fig. 1B**) is obtained using CD45 immunoprecipitated from $2–5 \times 10^4$ cells. Immunoprecipitations from BW5147 CD45⁻ cells, using the CD45 MAb, can be used to obtain background readings for the PTP assay.

9. Measure the absorbance at 650 nm using a multiwell microtiter plate reader to detect the release of inorganic phosphate. Convert values to nmoles using the standard curve generated with KH_2PO_4. Typical readings for 0–20 nmoles phosphate are shown in **Fig. 1A**. **Fig. 1B** represents the linear range of the standard curve, typically ranging from 0.1–2 nmoles and generating OD_{650nm} values between 0.05 and 1.0. The initial rate of phosphatase activity should be linear and from this one can calculate the rate of hydrolysis in nmoles hydrolyzed/min/CD45 isolated from X no. of cells. **Fig. 2** shows the initial reaction rates for CD45 isolated from different numbers of BW5147 T cells. From these measurements, the phosphatase activity of CD45 was found to be 0.5 nmoles/min/1×10^5 cell equivalents, using the src pY416 peptide as the substrate.

3.3. Western Blot (Quick Method)

When comparing the activity of CD45 between different samples, it is often useful to compare the amount of CD45 present in each sample. Although precise quantitation is difficult, a comparison of relative amounts can be made by Western blot analysis (*see* **Note 13**).

1. Take an aliquot of immunoprecipitated CD45 (typically from 1–5×10^5 BW5147 T cells), electrophorese on a 7.5% SDS gel and transfer to Immobilon P membrane. Allow the membrane to dry completely (for at least 1 h).
2. Dilute anti-CD45 rabbit antiserum in 10 mL of 5% skim milk powder in TTBS buffer (typically 1/1000–1/5000) and add to dry membrane. Incubate at room temperature, shaking for 45 min to 1 h.
3. Wash membrane 3 times with TTBS, 15 s each wash.
4. Add 10 mL of protein A conjugated to horseradish peroxidase diluted 1/10,000 in 5% skim milk powder in TTBS buffer, and incubate at room temperature, shaking for 20–30 min.
5. Wash 3 times, 15 s with TTBS buffer, then a final wash for approx 2 min.
6. Develop blot using enhanced chemiluminesence (ECL kit, Amersham, Arlington Heights, IL) as per manufacturer's instructions. A typical blot showing the amount of CD45 immunoprecipitated from different numbers of BW5147 T cells is presented in **Fig. 3A**.
7. Scan the blot using a densitometer. **Fig. 3B** shows the relationship between the band values ($ODmm^2$) and the amount of cells that CD45 was immunoprecipitated from.

4. Notes

1. It is possible that various MAbs used in the immunoprecipitation procedure, which bind to different epitopes of CD45, may differentially affect the enzymatic activity of CD45. In view of this possibility, we compared the phosphatase activity of CD45 immunoprecipitated either by I3/2 or Ly5.2 and found no significant differences in the phosphatase activity of CD45. However, as suggested by others, it is still possible that other anti-CD45 antibodies may modulate phosphatase activity *(22)*.
2. The pH optimum for immunoprecipitated CD45 has been previously determined to be pH 7.2 *(14)*. The pH of the PTP buffer can be adjusted according to the optimum pH of the phosphatase being assayed.
3. Any substrate that generates free phosphate upon hydrolysis can be measured using the malachite green assay. However, 9–13-mer phosphopeptide substrates have been shown to have the best K_m and k_{cat} values compared to other nonphysiological substrates. It is worthy to note that a phosphopeptide corresponding to the p56^{lck} C-terminal region is technically difficult to synthesize in large amounts.
4. Recent optimization of this procedure has found that addition of 0.01% Triton X-100 to the PTP buffer results in a 2–3-fold increase in enzymatic activity. Thus, we recommend that this should be included in assays where a higher level of sensitivity is required.
5. We have only tried Immobilon P (Millipore) PVDF membrane using the quick Western blot technique *(23)*. Other membranes may or may not be suitable.

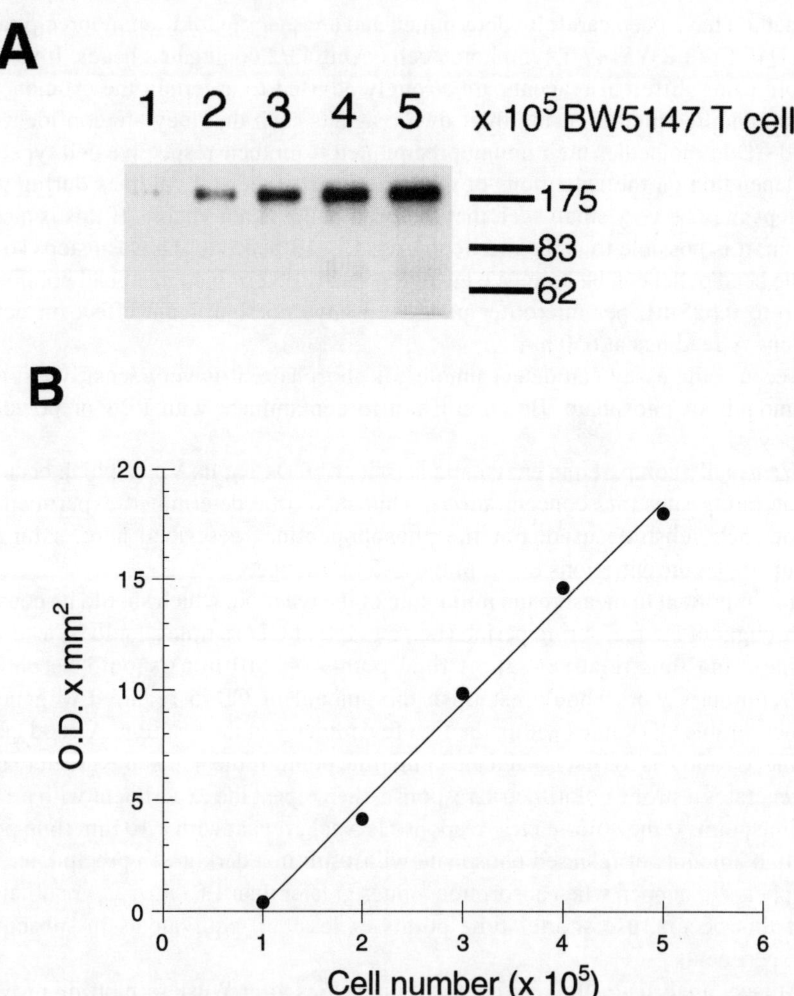

Fig. 3. (**A**) Western blot analysis of CD45 immunoprecipitated from (1) 1×10^5, (2) 2×10^5, (3) 3×10^5, (4) 4×10^5, and (5) 5×10^5 BW5147 T lymphoma cells. Primary antibody used was 1/5000 antimouse CD45 cytoplasmic domain rabbit antiserum (R02.2). (**B**) Graph showing relative amounts of CD45 immunoprecipitated from increasing amounts of BW5147 T cells. Relative amounts of CD45 (ODmm²) were obtained by densitometric scanning of the Western blot in A.

6. Immunoprecipitation of CD45 from cells will take approx 3.5 h. The malachite green assay should take approx 30 min, if only one plate is being used. The Western blot procedure can be performed later and takes approx 1.5 h after drying.
7. The amount of antibody required to immunoprecipitate CD45 will depend on the antibody and the expression levels of CD45 in the cell. The amounts given in this

method have been carefully determined and are specific for immunoprecipitating CD45 from BW5147 T lymphoma cells using I3/2 conjugated beads. Investigators using different reagents are strongly advised to ascertain the efficiency of immunoprecipitation using their own reagents such that they are confident that all CD45 molecules are immunoprecipitated from their respective cell type(s).

8. Depending on the conditions of the experiment, the bead volumes during wash steps may be very small such that the bead pellet is not visible. If this is a problem, it is possible to add extra Sepharose CL-4B beads to the wash steps so that the bead pellet can be seen. We have previously determined that bead volumes of up to 0.625 µL per microtiter plate well have no significant effect on optical density readings at 650 nm.

9. Because the assay can detect pmoles of phosphate, it is very sensitive to trace amounts of phosphate. Be careful not to contaminate with PBS or powdered gloves!

10. We usually compare the enzymatic activity of CD45 at its V_{max}, which occurs at saturating substrate concentrations. This should be determined experimentally for each substrate used. For the phosphopeptides described here, saturating substrate concentrations occur in the 1–5 mM range.

11. It is important to measure the initial rate of the reaction, which should be constant throughout the measuring period (i.e., a graph of OD vs time should be a straight line). and thus relatively short time points (~1–10 min) should be chosen. Preliminary work should establish the amount of CD45 required to generate measurable OD values within the first few minutes of the reaction. A good guideline to follow is to first conduct a 3 min time point. If the malachite green reagent generates a strong colorimetric response, then repeat the experiment with a 1 min time point. If the colorimetric response is weak, repeat with a 10 min time point.

12. High amounts of released phosphate will result in a dark green precipitate. This appears to happen when absorption values greater than 1.0 OD_{650nm} are obtained. If this occurs, use shorter time points or less cell equivalents in subsequent experiments.

13. At best, analysis of the relative band intensities after Western blotting provides an ESTIMATE of comparative amounts, as both ECL and X-ray film have a limited linear range and can be easily saturated. A series of standards (such as shown in **Fig. 3**) can be electrophoresed to help assess whether the bands fall within a linear range or not.

References

1. Trowbridge, I. S. and Thomas, M. L. (1994) CD45: An emerging role as a protein tyrosine phosphatase required for lymphocyte activation and development. *Annu. Rev. Immunol.* **12,** 85–116.

2. Justement, L. B. (1997) The role of CD45 in signal transduction. *Adv. Immunol.* **66,** 1–65.

3. Johnson, P., Maiti, A., and Ng, D. H. W. (1997) CD45: A family of leukocyte specific cell surface glycoproteins, in *Weir's Handbook of Experimental Immu-*

nology vol. II, 5th ed. (Herzenberg, L. A., Weir, D. M., Herzenberg, L. A., and Blackwell, C., eds.), Blackwell Science Inc., Malden, MA, pp. 62.1–62.16.

4. Ostergaard, H. L., Shackelford, D. A., Hurley, T. R., Johnson, P., Hyman, R., Sefton, B. M., and Trowbridge, I. S. (1989) Expression of CD45 alters phosphorylation of the lck-encoded tyrosine protein kinase in murine lymphoma T-cell lines. *Proc. Natl. Acad. Sci. USA* **86,** 8959–8963.

5. Mustelin, T., Coggeshall, K. M., and Altman, A. (1989) Rapid activation of the T-cell protein tyrosine kinase pp56^{lck} by the CD45 phosphotyrosine phosphatase. *Proc. Natl. Acad. Sci. USA* **86,** 6302–6306.

6. Mustelin, T., Pessa-Morikawa, T., Autero, M., Gassmann, M., Andersson, L. C., Gahmberg, C. G., and Burn, P. (1992) Regulation of the p59^{fyn} protein tyrosine kinase by the CD45 phosphotyrosine phosphatase. *Eur. J. Immunol.* **22,** 1173–1178.

7. Cahir McFarland, E. D., Hurley, T. R., Pingel, J. T., Sefton, B. M., Shaw, A., and Thomas, M. L. (1993) Correlation between src family member regulation by the protein-tyrosine-phosphatase CD45 and transmembrane signaling through the T-cell receptor. *Proc. Natl. Acad. Sci. USA* **90,** 1402–1406.

8. Hurley, T. R., Hyman, R., and Sefton, B. M. (1993) Differential effects of expression of the CD45 tyrosine protein phosphatase on the tyrosine phosphorylation of the lck, fyn and c-src tyrosine protein kinases. *Mol. Cell Biol.* **13,** 1651–1656.

9. Itaya, K. and Ui, M. (1966) A new micromethod for the colorimetric determination of inorganic phosphate. *Clin. Chim. Acta* **14,** 361–366.

10. Lanzetta, P. A., Alvarez, L. J., Reinach, P. S., and Candia, O. A. (1979) An improved assay for nanomole amounts of inorganic phosphate. *Anal. Biochem.* **100,** 95–97.

11. Cho, H., Ramer, S. E., Itoh, M., Winkler, D. G., Kitas, E., Bannwarth, W., Burn, P., Saito, H., and Walsh, C. T. (1991) Purification and characterization of a soluble catalytic fragment of the human transmembrane leukocyte antigen related (LAR) protein tyrosine phosphatase from an *Esherichia coli* expression system. *Biochem.* **30,** 6210–6216.

12. Harder, K. W., Owen, P., Wong, L. K. H., Aebersold, R., Clark-Lewis, I., and Jirik, F. R. (1994) Characterization and kinetic analysis of the intracellular domain of human protein tyrosine phosphatase beta (Hptp beta) using synthetic phosphopeptides. *Biochem. J.* **298,** 395–401.

13. Fisher, D. K. and Higgins, T. J. (1994) A sensitive, high-volume, colorimetric assay for protein phosphatases. *Pharmaceut. Res.* **11,** 759–763.

14. Ng, D. H. W., Harder, K. W., Clark-Lewis, I., Jirik, F., and Johnson, P. (1995) Nonradioactive method to measure CD45 protein tyrosine phosphatase activity isolated directly from cells. *J. Immunol. Methods* **179,** 177–185.

15. Streuli, M., Krueger, N. X., Thai, T., Tang, M., and Saito, H. (1990) Distinct functional roles of the two intracellular phosphatase like domains of the receptor-linked protein tyrosine phosphatases LCA and LAR. *EMBO J.* **9,** 2399–2407.

16. Zhao, Z. Z., Zander, N. F., Malencik, D. A., Anderson, S. R., and Fischer, E. H. (1992) Continuous spectrophotometric assay of protein tyrosine phosphatase using phosphotyrosine. *Anal. Biochem.* **202,** 361–366.

17. Zhang, Z. Y., Maclean, D., Thiemesefler, A. M., Roeske, R. W., and Dixon, J. E. (1993) A continuous spectrophotometric and fluorimetric assay for protein tyrosine phosphatase using phosphotyrosine-containing peptides. *Anal. Biochem.* **211,** 7–15.
18. Trowbridge, I. S. (1978) Interspecies spleen-myeloma hybrid producing monoclonal antibodies against mouse lymphocyte surface glycoprotein, T200. *J. Exp. Med.* **148,** 313–323.
19. Hasegawa, H., Parniak, M., and Kaufman, S. (1982) Determination of the phosphate content of purified proteins. *Anal. Biochem.* **120,** 360–364.
20. Chui, D., Ong, C. J., Johnson, P., Teh, H. S., and Marth, J. D. (1994) Specific CD45 isoforms differentially regulate T-cell receptor signaling. *EMBO J.* **13,** 798–807.
21. Ng, D. H. W., Jabali, M. D., Maiti, A., Borodchak, P., Harder, K. W., Brocker, T., Malissen, B., Jirik, F. R., and Johnson, P. (1997) CD45 and RPTPalpha display different protein tyrosine phosphatase activities in T lymphocytes. *Biochem. J.* **327,** 867–876.
22. Goldman, S. J., Uniyal, S., Ferguson, L. M., Golan, D. E., Burakoff, S. J., and Kiener, P. A. (1992) Differential activation of phosphotyrosine protein phosphatase activity in a murine T-cell hybridoma by monoclonal antibodies to CD45. *J. Biol. Chem.* **267,** 6197–6204.
23. Mansfield, M. A. (1995) Rapid immunodetection on polyvinylidene fluoride membrane blots without blocking. *Anal. Biochem.* **229,** 140–143.

25

Measurement of Protein Tyrosine Phosphorylation in T-Cell Subsets by Flow Cytometry

Dariush Farahi Far and Bernard Rossi

1. Introduction

Stimulation of T lymphocytes, as induced by the interaction of their T-cell receptor with a peptide/MHC complex or by the use of anti-CD3 antibodies, triggers the activation of tyrosine kinases activities within a few seconds. This very early step leads to a series of biochemical events that include the expression of cytokine receptors (1–2 h), secretion of cytokines (5–6 h), DNA replication (24 h), and cell division (48 h). Phosphorylation of cellular substrates on tyrosine residues appears as the first detectable molecular event that hallmarks T-cell activation. It has been established that three nonreceptor protein kinases are implicated in this process. The first of these kinases to be identified is $p56^{lck}$, which interacts physically and functionally with the CD4 and CD8 coreceptors. Indeed, T cells from mice deficient in the expression of this enzyme fail to display a biochemical response in response to antigen-receptor crosslinking *(1,2)*. The second kinase identified is $p59^{fyn}$, as demonstrated by the lack of TCR response when $p59^{fyn}$ activity is abrogated *(3)*. Both Lck and Fyn are members of the src-family that are abundantly expressed in T lymphocytes. A third kinase belonging to the Syk-familly, ZAP-70, was shown to associate with the TCRζ homodimer through its SH2 domains *(4,5)*. This association necessitates the previous phosphorylation of ITAMs (immuno-receptor tyrosine-based activation motifs) by both Lck *(6)* and Fyn *(7)*. Activation of ZAP-70 is also of crucial importance for T-cell signaling as exemplified by the severe combined immunodeficiency observed on patients suffering from mutations in the ZAP-70 gene *(8)*.

Tyrosine kinases that are implicated in the activation of T cells are not only under the control of the aggregation status of the TCR, but also depend on

From: *Methods in Molecular Biology, Vol. 134: T Cell Protocols: Development and Activation*
Edited by: K. P. Kearse © Humana Press Inc., Totowa, NJ

tyrosine phosphatase (PTPase) activities. CD45 is a receptor-type PTPase that is expressed at high levels on the surface of all hematopoietic cells. The tyrosine phosphatase activity of CD45 is necessary to trigger T-cell activation, as demonstrated by the lack of response to TCR crosslinking in cell lines defective in expression of this type of PTPase *(9,10)*. The major target of CD45 lies most probably in the C-terminal Y505 site of Lck, which exerts a negative control on the enzymatic activity of this kinase when it is phosphorylated. Relief of this negative control would allow activation of Lck and Fyn. At variance to CD45, the SH2-domain containing PTPases SHP-1 and SHP-2 behave as negative regulators of the TCR-triggered tyrosine kinase cascade, especially by dephosphorylating ZAP-70 after T-cell stimulation *(11)*. The delayed tyrosine kinase-mediated recruitment of SHP-1 is likely responsible of the transient aspect of cellular substrates tyrosine phosphorylation that follows TCR crosslinking.

Estimation of the intracellular tyrosine phosphorylation content is usually performed by Western blot. However, this technique is time consuming, and is not convenient for studies aimed at comparing different T-cell subsets, inasmuch as it requires a previous purification of the investigated cell populations. For these reasons, the authors *(12,13)* and others *(13,14)* have developed a flow cytometry technique to estimate the level of cellular tyrosine phosphorylated proteins using conditions that are compatible with a second or a third labeling of surface antigens or parameters related to apoptosis *(15)*.

2. Materials

1. Venous blood from healthy donors.
2. EDTA Vacutainer tubes (Becton-Dickinson, San Jose, CA).
3. Complete RPMI 1640, 10 m*M* HEPES (Gibco-BRL Laboratories, Grand Island, NY).
4. Ficoll-Hypaque (Pharmacia, Uppsala, Sweden).
5. Antibodies: MAb against CD3, CD4 and CD8, polyclonal rabbit antimouse IgG, and MAb FITC-conjugated antiphosphotyrosine (alternatively conjugated with biotin for a two-step labeling with streptavidin coupled to FITC).
6. Washing buffer 1: PBS, pH 7.4, 0.1% BSA, 0.1% NaN_3.
7. Fixing buffer: PBS, pH 7.4, 1% formaldehyde, 0.1% NaN_3.
8. Labeling buffer 1: PBS, pH 7.4, 1% calf serum; 0.1% NaN_3.
9. Labeling buffer 2: PBS, pH 7.4, 0.1% BSA, 0.1% saponin.
10. Permeabilizing buffer: PBS, pH 7.5, 0.2% saponin.

3. Procedures

3.1. Cell Preparation

1. Collect venous blood into a test tube containing an anticoagulant.
2. Isolate the mononuclear cells from heparinized venous blood by underlying 30 mL of blood onto 15 mL of Ficoll-Hypaque. Centrifuge for 20 min at 600*g* at room temperature.

3. Collect mononuclear cells at the medium/Ficoll interface by slowly moving the tip of a Pasteur pipet at the surface of the high density layer. Harvested cells are centrifuged at 500g for 3 min. Discard the supernatant.

4. Resuspend cells in 40 mL of RPMI 1640, 10 mM HEPES and wash three times in the same medium (for centrifugation proceed as in **step 3**). Resuspend the cell pellet in RPMI 1640, 10 mM HEPES supplemented with 2% SVF at a final density of 2×10^7 cells/mL.

3.2. Lymphocyte Stimulation

1. Transfer 100 µL of the cell suspension to a test tube and keep on ice for 5–10 min.

2. Add the purified stimulating antibody at a concentration recommended by the manufacturer (e.g., 10 µg/mL of the anti-CD3 MAb Clone X-35 IgG2a, Coulter-Immunotech, Marseille, France). Incubate for 5 min at 4°C.

3. Add the crosslinking secondary anti-mouse IgG antibody at the optimal saturating concentration (e.g., polyclonal rabbit anti-mouse IgG, Dako 20 µg/mL) and stir gently.

4. Transfer the tube into a water bath at 37°C and incubate for various time periods to determine the optimal time of stimulation (typically 1–5 min).

5. Add 2 mL of ice-cold washing buffer and centrifuge at 500g for 3 min. Repeat this washing procedure once.

6. Resuspend cells in 100 µL of PBS pH 7.4, 1% SVF, 0.1% NaN3 containing phycoerythrine-conjugated anti-CD4 or anti-CD8 antibodies at a saturating concentration recommended by the manufacturer. Incubate in the dark for 30 min at 4°C.

7. Wash cells with 2 mL of ice-cold washing buffer, and centrifuge at 500g for 3 min. Repeat this procedure once.

3.3. Surface Antigen Staining

1. Resuspend the pellet in fixing buffer containing 1% formaldehyde for 15 min at 4°C. Centrifuge at 500g for 3 min to remove formaldehyde. Discard the supernatant.

2. Wash cells once with 2 mL of ice-cold washing buffer, and centrifuge at 500g for 3 min. Discard the supernatant.

3. Resuspend the cell pellet in 100 µL of washing buffer, and permeabilize cells by adding an equal volume of PBS, pH 7.4, 0.2% saponin. Incubate for 5 min. Centrifuge at 500g for 3 min. Discard the supernatant.

4. Resuspend in 100 µL of PBS, pH 7.4, 0.1% BSA, 0.1% saponin, containing 10 µg/mL of FITC-conjugated anti-phosphotyrosine MAb mouse IgG1, clone PT-66 (Sigma, St. Louis, MO) (use the concentration recommended by the manufacturer of each source). Incubate in the dark for 30 min at 4°C.

5. Centrifuge cells as in **step 3** and wash the sample with 2 mL of PBS pH 7.4, 0.1% BSA, 0.1% saponin. Centrifuge and resuspend in 2 mL of washing buffer. Centrifuge again and resuspend in 500 µL of washing buffer for FACS analysis.

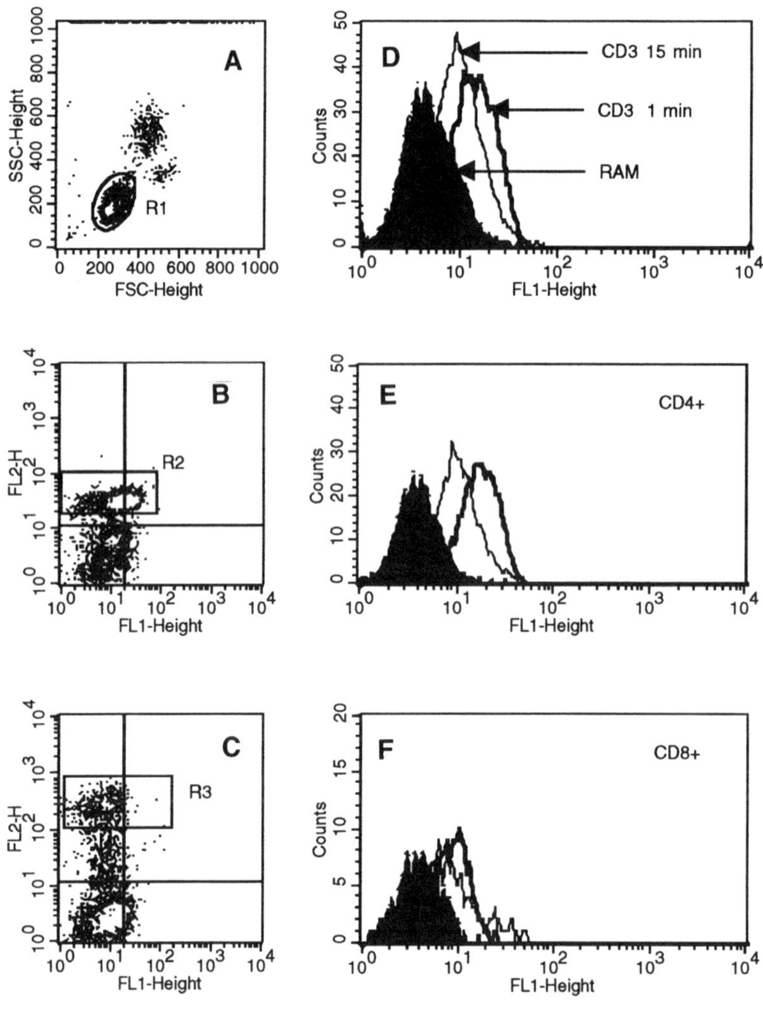

Fig. 1. Phosphotyrosine analysis of CD3-stimulated CD4 and CD8 T-cell subpopulations by flow cytometry. Normal PBMC were stimulated in a two step fashion with X-35 (anti CD3) and rabbit anti-mouse (RAM) or with RAM alone. Cells were then labeled with anti CD4 or CD8 MAbs conjugated to PE. After fixation and permeabilization with saponin intracellular tyrosine phosphorylated proteins were revealed by anti-phosphotyrosine MAb coupled to FITC. Total lymphocytes are gated (gate 1) on double scatter plot (**A**) and the time-course of their tyrosine phosphorylated content under CD3 stimulation is presented in (**D**). (**B,C**) CD4[+] and CD8[+] subpopulation, as gated in the R2 and R3 windows, respectively. Time-courses of tyrosine phosphorylation of CD4[+] and CD8[+] subsets are presented in (**E**) and (**F**), respectively. (D–F) Phosphotyrosine labeling in unstimulated cells (RAM alone), (solid peak), CD3[+] RAM stimulated cells for 1 min (thick line), and CD3[+] RAM stimulated cells for 15 min (thin line).

3.4. Flow Cytometry

Protein tyrosine phosphorylation was analyzed by flow cytometry (FACScan analyzer Becton-Dickinson) fitted with a 15-mW air-cooled argon-ion laser emitting at 488 nm as shown in **Fig. 1**. Forward scatter, side scatter, FITC and PE fluorescence were analyzed following standard procedures with CellQuest software (Becton-Dickinson). In a first instance, lymphocytes were gated following a double scatter. Then, phosphotyrosine-FITC (FL-1) and CD4 or CD8 conjugated to PE (FL-2) were analyzed by dot plot (*see* **Note 1**). Finally, CD4+ or CD8+ cells were gated, and the intensity of the fluorescence associated with tyrosine phosphorylated proteins in each T-cell subset was quantitated on a histogram plot. Ten thousand events were analyzed for each sample.

4. Notes

1. Intracellular anti-phosphotyrosine staining must be performed with a low molecular weight fluorochrome. Fluorescein isothiocyanate (FITC) is suitable for this type of labeling, but depending on the nature of the labeled antibodies that are available for bi- or tri-labeling, other dyes, such as 7-amino-4-methylcumarin-3-acetic acid (AMCA) or Cascade Blue may be used. However, one has to consider that these dyes require excitation in the UV range. If necessary, the antiphosphotyrosine signal might be enhanced by using biotinylated anti-phosphotyrosine (10 µg/mL) mAb, with fluorescein-conjugated streptavidin in the second step.

References

1. Straus, D. B. and Weiss, A. (1992) Genetic evidence for the involvement of the lck tyrosine kinase in signal transduction through the T cell antigen receptor. *Cell* **70,** 585–593.
2. Molina, T. J., Kishihara, K., Siderovski, D. P., vanEwijk, W., Narendran, A., Timms, E., Wakeham, A., Paige, C. J., Hartmann, K. U., Veillette, A., Davidson, D., and Mak, T. W. (1992) Profound block in thymocyte development in mice lacking p^{56lck}. *Nature* **357,** 161–164.
3. Appleby, M. W., Gross, J. A., Cooke, M. P., Levin, S. D., Qian, X., and Perlmutter, R. M. (1992) Defective T cell receptor signaling in mice lacking the thymic isoform of p^{59fyn}. *Cell* **70,** 751–763.
4. Chan, A. C., Iwashima, M., Turck, C. W., and Weiss, A. (1992) ZAP-70 a 70 kd protein-tyrosine kinase that associates with the TCR ζ chain. *Cell* **71,** 649–662.
5. Wange, R. L., Kong, A. T., and Samelson, L. E. (1992) A tyrosine phosphorylated 70 kDa protein binds a photoaffinity analogue of ATP and associates with both the ζ chain and CD3 components of the activated T cell antigen receptor. *J. Biol. Chem.* **267,** 11,685–11,688.
6. vanOers, N. S. C., Killeen, N., and Weiss, A. (1996) Lck regulates the tyrosine phosphorylation of the T cell receptor subunits and ZAP-70 in murine thymocytes. *J. Exp. Med.* **183,** 1053–1062.

7. Ganen, L. K., Zhu, Y., Letourneur, F., Hu, Q., Bolden, J. B., Matis, L. A., Klausner, R. D., and Shaw, A. S. (1994) Interaction of p^{59fyn} and ZAP-70 with T-cell receptor activation motifs defining the nature of a signaling motif. *Mol. Cell. Biol.* **14,** 3729–3741.

8. Arpaia, E., Shahar, M., Dadi, H., Cohen, A., and Roitman, C. M. (1994) Defective T cell receptor signaling and $CD8^+$ thymic solution in humans lacking ZAP-70 kinase. *Cell* **76,** 947–958.

9. Pingel, J. T. and Thomas, M. L. (1989) Evidence that the leukocyte-common antigen is required for antigen-induced T lymphocyte proliferation. *Cell* **58,** 1055–1065.

10. Koretzky, G. A., Piens, J., Thomas, M. L., and Weiss, A. (1990) Tyrosine phosphatase CD45 is essential for coupling T-cell antigen receptor to the phosphatidyl-inositol pathway. *Nature* **346,** 66–68.

11. Sells, S. F., Muthukumar, S., Sukhatm, V. P., Crist, S. A., and Rangnekar, V. M. (1995) The zinc finger transcription factor EGR-1 impedes interleukin-1 inducible tumor growth arrest. *Mol. Cell. Biol.* **15,** 682–692.

12. Farahi Far, D., Peyron, J. F., Imbert, V., and Rossi, B. (1994) Immunofluorescent quantification of tyrosine phosphorylation of cellular proteins in whole cells by flow cytometry. *Cytometry* **15,** 327–334.

13. Vuiller, F., Scott-Algara, D., Cayota, A., Siciliano, J., Nugeyre, M. T., and Dighiero, G. (1995) Flow cytometric analysis of protein-tyrosine phosphorylation in peripheral T cell subsets. Application to healthy and HIV-positive subjects. *J. Immunol. Methods* **185,** 43–56.

14. Hubert, P., Grenot, P., Autran, B., and Debré, P. (1997) Analysis by flow cytometry of tyrosine-phosphorylated proteins in activated T-cell subsets on whole blood samples. *Cytometry* **29,** 83–91.

15. Lund-Johansen, F., Frey, T., Ledbetter, J. A., and Thomson, P. A. (1996) Apoptosis in hematopoietic cells is associated with an extensive decrease in cellular phosphotyrosine content that can be inhibited by the tyrosine phosphatase antagonist pervanadate. *Cytometry* **25,** 182–190.

26

Biochemical Analysis of Activated T Lymphocytes

*Protein Phosphorylation and Ras, ERK,
and JNK Activation*

Patrick E. Fields and Thomas F. Gajewski

1. Introduction

One of the earliest detectable responses following TCR ligation is the phosphorylation of cellular proteins on either serine, threonine, or tyrosine residues. These covalent modifications are mediated by kinases, and are thought to facilitate various cellular functions, including enzyme activation and protein–protein interactions necessary for the initiation and propagation of catalytic cascades. The coordinated activation of several of these enzymatic cascades following TCR ligation is thought to be necessary for the synthesis and/or activation of the transcription factors that initiate cytokine gene expression, as well as for mediating cell-cycle progression and other T-cell effector functions.

Two tyrosine kinases of the Src family, Lck and Fyn, and an additional tyrosine kinase of the Syk family, ZAP-70, are critical for initial TCR-mediated signaling events *(1)*. Tyrosine phosphorylation of several early substrates has been defined, including PLC-γ1, SLP-76, p36/LAT, Vav, and the adapter Shc *(2)*. Phosphorylation of these and other proteins can be detected by immunoprecipitation followed by Western blotting with antiphosphotyrosine antibodies, or by labeling the cells with ^{32}P-orthophosphate prior to immunoprecipitation. In addition, antibodies have been generated recently that recognize only the phosphorylated form of particular proteins, making them usable directly in Western blotting without a need for first immunoprecipitating the molecule of interest.

From: *Methods in Molecular Biology, Vol. 134: T Cell Protocols: Development and Activation*
Edited by: K. P. Kearse © Humana Press Inc., Totowa, NJ

One pathway downstream from TCR-mediated tyrosine kinases is controlled by the small guanine nucleotide-binding protein, Ras *(3)*. Ras is thought to become activated when the guanine nucleotide exchanger, SOS, bound to its adapter, Grb2, is recruited to the membrane where it can load guanosine triphosphate (GTP) onto Ras. Once bound to GTP, Ras assumes an activated conformation, enabling its binding to downstream effectors, such as Raf-1. This interaction triggers a cascade ultimately leading to the activation of the MAP-kinase family members, ERK-1 and ERK-2, which phosphorylate the transcription factor Elk-1, a transactivator of the *c-fos* gene. Fos proteins comprise one component of the AP-1 transcription factor complex that contributes to the initiation of *IL-2* gene transcription *(4)*. A parallel and possibly intersecting pathway leads to activation of another MAP-kinase family member, JNK, which may require costimulation through CD28 for optimal activation *(5)*. C-Jun-N-terminal kinase (JNK) phosphorylates c-Jun, and teams up with Fos family members as a second component of AP-1. One hypothetical signaling cascade leading to both extracellular signal-regulated kinase (ERK) and JNK activation is depicted in **Fig. 1**. According to this model, activation of both ERK and JNK is dependent on Ras activation. However, ERK lies in a pathway that is directly downstream of Ras, whereas JNK activation occurs in a parallel pathway initiated by Ras-dependent activation of the Ras-superfamily member, Rac. The importance of AP-1 for expression of several genes, and the fact that AP-1 transactivation is defective in anergic T cells, have generated heightened interest in these signaling pathways *(6)*.

In this chapter, methods of murine T-cell activation using either monoclonal antibodies specific for the TCR/CD3 complex and the costimulatory receptor CD28, or specific antigen presented by antigen-presenting cells (APC), are described first. Subsequently, methods for detection of activation-induced protein phosphorylation and activation of the Ras pathway are outlined. Although the techniques described have been optimized using ovalbumin (OVA)-reactive, murine Th1 T-cell clones *(7)*, they may be applied to other cell types, such as splenic or lymph node T cells from wild-type or TCR-transgenic mice, peripheral blood T lymphocytes from humans, or T-cell hybridomas or tumor cell lines.

2. Materials

2.1. Antibody-Mediated Stimulation of T Cells

1. Biotinylated anti-CD3 (145-2C11) and anti-CD28 (37.5.1) can be purchased (PharMingen, San Diego, CA). Alternatively, these or other noncommercially available antibodies can be biotinylated using a protein biotinylation kit (Boeringer Mannheim, Mannheim, Germany). These antibodies will be

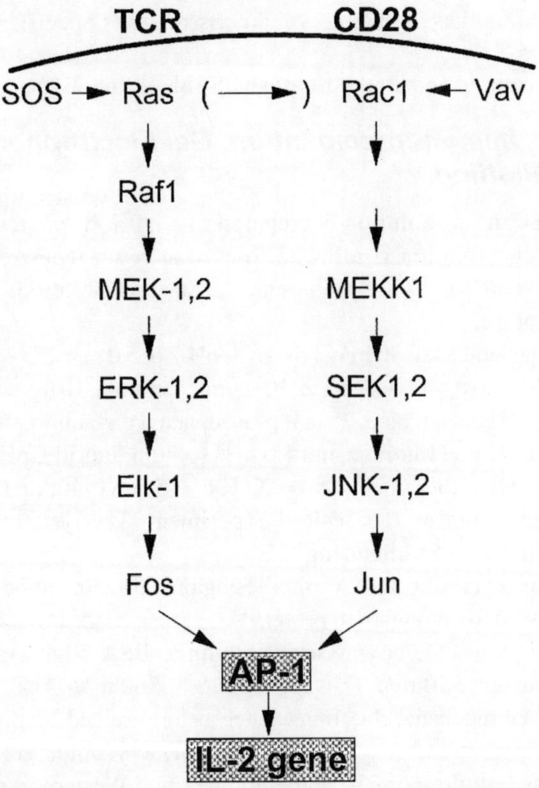

Fig. 1. Schematic diagram of a putative Ras activation pathway leading to AP-1 activation.

bound to streptavidin-coupled beads (Dynal, Oslo, Norway) and used to stimulate T cells (*see* **Note 5**).

2. Bead binding buffer: 0.5% bovine serum albumin (BSA; Sigma, Inc., St. Louis, MO) in Dulbecco's phosphate-buffered saline (DPBS; Gibco-BRL, Gaithersburg, MD).

3. Stimulation medium: T cells are stimulated in Dulbecco's modified eagle's medium (DMEM; Gibco-BRL) containing 1 mM morpholinopropanesulfonic acid (MOPS).

4. Stop buffer: T-cell stimulation is stopped by addition of DPBS containing 10 mM sodium pyrophosphate (Sigma, Inc.).

2.2. Antigen/APC Stimulation of T Cells

1. Stimulator cell line: For OVA-reactive, I-A^d-restricted T-cell clones, use the B cell hybridoma, LK35.2 (ATCC). Other tumor cells transfected with the relevant major histocompatability complex (MHC) molecules and other ligands also have been used successfully.

2. Antigen: Ovalbumin (Sigma, Inc.). T cells of other specificities will require other antigens.
3. Stimulation medium and stop buffer as in **Subheading 2.1.**

2.3. Cell Lysis, Immunoprecipitation, Gel Electrophoresis, and Western Blotting

1. Detergents: Digitonin solution is prepared as a 2.0% (w/v) stock by boiling for 10–15 min. The solution is allowed to cool at room temperature before use. Triton X-100 and NP-40 are prepared as 20% stock solutions by dissolving at room temperature.
2. Lysis buffer (general use): 50 mM Tris-HCl, pH 7.6, 5.0 mM EDTA, 150 mM NaCl, 1.0 mM Na$_3$VO$_4$, 10 μg/mL leupeptin, 10 μg/mL aprotinin, 10 μg/mL soybean trypsin inhibitor, 1.0 mM benzamidine, 25 mM p-nitrophenyl p-guanidinebenzoate, 1.0 mM phenylmethylsulfonyl fluoride, and 1.0 mM sodium fluoride, pH 7.4. This buffer also must include either 0.5% Triton X-100, 0.5% NP-40, or 1% digitonin as a detergent, depending on the desired experiment. The lysis buffer used in the Ras assay is listed in **Subheading 2.5.**
3. Antibody/agarose conjugates: Antibodies against proteins to be immunoprecipitated are allowed to conjugate to protein A-agarose beads (Gibco-BRL, prepared as a 50% slurry) in 0.5% bovine serum albumin (BSA; Sigma) in DPBS.
4. 5X sample buffer: 250 mM Tris-HCl, pH 6.8, 500 mM DTT, 10% SDS, 50% glycerol, 0.5% bromophenol blue. Immediately before use, add 2% β-mercaptoethanol.
5. Standard equipment and reagents for SDS-polyacrylamide gel electrophoresis, transfer to nitrocellulose or PVDF membranes, and Western immunoblotting are required for resolving and detecting proteins.
6. Antibodies for detection of phosphorylation: antiphosphotyrosine, 4G10 (Upstate Biotechnology [UBI], Lake Placid, NY); antiphospho-Erk and antiphospho-Jnk are available from Promega (Madison, WI). Commercial sources for antibodies against other proteins for immunoprecipitation and/or Western blotting include Santa Cruz Biotechnology (Santa Cruz, CA) and Transduction Laboratories (Lexington, KY).

2.4. ^{32}P-Labeling of T Cells

1. ^{32}P-orthophosphate: ICN Biochemicals.
2. Labeling buffer: Phosphate-free DMEM (Gibco-BRL) supplemented with 10% FCS dialyzed against phosphate-free DMEM (to remove free phosphate).

2.5. Ras Assay

1. Ras assay lysis buffer: 50 mM HEPES, pH 7.4, 1.0% Triton X-100, 100 mM NaCl, 20 mM MgCl$_2$, 1 mg/mL BSA (fatty acid-free), 0.1 mM GTP, 0.1 mM GDP, 1 mM ATP, 1 mM sodium phosphate, pH 7.4, 0.4 mM PMSF, 10 μg/mL aprotinin, 10 μg/mL soybean trypsin inhibitor, 10 μg/mL leupeptin, and 10 mM benzamidine.

2. Ras immunoprecipitation antibody: Y13-259 (ATCC).
3. Anti-Rat-conjugated agarose beads (Sigma) or protein G-agarose beads, for immunoprecipitation.
4. Immunoprecipitation wash buffer: 50 mM Tris-HCl, pH 7.4, 20 mM MgCl$_2$, 150 mM NaCl.
5. Elution buffer: 2.0 mM EDTA, 2 mM DTT, 0.2% SDS, 0.5 mM GTP, 0.5 mM GDP.
6. Thin layer chromatography (TLC) polyethyleneimide cellulose plates: Baker-Flex cellulose PEI-F plates (20 × 20 cm) (J. T. Baker, Inc., Phillipsburg, NJ).
7. TLC running buffer: 1 M KH$_2$PO$_4$, pH 3.41.

3. Methods

3.1. Antibody-Mediated Stimulation of T Cells

1. T-cell clones are prepared for stimulation by centrifugation (1800g for 15 min) over a Ficoll-Hypaque gradient *(8)* followed by washing twice in stimulation buffer. The cells are resuspended at a final concentration of 4×10^7 cells/mL in stimulation medium.
2. The streptavidin-coated beads are washed once with 1 mL of bead-binding buffer. Biotinylated anti-CD3 (10 µg/mL) and anti-CD28 (1 µg/mL) MAbs diluted in bead-binding buffer are added and allowed to bind for 1 h while rocking gently at 4°C. Generally, beads are coated at a concentration of 10^8 beads/mL of antibody solution in microcentrifuge tubes.
3. The antibody-coated beads are washed twice with 1 mL of stimulation medium and resuspended in stimulation medium at a concentration of 2×10^8 beads/mL.
4. The T cells (0.25 mL) are added to an aliquot of beads (0.25 mL) in microcentrifuge tubes and vortexed for 1 s. The tubes are either placed directly into a 37°C water bath, or are first centrifuged at high speed (12,000g) in a microcentrifuge for 8 s to force contact between beads and cells, and then are placed in a 37°C water bath for the duration of the stimulation time. Signaling events can usually be observed between 5 s and 20 min following stimulation (*see* **Note 1**).
5. The stimulation is stopped by placing the samples on ice and immediately adding 0.5 mL stop buffer. Samples are then centrifuged at high speed for 8 s, the supernatant is removed, and the pellet is lysed by addition of ice-cold lysis buffer. For immunoprecipitations, 0.5 mL lysis buffer is generally used. For whole cell lysates, 50–100 µL lysis buffer is sufficient.

3.2. Antigen/APC Stimulation of T Cells

1. Incubate the stimulator cell line with antigen for 4–12 h at 37°C in the usual culture medium for that cell line.
2. Wash the stimulator cell line three times with stimulation medium and resuspend at a final concentration of 2×10^7 cells/mL in stimulation medium.
3. Prepare T cells for stimulation as in **Subheading 3.1.**
4. Add T cells (0.25 mL) to stimulator cells (0.25 mL) in microcentrifuge tubes, and vortex briefly.

5. Place tubes in a 37°C water bath and allow cells to settle during the stimulation. Optimal times range from 1 to 20 min for various signaling events.

6. Stop the stimulation by placing the samples on ice and immediately adding 0.5 mL stop buffer. Samples are then centrifuged at high speed for 8 s, the supernatant is removed, and the pellet is lysed by addition of ice-cold lysis buffer. For immunoprecipitations, 0.5 mL lysis buffer is generally used. For whole cell lysates, 50–100 µL lysis buffer is usually sufficient.

3.3. Immunoprecipitation

1. For immunoprecipitations, preadsorb 25 µL protein-A agarose beads with immunoprecipitating antibody for 1 h at 4°C. Generally, 1 µg/mL antibody is sufficient, but this should be optimized for each antibody used.
2. Stimulate cells as in **Subheading 2.**, and add 0.5 mL desired ice-cold lysis buffer.
3. Vortex vigorously, and allow cells to lyse for 30 min on ice.
4. Centrifuge 10 min at 4°C to pellet nuclei and insoluble material.
5. While lysates are centrifuging, wash agarose beads twice with lysis buffer, and remove supernatant. Keep samples on ice at all possible times.
6. Transfer the supernatant from the cell lysates to the pelleted antibody/agarose conjugates, and mix by tapping. Incubate 1–16 h at 4°C while gently rocking.
7. Wash immunoprecipitates three times with lysis buffer and elute proteins by addition of 50 µL lysis buffer plus 13 µL of 5X sample buffer. Boil samples immediately for 5 min. Immunoprecipitated proteins can be analyzed with anti-phosphotyrosine or conventional antibodies.
8. For analysis of whole cell-lysates, lyse cell pellets in 50 µL of lysis buffer for 30 min on ice. Centrifuge at high speed at 4°C for 10 min to remove nuclei. Transfer lysate to a tube containing 13 µL of 5X reducing sample buffer, and boil for 5 min. Whole-cell lysates can be analyzed by Western blotting using phospho-specific or conventional antibodies (*see* **Notes 3** and **4**).
9. Resolve proteins using standard SDS-PAGE and Western immunoblotting techniques. Generally, between 8 and 15% polyacrylamide gels are used, depending on the size of the proteins of interest.
10. Following transfer, the blot is typically blocked with 5% milk buffer in TBST. However, high background can be seen with some antibodies, such as the antiphosphotyrosine antibody 4G10. For those cases, 1–6% BSA in TBST is used to block. Western blotting is then performed using standard methods, and developed using commercial chemiluminescence reagents.
11. The detection of activated ERK and JNK with phospho-specific antibodies is shown in **Fig. 2**. Murine Th1 and Th2 clones were stimulated with anti-CD3 plus anti-CD28 MAbs bound to streptavidin beads as described. Whole-cell lysates were divided and then resolved by SDS-PAGE. Western immunoblotting was performed using antiphospho-ERK (upper panels) or antiphospho JNK (lower panels) Abs.
12. The detection of tyrosine phosphorylation of PLC γ-1 is shown in **Fig. 3**. After stimulation of T cells with anti-CD3 MAb for the indicated times,

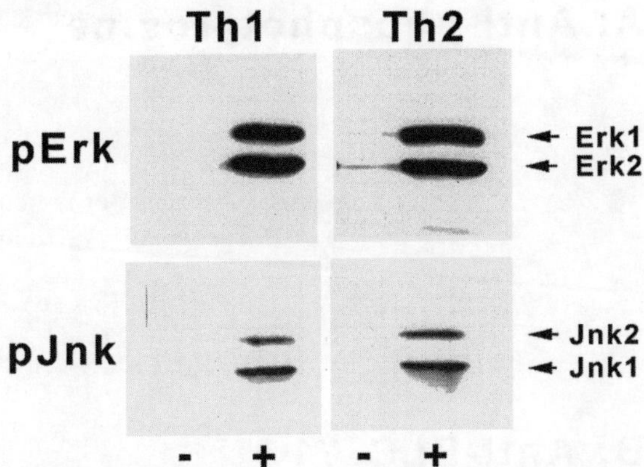

Fig. 2. The activation of ERK and JNK in mouse Th1 and Th2 clones as determined by phosphospecific antibody detection. In this experiment, 1×10^7 cells were stimulated for 5 min with streptavidin beads bound to anti-CD3 and anti-CD28 Abs. The cells were lysed in 100 µL lysis buffer containing 0.5% Triton X-100, and the lysate was divided blotted with anti-phospho ERK (upper panels) or anti-phospho-JNK (lower panels) Ab following separation on a 10% SDS-PAGE gel.

PLC γ-1 was immunoprecipitated and the eluted proteins were split and resolved by SDS-PAGE. The proteins were transferred onto nitrocellulose membranes, and the membranes were probed with anti-phosphotyrosine to detect phosphorylated PLC γ-1 (top panel) or anti-PLC γ-1 to determine relative amount of the enzyme in each immunoprecipitate (bottom panel) (*see* **Note 6**).

3.4. ^{32}P-Labeling of T Cells

1. Labeling is performed prior to T-cell stimulation.
2. Wash T cells in labeling buffer and resuspend at a final concentration of 1.5×10^7 cells/mL.
3. Incubate T cells in labeling buffer with ^{32}P-orthophosphate at 1 mCi ^{32}P/1.5×10^7 T cells/mL for 4–6 h at 37°C.
4. Wash labeled T cells three times with labeling buffer to remove excess ^{32}P.
5. Following stimulation of cells, Ras can be immunoprecipitated to elute radiolabeled guanine nucleotides. Alternatively, other proteins can be immunoprecipitated and analyzed by SDS-PAGE to assess their phosphorylation status.

3.5. Ras Assay

1. ^{32}P-label T cells as described in **Subheading 3.3.**, and stimulate as in **Subheading 3.1.**
2. Preadsorb anti-Ras antibody onto anti-Rat agarose or protein G-agarose beads, and wash twice with Ras lysis buffer, similar to **Subheading 3.2.**

A: Anti-phosphotyrosine

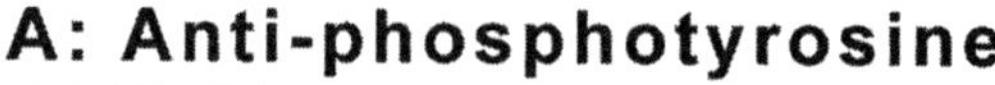

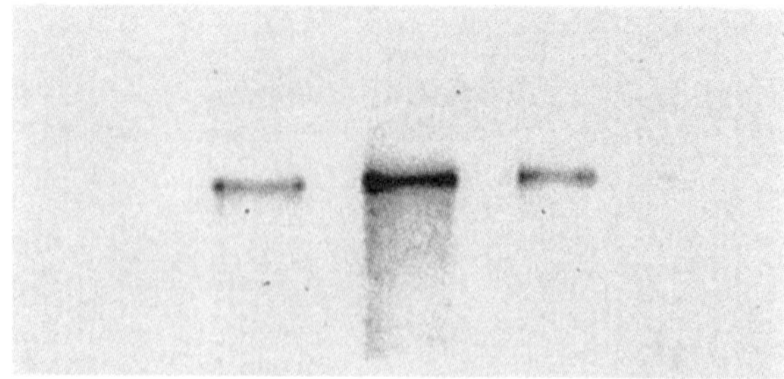

B: Anti-PLC-γ1

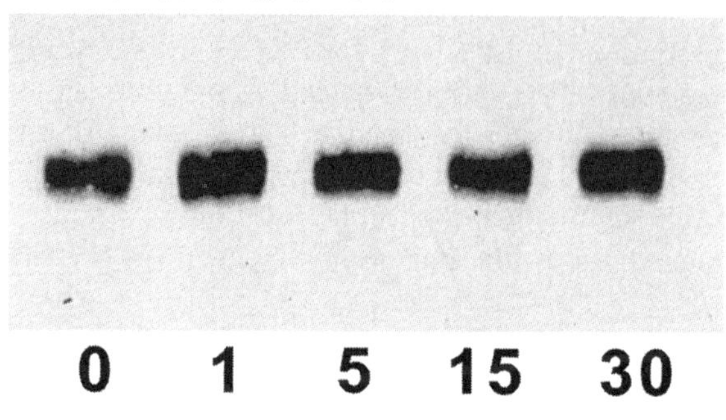

Time (minutes)

Fig. 3. The TCR stimulation-induced tyrosine phosphorylation of the enzyme, phospholipase C γ-1 (PLC γ-1): In this experiment, 3×10^7 cells were stimulated for the indicated times with anti-CD3 MAb. The cells were lysed in 0.5 mL lysis buffer and PLC γ-1 was immunoprecipitated with anti-PLC γ-1-specific antibodies (UBI) as described in **Subheading 3.2.** The immunoprecipitates were washed three times with lysis buffer and PLC γ-1 was eluted from the protein-A agarose beads as described. The eluted proteins were divided and resolved by SDS-PAGE and Western immunoblotting. 2.5×10^7 cell equivalents were blotted with the antiphosphotyrosine MAb, 4G10 (**A**) and 5×10^6 cell equivalents were blotted with anti-PLC γ-1 Ab (**B**).

3. Lyse T cells in Ras assay lysis buffer (10^8 T-cell equivalents/mL), and incubate on ice for 30 min. Centrifuge for 10 min in a microfuge and transfer supernatants to the antibody/bead conjugates.
4. Immunoprecipitate Ras from 10^7 T-cell equivalents in a final volume of 0.5 mL for 1 h at 4°C.
5. Wash immunoprecipitates 3–4 times with Ras assay lysis buffer and 3 times with immunoprecipitation wash buffer. Remove remaining supernatant.
6. Elute labeled nucleotides with 25 μL of nucleotide elution buffer at 68°C for 20 min.

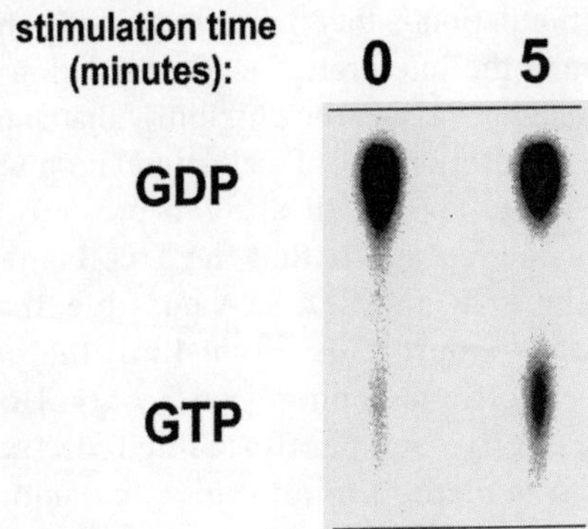

Fig. 4. Ras activation following TCR stimulation. In this experiment, 1×10^7 T cells were ^{32}P-labeled as described. The labeled cells were stimulated with anti-CD3 for the times indicated and lysed with Ras assay lysis buffer. Ras protein was immunoprecipitated and the radiolabeled nucleotides were eluted and resolved by TLC and autoradiography as described. The film was exposed for 24 h at −70°C.

7. Spot samples onto polyethylene imids (PEI) cellulose TLC plate at 1.5 cm intervals approx 2 cm from the bottom of the plate. Allow spots to dry thoroughly.
8. Wash plate twice with absolute methanol, drying between each wash.
9. Prerun TLC in water for approx 4–6 cm.
10. Run TLC by placing plate in a TLC chamber containing 1 cm of 1 M KH$_2$PO$_4$. Allow solvent front to reach the top of the plate (approx 2–4 h).
11. Expose plate to film at −70°C and develop. Overnight exposure usually is sufficient, but this should be optimized for individual experiments.
12. Ras activation is calculated as the ratio of radiolabeled GTP to GDP + GTP eluted from immunoprecipitated Ras protein. The relative amounts of eluted nucleotides can be determined by direct scanning of the TLC plate with a β-scanner.
13. The activation of Ras in a murine Th1 T-cell clone stimulated with anti-CD3 MAb is depicted in **Fig. 4**. T cells were ^{32}P-labeled as described. They were then stimulated with anti-CD3 MAb and lysed in Ras assay lysis buffer. Ras protein was immunoprecipitated and the radiolabeled GDP and GTP were eluted from immunoprecipitates. These were resolved by TLC and visualized by autoradiography (*see* **Note 7**).

4. Notes

1. The principle behind antibody-mediated T-cell activation is that co-crosslinking of CD3ε with the costimulatory receptor, CD28, on the T-cell surface, mimics the crosslinking of the TCR and CD28 by the natural ligands on the antigen presenting cell (APC). This crosslinking is accomplished using monoclonal antibodies specific for these cell surface receptors. The principal advantage to

using this mode of stimulation is that there are no APC phosphoproteins present to potentially confound the interpretation of stimulation-induced phosphorylation events. Disadvantages include the possibility that antibody-mediated T-cell activation might not precisely mimic T-cell stimulation with antigen.

2. When T cells are stimulated with antigen-presenting cells loaded with antigen, the obvious advantage is that the T cells are stimulated with the natural ligands to the TCR and CD28. A possible disadvantage is that the presence of APC phosphoproteins might limit the use of this method to the study of T cell-specific phosphoproteins only. However, several laboratories have successfully used paraformaldehyde fixation or inactivation with mitomycin-C as a method to minimize the amount of contaminating APC phosphoproteins *(9,10)*. Alternatively, ^{32}P-labeled T cells can be used in order to limit detection to phosphorylated proteins present in the T cells only. This can be performed as for the Ras assay, as described in **Subheading 3.4.**

3. For determination of phosphorylation of proteins in whole-cell lysates or of immunoprecipitated proteins, cells are usually lysed in buffer containing either 0.5% Triton X-100 or 0.5% NP-40. For optimal detection of coassociated proteins, cells often are lysed in buffer containing 1.0% digitonin. Many tightly interacting proteins can be analyzed using the harsher detergents as well.

4. All lysis buffers and cell lysates should be prepared immediately before use on ice and kept ice-cold. In addition, cell lysates should be kept on ice throughout the experiment.

5. The antibody concentrations and bead:cell ratios for T-cell stimulations may need to be varied depending on the source of T cells, the quality of the antibodies, and so forth. A bead:cell ratio of 5:1 has worked well, but a range of bead numbers should be tested to optimize results for the particular cell system used.

6. Immunoprecipitated kinases, such as Fyn or Lck, can be assayed for kinase activity in vitro. This involves resuspending the washed immunoprecipitates in kinase buffer containing ^{32}P-ATP, which also can include a phosphorylatable substrate. Details on this procedure are available in several references *(11)*.

7. GDP and GTP can be identified on the TLC plates by viewing the plate with a short wave ultraviolet light source. GDP migrates faster than GTP under the TLC conditions described.

References

1. Chan, A. C., Desai, D. M., and Weiss, A. (1994) The role of protein tyrosine kinases and protein tyrosine phosphatases in T cell antigen receptor signal transduction. *Ann. Rev. Immunol.* **12,** 555–592.
2. Koretzky, G. A. (1997) The role of Grb2-associated proteins in T cell activation. *Immunol. Today.* **18(8),** 401–406.
3. Downward, J., Graves, J. D., Warne, P. H., Rayter, S., and Cantrell, D. A. (1990) Stimulation of p21ras upon T cell activation. *Nature* **346(6286),** 719–723.
4. Schwartz, R. H. (1997) T cell clonal anergy. *Curr. Opin. Immunol.* **9(3),** 351–357.

5. Su, B., Jacinto, E., Hibi, M., Kallunki, T., Karin, M., and Ben-Neriah, Y. (1994) JNK is involved in signal integration during costimulation of T lymphocytes. *Cell* **77(5)**, 727–736.

6. Kang, S. M., Beverly, B., Tran, A. C., Brorson, K., Schwartz, R. H., and Lenardo, M. J. (1992) Transactivation of AP-1 is a molecular target of T cell clonal anergy. *Science* **257(5073)**, 1134–1138.

7. Gajewski, T. F., Joyce, J., and Fitch, F. W. (1989) Anti-proliferative effect of IFN-γ in immune regulation. III. Differential selection of Th1 and Th2 murine helper T lymphocyte clones using recombinant IL-2 and recombinant IFN-γ. *J. Immunol.* **143,** 15–22.

8. Davidson, W. F. and Parish, C. R. (1975) A procedure for removing red cells and dead cells from lymphoid cells. *J. Immunol. Methods* **7,** 291–297.

9. Klasen, S., Pages, F., Peyron, J.-F., Cantrell, D. A., and Olive, D. (1998) Two distinct regions of the CD28 intracytoplasmic domain are involved in the tyrosine phosphorylation of Vav and GTPase activating protein-associated p62 protein. *Int. Immunol.* **10(4),** 481–490.

10. Boussiotis, V. A., Barber, D. L., Lee, B. J., Gribben, J. G., Freeman, G. J., and Nadler, L. J. (1996) Differential association of protein tyrosine kinases with the T cell receptor is linked to the induction of anergy and its prevention by B7 family-mediated costimulation. *J. Exp. Med.* **184,** 365–376.

11. Qian, D., Griswold-Prenner, I., Rosner, M. R., and Fitch, F. W. (1993) Multiple components of the T cell antigen receptor complex become tyrosine-phosphorylated upon activation. *J. Biol. Chem.* **268(6),** 4488–4493.

27

Activation of Heterotrimeric GTP-Binding Proteins Upon TCR/CD3 Engagement

Constantine D. Tsoukas, Jack Stanners, and Keith A. Ching

1. Introduction

Thymically derived lymphocytes perceive antigenic signals via the T-cell antigen receptor-CD3 molecular complex *(1,2)*. The TCR/CD3 is a multimeric complex of proteins composed of an α/β heterodimer that is responsible for the recognition of the antigenic signal (in the case of T cells a peptide in the context of self-MHC class I or II), and the associated CD3 ($\gamma,\delta,\varepsilon$) and ζ proteins that are responsible for transducing the signal into the intracellular environment *(3)*. It has been demonstrated that the signaling pathways involve protein tyrosine kinases and phosphatases *(4)*, the Rho family of small guanosine triphosphate (GTP)-binding proteins *(5)*, and the heterotrimeric GTP-binding proteins (G proteins) of the Gq family *(6,7)*. The involvement of G proteins in TCR/CD3-mediated signaling is of particular interest in view of recent reports suggesting a crosstalk between G protein coupled-receptors and tyrosine kinase receptors *(8,9)*, and the demonstration that Gαq and Gβ/γ subunits can activate lymphocyte-specific tyrosine kinases *(10,11)*. Thus, an assay that would measure the activation of heterotrimeric G proteins upon TCR/CD3 engagement would be a useful technique.

1.1. Activation of Heterotrimeric GTP-Binding Proteins

At their resting state, heterotrimeric GTP-binding proteins exist as a complex of α, β, and γ subunits, having bound to the α subunit a molecule of GDP; *12)*. Upon ligand binding to a receptor that is coupled to heterotrimeric GTP-binding proteins, the Gα subunit is induced to exchange GDP for GTP and in doing so dissociates from its β/γ partners *(12)*. In this active conformation, the α subunit interacts with and activates effector molecules, such as PLCβ, adenylate cyclase, and ion channels *(12)*. The β and γ subunits associate with each other with very high affinity, and they also have effector functions, including activation of certain isoforms of adenylate cyclase, PLCβ, PLA$_2$, as well as Ca^{2+} channels *(13)*. The system becomes 'deactivated' owing to the fact that the α subunit possesses intrinsic GTPase activity and thus, in a timely manner, hydrolyzes the bound GTP to GDP. Following GTP hydrolysis the α subunit reverts back to an inactive conformation and regains its β/γ partners *(12)*.

1.2. Heterotrimeric GTP-Binding Proteins and T-Cell Activation

Several lines of evidence have argued for the involvement of heterotrimeric GTP-binding proteins in the activation of T cells via the TCR/CD3. Data that have been obtained by utilizing bacterial toxins to modify GTP-binding protein function suggest that a GTP-binding protein-TCR/CD3 coupled mechanism might be involved in the initial events leading to T-cell activation *(14–18)*. The involvement of GTP-binding proteins in TCR/CD3-mediated signaling is also suggested by the results of several other investigators. Mustelin and his coworkers showed that addition of GTP-γ-S to permeabilized human T cells induces the rapid activation of ornithine decarboxylase in a manner analogous to mitogen stimulation *(19)*. Addition of IP$_3$ to permeabilized cells produced a similar response, suggesting that an activated GTP-binding protein was a possible mediator for the IP$_3$ production necessary for ornithine decarboxylase activity *(19)*. O'Shea and colleagues demonstrated that treatment of murine T cells with AlF$_4^-$, a nonspecific activator of GTP-binding proteins, resulted in the release of intracellular Ca^{2+}, the breakdown of polyphosphoinositides and production of phosphoinositols, the activation of PKC, and the serine/threonine phosphorylation of the γ and ε chains of the CD3 complex in a fashion identical to that resulting from TCR/CD3 stimulation *(20)*. Interestingly, Cenciarelli et al. have shown that GTP-γ-S and Gpp(NH)p, activators of Gα subunits, enhance the tyrosine phosphorylation of the CD3-ζ chain upon TCR/CD3 antibody crosslinking in a protein kinase C (PKC)-independent manner *(21)*.

Our laboratory has provided more direct biochemical and genetic evidence for the involvement of GTP-binding proteins of the Gq family in TCR/CD3-mediated T-cell signaling. Stimulation of T cells through the TCR/CD3 induces guanine nucleotide exchange among the 42 kDa G protein α subunits of the Gq family *(6)*. Interestingly, protein tyrosine kinase inhibitors abrogate this nucleotide exchange *(6)*. Expression of function-deficient mutants of Gαq family members in T cells interferes with TCR/CD3-mediated events, including tyrosine phosphorylation of TCR/CD3 ζ and ε chains, intracellular Ca^{2+} mobilization, and cytokine production *(6,7)*.

If heterotrimeric GTP-binding proteins are involved in the signaling events that follow TCR-CD3 ligation, then one may proceed from the classic paradigm that ligand occupancy by the coupled receptor initiates the exchange of bound GDP for GTP, thus activating the α subunit of the responding GTP-binding protein *(12)*. We reasoned that if GTP-binding proteins are coupled to T-cell activation, then stimulation through the TCR/CD3 complex should induce nucleotide exchange. In this chapter, we describe a technique for the photolabeling of GTP-binding protein α subunits with ^{32}P-GTP. This technique uses purified T-cell membranes that are incubated under conditions that initiate the TCR/CD3-induced signaling events.

2. Materials

1. PBS: 1.47 mM KH$_2$PO$_4$, 0.84 mM Na$_2$HPO$_4$, 137 mM NaCl, 2.7 mM KCl, 0.9 mM CaCl$_2$, 0.49 mM MgCl$_2$, pH 7.4–7.8.
2. Homogenization buffer: 50 mM Tris-HCl, 100 mM NaCl, 5 mM MgCl, 1 mM EDTA, 1 mM DTT, 1 mM PMSF, 2 µg/mL pepstatin A, pH 7.4.
3. Percoll gradient solution was made in Tris-sucrose (50 mM Tris, 250 mM sucrose, 1 mM EDTA, 1 mM PMSF, pH 7.4) following the supplier's instructions (cat. no. P1644; Sigma, St. Louis, MO).
4. Storage buffer: 50 mM Tris-HCl, 100 mM NaCl, 1 mM EDTA, 1 mM DTT, 1 mM PMSF, 2 µg/mL pepstatin A, 2 µg/mL leupeptin, 10% glycerol, pH 7.4.
5. Photolabeling buffer: 25 mM HEPES, 100 mM NaCl, 1 mM EDTA, 5 mM MgCl$_2$, 5 mM MnCl$_2$, 10% glycerol, 1 mM PMSF, 5 µg/mL pepstatin A, 5 µg/mL leupeptin, 2.5 µM ATP, 30 µM GDP, pH 7.4.
6. Monoclonal anti-CD3ε antibody OKT3 was produced in the laboratory from a hybridoma cell line (cat. no. CRL 8001) obtained from ATCC (Manolssos, VA).
7. UPC 10 control antibody was obtained from Bionetics (Charleston, SC).
8. [α-^{32}P]GTP 800 Ci/mmol was obtained from New England Nuclear (Boston, MA).
9. UV short wave length light source: Model UVG-11 Mineralight lamp, short wave UV-254 NM from Ultra-Violet Products Inc. (San Gabriel, CA).

3. Methods
3.1. Preparation of Plasma Membranes *(see Note 1)*

1. Collect cells by centrifugation of the culture at 200*g* (*see* **Notes 2** and **3**).
2. Wash twice in 10 mL of PBS.
3. Resuspend in 10 mL of homogenization buffer and incubate on ice for 30 min.
4. Freeze in ethanol-dry ice bath to rupture cells (cells may be ruptured by freezing at –70°C overnight, instead).
5. Homogenize in a Dounce homogenizer using 30 strokes (*see* **Note 4**).
6. Remove cellular debris and nuclei by centrifugation at 600*g* for 10 min.
7. Collect the membranes by centrifugation at 12,000*g* for 30 min.
8. Resuspend the membranes in Percoll solution and centrifuge at 35,000*g* for 30 min.
9. Collect the membranes that are on the top of the Percoll gradient (*see* **Note 5**).
10. Resuspend in 50 mL of Tris-sucrose solution (**Subheading 2.3.**).
11. Spin at 12,000*g* for 30 min.

12. Resuspend in 5 mL of storage buffer (**Subheading 2.4.**).
13. Assay protein content of preparation using any standard protein determination assay.
14. Aliquot and store at –70°C until needed.

3.2. Photolabeling of Membrane Proteins

1. Thaw stored aliquot and isolate membranes by centrifugation at 12,000g at 4°C for 10 min (*see* **Note 6**).
2. Resuspend membranes in cold photolabeling buffer (**Subheading 2.5.**) and incubate on ice for 30 min (*see* **Note 7**).
3. Add 10 µg of anti-CD3ε antibody OKT3 or isotype control antibody UPC10 and incubate for 3 min at 30°C (*see* **Note 8**).
4. Add [α-^{32}P]GTP to 0.05 µM and incubate an additional 3 min at 30°C (*see* **Note 9**).
5. Terminate reaction by rapidly cooling the samples on ice, followed by centrifugation at 12,000g for 10 min at 4°C to collect the membranes.
6. Resuspend the membrane pellet in 50 µL nucleotide-free photolabeling buffer (**Subheading 2.5.**) containing 2 mM DTT.
7. Transfer sample to a section of parafilm overlaying a glass plate on ice, and irradiate for 12 min in the dark with short wavelength UV light source at a distance of 3 cm.
8. Collect membranes by centrifugation at 12,000g for 10 min at 4°C.
9. Analysis of the photolabeled membranes can be performed either by SDS-PAGE and autoradiography using standard gel electrophoresis techniques (*see* **Note 10**), or by immunoprecipitation with specific anti-Gα subunit antibodies followed by SDS-PAGE analysis or scintillation counting (*see* **Note 11**).

4. Notes

1. All procedures in this section should be performed at 4°C in order to minimize protein degradation.
2. The protocol described here was developed using Jurkat T cells. However, any T-cell line that expresses TCR/CD3 and can be stimulated by anti-CD3ε antibodies may be used. The cells can be grown in any suitable tissue culture medium, such as RPMI-1640 supplemented with 10% heat inactivated FBS, 2 mM L-glutamine, and 1 mM HEPES buffer.
3. In order to obtain a reasonable yield of membranes, a minimum of 1×10^9 cells should be processed.
4. Cell suspension should be kept chilled during homogenization to minimize protein degradation. It is recommended that cells be rested on ice for 2 min after each 10 homogenization strokes.
5. Purification of membranes can also be performed with any other standard gradient purification technique.
6. Aliquot should contain the equivalent of 50–100 µg of protein.
7. Volume depends on concentration of stock solutions of antibody and [α–^{32}P]GTP. Final reaction volume should be 50–70 µL.

8. If antibody OKT3 is not available, any other anti-CD3ε antibody that can stimulate T cells similar to OKT3 can be used. However, if the substituting antibody is not of the IgG2a subclass, an appropriate control antibody, other than UPC10, should be also used.
9. Radioactive GTP should be freshly labeled for best results.
10. Considering the relative molecular size of Gα subunits, a 10% SDS-PAGE gel is recommended.
11. If immunoprecipitation is used to analyze the photolabeled membranes, a higher specific activity preparation of [α-^{32}P]GTP (3000 Ci/mmol) should be used to increase the sensitivity of the signal.

Acknowledgment

This work was supported by grants from the National Institutes of Health (GM39518, GM56374, AI38448).

References

1. Weiss, A., Imboden, J., Hardy, K., Manger, B., Terhorst, C., and Stobo, J. (1986) The role of the T3/antigen receptor complex in T-cell activation. *Ann. Rev. Immunol.* **4,** 593–619.
2. Tsoukas, C. D., Valentine, M., Lotz, M., Vaughan, J. H., and Carson, D. A. (1984) The role of the T3 molecular complex in antigen recognition and subsequent activation events. *Immunol. Today* **5,** 311–313.
3. Allison, J. P. and Lanier, L. L. (1987) Structure, function, and serology of the T-cell antigen receptor complex. *Ann. Rev. Immunol.* **5,** 503–540.
4. Chan, A. C., Desai, D. M., and Weiss, A. (1994) The role of protein tyrosine kinases and protein tyrosine phosphatases in T cell antigen receptor signal transduction. *Annu. Rev. Immunol.* **12,** 555–592.
5. Reif, K. and Cantrell, D. A. (1998) Networking Rho family GTPases in lymphocytes. *Immunity* **8,** 395–401.
6. Stanners, J., Kabouridis, P. S., McGuire, K., and Tsoukas, C. D. (1995) Interaction between G proteins and tyrosine kinases upon T cell receptor-CD3-mediated signaling. *J. Biol. Chem.* **270,** 30,635–30,642.
7. Zhou, J., Stanners, J., Kabouridis, P., Han, H., and Tsoukas, C. D. (1998) Inhibition of TCR/CD3-mediated signaling by a mutant of the hematopoietically expressed G16 GTP-binding protein. *Eur J Immunol.* **28,** 1645–1655.
8. Della Rocca, G. J., van Biesen, T., Daaka, Y., Luttrell, D. K., Luttrell, L. M., and Lefkowitz, R. J. (1997) Ras-dependent mitogen-activated protein kinase activation by G protein-coupled receptors. Convergence of Gi- and Gq-mediated pathways on calcium/calmodulin, Pyk2, and Src kinase. *J. Biol. Chem.* **272,** 19,125–19,132.
9. Luttrell, L. M., Della Rocca, G. J., van Biesen, T., Luttrell, D. K., and Lefkowitz, R. J. (1997) G βγ subunits mediate Src-dependent phosphorylation of the epidermal growth factor receptor. A scaffold for G protein-coupled receptor-mediated Ras activation. *J. Biol. Chem.* **272,** 4637–4644.

10. Bence, K., Ma, W., Kozasa, T., and Huang, X. Y. (1997) Direct stimulation of Bruton's tyrosine kinase by Gq-protein α-subunit. *Nature* **389,** 296–299.

11. Langhans-Rajasekaran, S. A., Wan, Y., and Huang, X. Y. (1995) Activation of Tsk and Btk tyrosine kinases by G protein βγ subunits. *Proc. Natl. Acad. Sci. USA* **92,** 8601–8605.

12. Gilman, A. G. (1987) G proteins: Transducers of receptor-generated signals. *Ann. Rev. Biochem.* **56,** 615–649.

13. Clapham, D. E. and Neer, E. J. (1993) New roles for G-protein βγ-dimers in transmembrane signalling. *Nature* **365,** 403–406.

14. Imboden, J. B., Shoback, D. M., Pattison, G., and Stobo, J. D. (1986) Cholera toxin inhibits the T-cell antigen receptor-mediated increases in inositol triphosphate and cytoplasmic free calcium. *Proc. Natl. Acad. Sci. USA* **83,** 5673–5677.

15. Anderson, D. L. and Tsoukas, C. D. (1989) Cholera toxin inhibits resting human T cell activation via a cAMP-independent pathway. *J. Immunol.* **143,** 3647–3652.

16. Gray, L. S., Huber, K. S., Gray, M. C., Hewlett, E. L., and Engelhard, V. H. (1989) Pertussis toxin effects on T lymphocytes are mediated through CD3 and not by pertussis toxin catalyzed modification of a G protein. *J. Immunol.* **142,** 1631–1638.

17. Graves, J. D. and Cantrell, D. A. (1991) An analysis of the role of nucleotide binding proteins in antigen receptor/CD3 antigen coupling to phospholipase C. *J. Immunol.* **146,** 2102–2107.

18. Bonvini, E., Debell, K. E., Taplits, M. S., Brando, C., Laurenza, A., Seamon, K., and Hoffman, T. (1991) A role for guanine-nucleotide-binding proteins in mediating T cell receptor coupling to inositol phospholipid hydrolysis in a murine T-helper (type II) lymphocyte clone. *Biochem. J.* **275,** 689–696.

19. Mustelin, T., Poso, H., and Andersson, L. C. (1986) Role of G-proteins in T cell activation: non-hydrolyzable GTP analogs induce early ornithine decarboxylase activity in human T lymphocytes. *EMBO J.* **5,** 3287–3290.

20. O'Shea, J. J., Urdahl, K. B., Luong, H. T., Chused, T. M., Samelson, L. E., and Klausner, R. D. (1987) Aluminum fluoride induces phosphatidylinositol turnover, elevation of cytoplasmic free calcium, and phosphorylation of the T-cell antigen receptor in murine T-cells. *J. Immunol.* **139,** 3463–3469.

21. Cenciarelli, C., Hohman, R. J., Atkinson, T. P., Gusovsky, F., and Weissman, A. M. (1992) Evidence for GTP-binding protein involvement in the tyrosine phosphorylation of the T cell receptor zeta chain. *J. Biol. Chem.* **267,** 527–530.

28

Generation of Human T Helper 1 and T Helper 2 Subsets from Peripheral Blood-Derived Naive CD4+ T Cells

Ellen M. Palmer, Roshanak Tolouei Semnani, Bradford L. McRae, and Gijs A. van Seventer

1. Introduction

CD4+ T helper (Th) cells are crucial for the generation of the antigen-specific immune response *(1)*. They regulate many different aspects of the immune response, both by the secretion of cytokines and through cell surface expressed molecules. CD4+ precursor (Thp) Th cells or naive Th cells are fully developed Th cells that have left the thymic environment and have not yet encountered the specific antigen for their unique antigen-specific T-cell receptor (TCR). Thp cells have the capacity to differentiate into effector and memory Th cells with a wide variety of functional capabilities. The differentiation status of human resting Th cells can be distinguished by the cell surface expression of distinct isoforms of the molecule CD45 *(1,2)*. Naive Th cells express high levels of the CD45RA form, in the absence of the CD45RO form, while previously activated Th cells (memory/effector Th cells) express high levels of the CD45RO form and low levels of the CD45RA form.

To allow for the generation of the most effective immune response Thp cells can upon activation differentiate into functionally distinct Th cell subsets, which at present are best defined by their cytokine secretion profile *(3–6)*. Although a whole spectrum of Th cell cytokine secretion profiles exists, the best characterized Th cell subsets are the Th1 and Th2 subsets. Th1 cells secrete interferon (IFN)-γ, tumor necrosis factor (TNF)-α and lymhotoxin (LT) or TNF-β, and provide help for inflammatory immune responses, e.g., help for the generation of cytotoxic CD8+ T cells, for delayed type hypersensitivity reactions, for activation of macrophages and for isotype switching of B cells to

From: *Methods in Molecular Biology, Vol. 134: T Cell Protocols: Development and Activation*
Edited by: K. P. Kearse © Humana Press Inc., Totowa, NJ

isotypes that can provide opsonization of antigen for macrophages. Th2 cells are involved in the induction of the humoral immune response and are also considered more anti-inflammatory in their effector functions. They secrete interleukin (IL)-4, IL-5, and IL-13, drive B cell activation and IgE antibody secretion, and regulate immune responses to helminths by stimulating the generation of eosinophils. A crucial distinction between murine and human Th cell subsets is the secretion of the anti-inflammatory cytokine IL-10, which can be secreted both by Th1- and Th2-like subsets, in the human *(7–10)*, but is restricted to the Th2-like subset in the mouse *(11)*.

Since the Thp cell has the full capacity to become either a Th1 or Th2 effector cell, much research has been focused on what factors regulate the differentiation towards a Th1 or a Th2 cell. Whereas many factors clearly play a role, including antigen-density and costimulatory signals from accessory pathways, the dominant influence is from cytokines present during initial antigen-specific activation of the Thp cells. These cytokines are either secreted by the antigen-presenting cell or otherwise derived in the local micro environment. The most important and best characterized of these cytokines are IL-4 and IL-12, which at the time of Thp cell activation strongly influence the differentiation to Th2 and Th1 cells, respectively *(12)*.

In this chapter, two closely related methods for the in vitro generation of T helper subsets from human naive CD4$^+$ T cells are described *(10,13)*. In these procedures, naive CD4$^+$ T cells are activated by antibody stimulation through TCR-associated signaling complex CD3 and by costimulation through cell surface molecules expressed on antigen-presenting cells, which in these systems function more as accessory cells. Skewing towards Th1- and Th2-like effector subsets is achieved through the manipulation of the available IL-12 and IL-4 in the cultures. This technique polyclonally activates Thp cells and generates T helper effector populations that can be used to study both the requirements for Th cell differentiation as well as the effector functions of T helper cell subsets in vitro.

2. Materials

2.1. Isolation of Peripheral Blood Mononuclear Cells (PBMC)

1. 25–50 mL buffy coat of 1 unit of human blood (*see* **Note 1**).
2. Dulbecco's phosphate buffered saline (DPBS) [0.0095 *M* (phosphate)] without calcium or magnesium.
3. Bead separation medium:
      500 mL Hank's balanced salt solution without calcium, magnesium, or phenol red
      4 mL 25% human serum albumin (HSA)
      5 mL Penicillin (10,000 units/mL) /Streptomycin (10,000 mg/mL)
4. Lymphocyte separation medium or Ficoll (density 1.077 g/mL) (Biowhittaker, Walkersville, MD).

5. 60 cc syringe, 18G $1^{1}/_{2}$ needle, sampling site coupler (Baxter HealthCare Corporation, Deerfield, IL).
6. 50 mL polypropylene conical tubes.
7. Trypan blue, hemacytometer, light microscope with phase contrast.

2.2. Isolation of Naive CD4$^+$ T Cells from PBMC

1. Mouse monoclonal antibody (MAb) cocktail for negative selection of naive CD4$^+$ T cells includes MAbs to human cell surface molecules *(14)*.
    a. CD14 (expressed on monocytes).
    b. Mac-1 (expressed on monocytes and subset of CD8$^+$ T cells).
    c. Class II (expressed on B cells, monocytes and activated T cells).
    d. CD16 (FcgRIII) (expressed on monocytes, B cells, and natural killer [NK] cells).
    e. CD19 (expressed on B cells).
    f. CD8 (expressed on CD8$^+$ T cells and subset of NK cells).
    g. Glycophorin (expressed on red blood cells).
    h. CD45RO (preferentially expressed on activated and primed CD4$^+$ T cells). Most of the hybridoma secreting MAbs with these specificities are available through the American Tissue Type Collection (ATTC, Manassas, VA). Alternatively, specific separation kits for the isolation of CD45RA$^+$RO$^-$ CD4$^+$ T cells are commercially available from Dynal, Inc. (Lake Success, NY).
2. BioMag goat antimouse IgG (H & L)-coated beads (PerSeptive Diagnostics, Cambridge, MA).
3. Rotator.
4. Rare earth magnet.
5. Bead separation medium (*see* recipe above).

2.3. Derivation of Dendritic Cells from Peripheral Blood Monocytes

1. CD14$^+$ elutriated monocytes from buffycoat of peripheral blood *(15)*.
2. Tissue culture treated 6-well plates.
3. Culture medium:
       500 mL RPMI 1640 with L-glutamine
       50 mL Fetal calf serum (FCS)
       5 mL Penicillin (10,000 U/mL)/Streptomycin (10,000 µg/mL)
4. Recombinant human cytokines: GM-CSF, IL-4, TNF-α (e.g., Pharmingen, San Diego, CA).
5. DPBS.
6. Versine /EDTA (BioWhittaker, Walkersville, MD).
7. 2 mL nonpyrogenic pipet.
8. 50 mL polypropylene conical tubes.
9. Dimethyl sulfoxide (DMSO).
10. Cryo tubes (Nunc cryopreservation vials with rubber O-ring).
11. Trypan blue, hemacytometer, light microscopy with phase contrast.

12. Liquid nitrogen tank.
13. 37°C Incubator.
14. –30°C freezer.
15. –80°C freezer.

2.4. Stimulation of Naive CD4+ T Cells

1. Tissue culture treated six-well and 24-well plates.
2. Culture medium.
3. PBS.
4. Antibody to human anti-CD3 (sterile), OKT3 hybridoma available from the ATTC.
5. Recombinant cytokines (*see* **Note 2**): Interleukin-1 (IL-1), IL-4, IL-6 and IL-12 (Protocol A) or IL-4 and anti-IL-12 (R&D, Minneapolis, MN) (Protocol B).
6. JY cells or other Epstein Bar virus (EBV) transformed human B-cell line (Protocol A) or Dendritic cells generated from elutriated monocytes (Protocol B).
7. γ-Irradiator.
8. 37°C Incubator.

3. Methods

3.1. Isolation of PBMC from Buffy Coat of Peripheral Blood

1. To remove buffy coat, place sampling site coupler in bag. With needle and syringe, remove cells from the bag through the sampling site coupler.
2. Distribute buffy coat evenly in 2–4 50-mL conical tubes (~12 mL per tube).
3. Add bead separation buffer to equalize volume in each tube at 35 mL.
4. Mix buffy coat and bead separation buffer well.
5. Layer 10 mL of ficoll under mixture, being careful to minimize mixing of blood with ficoll.
6. Centrifuge tubes for 20 min at room temperature, $700g$. Let centrifuge spin stop naturally without application of the brake.
7. Remove the PBMC that accumulate like a creamy white layer on top of the ficoll layer (*see* **Note 3**).
8. Wash PBMC 3× with 50 mL of bead separation medium. Centrifuge for 15 min at $180g$ at 4°C to remove platelets and lymphocyte separation medium.
9. Count PBMC with trypan blue in hemacytometer under microscope (*see* **Note 4**).

3.2. Isolation of Naive CD4+ T Cells from PBMC

1. Resuspend PBMC in bead separation medium at 20×10^6 cells/mL, less 1/10 of the volume.
2. Add 1/10 vol of negative selection antibody cocktail (*see* **Note 5**), e.g., 500×10^6 PBMC; for 20×10^6 cells/mL, resuspend PBMC in 25 mL–2.5 mL = 22.5 mL bead separation medium; add 2.5 mL antibody cocktail.
3. Rotate cells in 50 mL conical tube on rotator for 1 h at 4°C.
4. Wash cells 3× with 50 mL bead separation medium, $400g$, 10 min at 4°C.

5. During cell washes, calculate the volume of beads needed for negative selection (*see* **Note 6**):

$$\text{total no. of PBMC} \times 40 \text{ beads per cell/ no. of beads per mL} \tag{1}$$

6. Remove calculated volume of beads needed from stock and place in 50 mL conical tube.
7. Add bead separation medium to 50 mL.
8. Wash beads 3× by applying magnet until beads come out of suspension. Remove supernatant with aspirator while magnet is continually applied. Refill tube with bead separation medium.
9. After final wash of beads, resuspend beads in 20×10^6 cell/mL final volume for antibody incubation.
10. After final wash of cells, resuspend cells with beads.
11. Rotate cells in 50 mL conical tube on rotator for 1 h at 4°C.
12. Fill tube to 50 mL vol with bead separation medium, if necessary.
13. Apply magnet until beads come out of suspension. Do not allow for settling of cells in a pellet (i.e., no more then 10–15 min on the magnet).
14. Transfer supernatant with 25 mL pipet to new 50 mL conical, while magnet is continually applied. Repeat **steps 13** and **14** 3× to remove all beads.
15. Centrifuge transferred cells. Resuspend and count.
16. Repeat **steps 5–15** on remaining cells determined in **step 15**. Rotate cells and beads for 1 h or overnight at 4°C (*see* **Note 4**).

3.3. Derivation of Dendritic Cells from Peripheral Blood Elutriated Monocytes (For Protocol B)

3.3.1. Freezing Elutriated Monocytes

1. Human PBMC from buffy coats of normal healthy donors are separated by Ficoll density-γ radiant centrifugation (i.e., elutriation).
2. Make up the freezing medium I by adding 10% (v/v) heat inactivated FCS to the culture medium (final of FCS is 20% v/v).
3. Make up the freezing medium II by adding 20% (v/v) DMSO slowly to freezing medium I.
4. Count the cells to be frozen. Freeze $4–5 \times 10^7$ elutriated monocytes per vial.
5. Label the vials to be frozen.
6. Spin the cells, decant, and resuspend in 0.5 mL freezing medium I.
7. Place cell suspension in each tube on ice.
8. Add 0.5 mL of freezing medium II dropwise over 30 s period, mixing continuously.
9. Immediately transfer cells into –30C for 30 min followed by 1 h at –80C. Then transfer to liquid nitrogen tanks.

3.3.2. Thawing Elutriated Monocytes for Dendritic Cell Differentiation

1. Make up thawing medium by adding 10% heat inactivated FCS to the culture medium.
2. Prewarm water bath to 37°C and thawing medium to room temperature.

3. Set up 50 mL conical so that the vials can be immediately transferred when thawed.
4. Warm up the vial in a water bath by rapidly agitating it.
5. When the last ice crystals are melting, transfer to 50 mL conical.
6. Add 20 mL of thawing media drop-wise to the cells.
7. Centrifuge for 10 min at 400g.
8. Resuspend the cells in 12 mL culture media.
9. Count monocytes with trypan blue in hemacytometer under microscope (*see* **Note 8**).
10. Add recombinant GM-CSF and IL-4 at 30 ng/mL to the cells in **step 8** and mix.
11. Plate the cells in a 6-well plate by adding 2 mL to each well.
12. Incubate for 10 d at 37°C.
13. On d 4 and d 8, add 30 ng/mL of recombinant GM-CSF and IL-4 without changing the medium.
14. On d 6, add human TNF-α at 100 U/mL to each well without changing the medium (*see* **Notes 9** and **10**).

3.3.3. Harvesting Dendritic Cells from Six-Well Plate

1. At d 10 of culture, harvest dendritic cells from plate by collecting the media into a 50 mL conical.
2. Add 2 mL of PBS (without Ca^{2+}/Mg^{2+}) to each well.
3. Wash the wells twice, using 2 mL pipet gently pipeting up and down.
3. Collect the wash in the same 50 mL conical as in **step 1**.
4. Add 1 mL Versene (EDTA) to each well.
5. Incubate in 37°C incubator for 30 min or until the cells are not adherent.
6. Collect the cells/Versene by gently pipeting up and down in to the same 50 mL conical as in **step 1**.
7. Wash once with PBS (without Ca^{2+}/Mg^{2+}).
8. Again, add the wash to the 50 mL conical in **step 1**.
9. Centrifuge at 4°C, 400g for 10 min.
10. Resuspend cells in culture media.
11. Count cells with trypan blue under light microscope.

3.4. Stimulation of Naive CD4+ T Cells
with Anti-CD3 Antibody and Accessory Cells (see Note 11)

1. One the day prior to T-cell stimulation, dilute anti-CD3 antibody to 1 µg/mL in sterile phosphate-buffered solution (PBS). Add 0.5 mL to 24-well plate wells. Incubate at 4°C overnight (*see* **Note 12**).
2. On the day of T-cell stimulation, wash anti-CD3-coated wells 3× with sterile PBS.

3.4.1. Stimulation of Naive T Cells
with JY B Cells (Protocol A) (see **Note 13**)

1. Harvest JY accessory cells from tissue culture; count cells and irradiate 4000 Rads.

2. Add 1×10^6 irradiated accessory cells, 1×10^6 T cells and recombinant cytokines to 24-well plate well coated with anti-CD3 antibody. IL-1 and IL-6 are added to all T-cell stimulation cultures at a final concentration of 2.5 U/mL, in combination with either 1 ng/mL IL-4 to generate Th2 cells or 1 ng/mL IL-12 to generate Th1 cells.
3. Incubate for 2 d at 37°C.
4. On d 2, collect supernatants from T-cell cultures for cytokine analysis. Supernatants should be aliquoted into multiple vials and frozen (*see* **Notes 14 and 15**). Transfer T cells to a larger well (six-well plate) and add fresh culture media (CM). Incubate for 5 d at 37°C. Add CM as cells expand, if necessary.
5. On d 7, collect T cells from culture and count.
6. Isolate live cells with lymphocyte separation medium. Repeat **steps 1–7** for second and third stimulation (*see* **Note 16**).

3.4.2. Stimulation of Naive T Cells with DC (Protocol B) (see **Note 17**)

1. Irradiate harvested DC with 2500 rads.
2. The ratio of T cell: DC is 10:1. Add 1×10^6 T cells and 0.1×10^6 DC in a 24-well plate coated with anti-CD3 antibody (*see* **Note 12**).
3. Stimulation of T cells with anti-CD3 and DC without any exogenous cytokines results in generation of Th1 cells.
4. Stimulation of T cells with anti-CD3 and DC with recombinant IL-4 (final 1 ng/mL) and neutralizing anti-IL-12 (final 10 µg/mL) results in generation of Th2 cells.
5. On d 2, collect supernatant from T cell for cytokine analysis, aliquot, and freeze at –70°C (*see* **Notes 14** and **15**).
6. Do not collect all supernatant; leave ~0.2 mL/well. Transfer T cells in 0.2 mL media back to the same 24-well plate add more culture media and incubate at 37°C.
7. On d 3, transfer T cells to six-well plate and add more media.
8. Repeat **steps 1–6** on d 7 for second stimulation (*see* **Note 16**).

4. Notes

1. Take necessary precautions when working with human blood products. Assume that all blood-derived products are to be considered potential hazards. This includes culture supernatants which are tested by ELISA for cytokines, as well as flow cytofluorometric analysis of Th cells.
2. Recombinant human cytokines are available from a number of vendors, including Pharmingen (San Diego, CA) and Life Technologies (Bethesda, MD). Titration of cytokines may be necessary for optimal Th cell response.
3. For easiest recovery of PBMC from the interface of lymphocyte separation medium, aspirate platelet containing supernatant to 5 mL above the dense layer of cells at the interface, then pipet PBMC out.
4. The expected yield of PBMC from a 25–50 mL buffy coat ranges from 0.2 to 1×10^9 cells. Yield of naive CD4$^+$ T cells is not more than 10% and often <5% of PBMC. Alternatively, one can try to obtain cordblood PBMC as source

for naive Th cells. This approach however, has two drawbacks: it is definitively harder to obtain cordblood, and even cordblood can contain a minor population of preactivated Th cells.

5. To determine the amount of each antibody necessary for the antibody cocktail, serial dilution of antibodies (as ascites fluid) are used to stain a known number of PBMC in a known volume. The antibody dilution used to stain is multiplied by the dilution of antibody in the staining volume for amount of antibody stock needed for the number of PBMC stained. This dilution of antibody can be extrapolated to 20×10^6 cells/mL for negative selection. We make our cocktail at a 10× concentration for easy dilution with PBMC. For information about possible sources for the hybridomas contact Dr. Gijs A. van Seventer.

6. The number of beads per cell used in negative selection of naive CD4$^+$ T cells may vary, depending on antibodies used to coat cells. Assessing purity of T cells is essential for determining the amount beads and all reagents needed for efficient T-cell isolation.

7. Purity of naive CD4$^+$ T cells can best be determined by two color flow cytofluorometric analysis with direct labeled antibodies to CD45RA and CD45RO.

8. The expected yield of elutriated monocytes from one frozen vial is 60–70%. On can expect further that the yield of dendritic cells after harvest from one vial of frozen elutriated monocytes is 20%. Thus, from 5×10^7 elutriated monocytes, $6–7 \times 10^6$ dendritic cells can be harvested at d 10 of culture.

9. Dendritic cells obtain an adherent morphology shortly after incubation with TNF-α that can be observed by electron microscopy. However, in some donors there are more floating cells even after incubation with TNF-α. On d 10 of culture monocyte-derived cells gain the morphology of dendritic cells. This can be confirmed by cytofluorometric analysis for CD1a and CD14 expression, as well as for a variety of costimulatory molecules. Dendritic cells at d 10 are CD1a$^+$ and CD14$^-$.

10. When analyzing endocytic activity of dendritic cells addition of TNF-α should be omitted. TNF-α induces maturation of immature dendritic cells and down regulates receptor-mediated and fluid phase antigen uptake *(16)*.

11. Alternative naive Th cell differentiation models that have been used are completely accessory cell independent, such as the combination of co-immobilized anti-CD3 and anti-CD28 MAbs with either exogenous IL-4 or IL-12 *(17)*. Another approach employs artificial accessory cells in the form of murine L-cells transfectants which express the low affinity FcγRII receptor CD32 (needed for the crosslinking of the anti-CD3 MAb), the CD28 ligand B7-1 (CD80) and the CD2 ligand LFA-3 (CD58) *(18)*. These artificial accessory cells also require exogenous IL-4 or IL-12 for polarization of the Th cells.

12. As an alternative to the anti-CD3 MAb stimulation with the DC protocol (Protocol B) one can use superantigen (SEA or SEB), which has the advantage that the antigen stimulation is directly by the accessory cell. The disadvantage is that one cannot easily generate Th2 cells with approach. For reasons not yet clarified the anti-IL-12 antibodies cannot prevent IFN-γ secretion by superantigen stimulated Th cells.

13. The big advantage of the model system with the JY cells as source of accessory cells is the easy access to a constant source of accessory cells. The major

disadvantage of the JY model is the requirement for exogenous cytokines for the generation of Th1 or Th2 cells. This latter will not allow for studies that are focused on the regulation of IL-12 by specific accessory pathways (e.g., CD40L-CD40) or by soluble factors (e.g., type-I IFNs or IL-10).

14. Determining the phenotype of Th-cell subsets generated is best done by sandwich cytokine enzyme linked immunosorbent assay (ELISA). The paired anti-cytokine MAb reagents available from Pharmingen are highly recommended (either as paired MAbs or as Optiset). Th2 cells generated by this method do not secrete IL-4, therefore detection of IL-5 can be used to determine phenotype of Th2 cells. IL-4 is detected by stimulating T cells with the pharmacological activators phorbolester (PMA)/ionomycin *(10)*. IFN-γ secretion is the best indicator of Th1 cells. The integrity of proteins is compromised by repeated freezing and thawing. For that reason, freezing small volumes of supernatant is recommended.

15. Dendritic cells produce high levels of IL-12, some TNF-α, IL-1 and IL-6. Therefore, in determining the phenotype of T-cell subsets generated with dendritic cells, the presence of TNF-α is not a good measure for the presence of Th1 cells. JY cells secrete LT and likewise the presence of LT in the culture supernatant is not a good indicator of Th1 cells.

16. Restimulation of the Th cells for the analysis of the cytokine secretion profile can be done either by stimulating under identical conditions as the initial stimulation or by stimulation in an accessory cell-free manner with immobilized anti-CD3 and anti-CD28 MAbs. The latter has the advantages that new accessory cells do not need to be generated and that all detected cytokines in the culture supernatant are derived from the Th cells. The disadvantage of the accessory cell-free restimulation is that one lacks the physiological multitude of accessory pathways and cytokines that help to regulate the cytokine secretion profile.

17. The use of dendritic cells as source of accessory cells clearly adds a more physiological aspect to the in vitro Th cell differentiation model, although one still needs to manipulate the system to obtain Th2 cells. Alternative protocols for acquiring precursor dendritic cells include isolation of CD34$^+$ cells from PBMC, isolation of dendritic cells from PBMC by a two-step adherence to plastic *(19)*. Both protocols require culture with GM-CSF/IL-4 and TNF-α, but the final cell culture is still phenotypically quite heterogenous compared to a starting population of elutriated monocytes. However, the effort of preparing the dendritic cells, both in labor and in the costs of reagents may make all of these models too advanced for the particular research question.

References

1. Fitch, F. W., Lancki, D. W., and Gajewski, T. F. (1993) T-cell-mediated regulation: help and suppression in *Fundamental Immunology* (Paul, W. E., ed.), Raven, New York, pp. 733–762.
2. Sanders, M. E., Makgoba, M. W., and Shaw, S. (1988) Human naive and memory T cells: reinterpretation of helper-inducer and suppressor-inducer subsets. *Immunol. Today* **9,** 195–199.

3. Merkenschlager, M. and Beverley, P. C. (1989) Evidence for differential expression of CD45 isoforms by precursors for memory-dependent and independent cytotoxic responses: human CD8 memory CTLp selectively express CD45RO (UCHL1). *Int. Immunol.* **1,** 450–459.

4. Romagnani, S. (1994) Lymphokine production by human T cells in disease states. *Annu. Rev. Immunol.* **12,** 227–257.

5. Mosman, T., Cherwinski, H., Bond, M. W., Giedlin, M. A., and Coffman, R. L. (1986) Two types of murine helper T cell clone. I. Definition according to profiles of lymphokine activities and secreted proteins. *J. Immunol.* **136,** 2348–2357.

6. Mosman, T. R. and Coffman, R. L. (1989) Th1 and Th2 cells: Different patterns of lymphokine secretion lead to different functional properties. *Ann. Rev. Immunol.* **7,** 145–173.

7. Del Prete, G., De Carli, M., Almerigogna, F., Giudizi, M. G., Biagiotti, R., and Romagnani, S. (1993) Human IL-10 is produced by both type 1 helper (Th1) and type 2 helper (Th2) T cell clones and inhibits their antigen-specific proliferation and cytokine production. *J. Immunol.* **150,** 353–360.

8. Gerosa, F., Paganin, C., Peritt, D., Paiola, F., Scupoli, M. T., Aste-Amezaga, M., Frank, I., and Trinchieri, G. (1996) Interleukin-12 primes human CD4 and CD8 T cell clones for high production of both interferon-gamma and interleukin-10. *J. Exp. Med.* **183,** 2559–2569.

9. Meyaard, L., Hovenkamp, E., Otto, S. A., and Miedema, F. (1996) IL-12-induced IL-10 production by human T cells as negative feedback for IL-12-induced immune responses. *J. Immunol.* **156,** 2776–2782.

10. Palmer, E. M. and van Seventer, G. A. (1997) Human T helper cell differentiation is regulated by the combined action of cytokines and accessory-cell dependent costimulatory signals. *J. Immunol.* **158,** 2654–2662.

11. Mosmann, T. R. and Moore, K. W. (1991) The role of IL-10 in crossregulation of Th1 and Th2 responses. *Immunol. Today* **12,** A49–A53.

12. Paul, W. E. and Seder, R. A. (1994) Lymphocyte responses and cytokines. *Cell* **76,** 241–251.

13. McRae, B. L., Semnani, R. T., Hayes, M. P., and van Seventer, G. A. (1998) Type I Interferons inhibit human dendritic cell IL-12 production and T helper 1 cell development. *J. Immunol.* **160,** 4298–4304.

14. Horgan, K. J. and Shaw, S. (1991) Immunomagnetic purification of T cell subpopulations. Section 7.4.1–7.4.5. *Current Protocols in Immunology* (Coligan, J. E., Kruisbeek, A. M., Margulies, D. H., Shevach, E. M., and Strober, W., eds.), Wiley Interscience, New York.

15. Gerrard, T. L., Jurgensen, C. H., and Fauci, A. S. (1983) Differential effect of monoclonal anti-DR antibody on monocytes in antigen- and mitogen-stimulated responses: mechanism of inhibition and relationship to interleukin 1 secretion. *Cell Immunol.* **82,** 394–402.

16. Sallusto, F. and Lanzavecchia, A. (1994) Efficient presentation of soluble antigen by cultured human dendritic cells is maintained by granulocyte/macrophage colony-stimulating factor plus interleukin-4 and down-regulated by tumor necrosis factor alpha. *J. Exp. Med.* **179,** 1109–1118.

17. Kalinski, P., Hilkens, C. M., Wierenga, E. A., van der Pouw-Kraan, T. C., van Lier, R. A., Bos, J. D., Kapsenberg, M. L., and Snijdewint, F. G. (1995) Functional maturation of human naive T helper cells in the absence of accessory cells. Generation of IL-4-producing T helper cells does not require exogenous IL-4. *J. Immunol.* **154,** 3753–3760.
18. Demeure, C. E., Wu, C. Y., Shu, U., Schneider, P. V., Heusser, C., Yssel, H., and Delespesse, G. (1994) In vitro maturation of human neonatal CD4 T lymphocytes II. Cytokines present at priming modulate the development of lymphokine production. *J. Immunol.* **152,** 4775–4782.
19. Cella, M., Sallusto, F., and Lanzavecchia, A. (1997) Origin, maturation, and antigen presenting function of dendritic cells. *Curr. Opin. Immunol.* **9,** 10–16.

29

Transcriptional Expression Analysis of T-Cell Activation by Multiplex Messenger Assay (MMA)

Karine Bernard, Samuel Granjeaud,
Geneviève Victoréro, and Catherine Nguyen

1. Introduction

Gene indices with many thousands of entries have been constructed by tag sequencing of randomly selected cDNA clones *(1–7)* and are widely available in repositories, such as the dbEST database *(16)*. As more and more genes are identified, efforts are redirected towards understanding the control of gene expression that occurs in a strictly ordered time and cell-dependent fashion. Expression measurements often constitute a first step in this direction, and can be performed on a reasonably large scale using highly parallel hybridization methods. Hybridization methods, using complex probes and large arrays of targets, derive their power from the fact that each individual experiment provides a very large amount of information. Unrivaled for large-scale measurement of gene expression, these methods are based on the hybridization of complex probes with high-density colony cDNA (or PCR product) filters followed by quantitative measurement of the amount of hybridized probe on each colony. There are three key elements indispensable for accomplishing this task: the robot (for spotting colonies), the phosphoimager (for analyzing exposure), and the image analysis software (**Fig. 1**).

Large-scale hybridization techniques to measure expression are presently available in three formats (for review *see* **ref.** *17*): high-density membranes to be hybridized with radioactive complex probes *(8–15)*, microarrays of DNA spots (a miniaturized version of the former technique) using fluorescent complex probes *(18–21)*, and oligonucleotide chips that, although developed for mutation detection *(22)*, can be adapted to perform expression measurements *(23,24)*.

From: *Methods in Molecular Biology, Vol. 134: T Cell Protocols: Development and Activation*
Edited by: K. P. Kearse © Humana Press Inc., Totowa, NJ

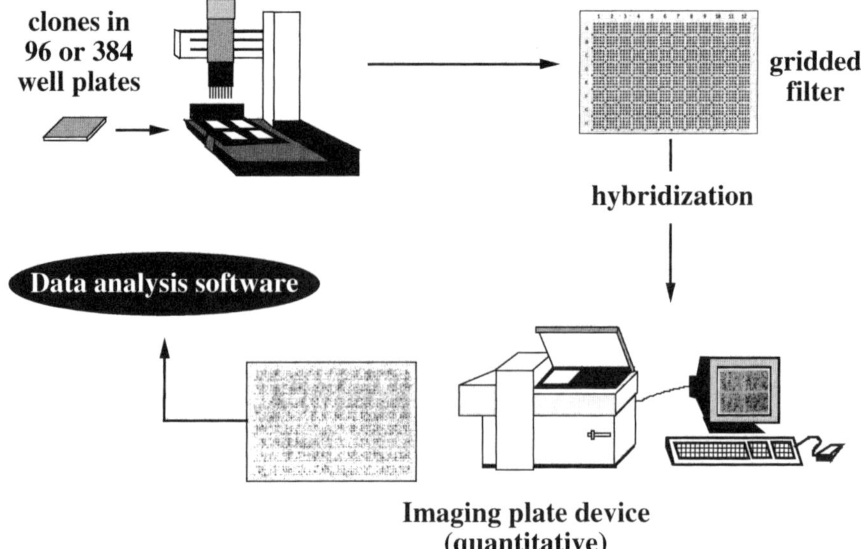

Fig.1. Technical approach: (**Upper left**) A robot to produce filters from 96- or 384-well plates. (**Upper right**) a filter hybrized with a vector probe showing the spotting patterns. The square A1 contains the clones at the position A1 from the 16 plates (96 wells). Spots localized at the bottom left of each square correspond to the control clone *A. thaliana* cytochrome c554 except for six spots toward the middle of the filter which contain the poly A control clones. Filters are exposed on a phosphor screen. (**Lower right**) the imaging plate device which transforms the hybridization signature into image files. (**Lower left**) the Bioimage software which quantifies intensity signals and assignes plate coordinates to each clone. Data are then transferred to EXCEL for further analysis.

1.1. The MMA Format and Its Application to Studies of T-Cell Activation

In the Multiplex Messenger Assay (MMA) approach, a set of known genes expected to be relevant to a given process are assembled on a membrane. This is facilitated by the freely available set of IMAGE cDNA clones *(25).*[*] The membrane is then used to assay expression levels for this chosen set of genes in a series of experimental or clinical situations. This approach is equivalent to a large series of Northern blots *(12)*. Commercial suppliers *(26,27)* now provide

---

[*] Unfortunately this very useful resource is not completely error-free: Discrepancies in the correspondence between physical clones and tag sequences range from 10 to 20%, imposing expensive and time-consuming verification when these entities are used as reagents.

a set of 588 human genes arrayed on Nylon membranes as PCR products from cDNA clones *(26)*.

We describe here the implementation of this method to follow the expression levels of 47 mouse genes in resting and activated T cells. The activation of T lymphocytes during an immune response is mediated by the T cell receptor (TCR) that recognizes peptide antigens bound to self major histocompatibility complex (MHC) molecules on the surface of an antigen-presenting cell. This stimulation initiates a cascade of biochemical events that culminate in cellular differentiation and proliferation *(28)*. The activation by an anti-CD3 antibody simulates the events observed after activation. The effect of the mechanisms used by cells at the transcriptional level to regulate the numerous genes involved in activation (including alterations of transcriptional rate, termination of transcription, and mRNA stability) are quantified in a single step by our method. Using fourfold spotting of colonies, imaging plate detection, and various correction and normalization procedures, the technique is sensitive enough to quantify expression levels for sequences present at 0.005% abundance in the probe *(12)*. Upon activation of a T-cell clone by an anti-CD3 antibody, variations ranging from two to 20-fold are measured, some of which have not been reported previously.

1.2. Measurement Parameters, Treatment of Artifacts, and Normalization

For probe sequences present in small amounts relative to their targets, the kinetics of the reaction (if both probe and target are in solution and if the reaction is far from completion) are described by Beltz et al. 1983 *(29)*. Projecting this to our experimental condition, the intensity of the hybridization signal can be used to estimate the abundance of the corresponding sequence in the probe, providing that the target is in great excess and that the probe concentration does not change during hybridization. In our MMA filters, approximate amounts are 100–200 ng of plasmid DNA per colony, i.e., 20–60 ng of insert material. For a mRNA species at 0.1% abundance, the amount of specific sequence in the probe is >1 ng, ensuring large target excess.

We have shown that the hybridization signal increases linearly with the target amount *(9)*. This result, which was not a *priori* obvious under these conditions, indicates that hybridization signals can, if necessary, be corrected for the differential growth of bacterial colonies using data obtained with a vector probe.

We have also shown that the hybridization signal increases linearly with the probe amount *(9)*. Under our experimental conditions, signal intensities are proportional to the abundance of corresponding sequences in the probe, both for colonies that give a strong signal (abundance sequences) and for colonies that are at the lower limit of detection. The signal observed therefore defines the abundance in the complex probe of the particular sequence hybridizing with a given clone and the expression level of the corresponding gene (**Fig. 2**).

A certain percentage of cDNA clones contain repeat sequences, and give a detectable signal with Cot1 mouse DNA. Annealing of the probe with Cot 1 DNA before hybridization can attenuate these signals. However, we prefer to tag these clones as "repeated" and exclude them from further analysis because they are too difficult to work with.

Reverse transcription of the poly(A+) RNA mixture from which the probe is generated and simultaneous labeling with $(^{32}P)dCTP$ produces many probe molecules beginning as (unlabeled) poly(T) and continuing as specific and labeled mRNA sequences. The abundance of such poly(T) containing molecules is high, and their hybridization to unrelated clones via the poly(A) stretch can be a significant problem. This is eliminated by our labeling protocol (**Fig. 3**). Elimination of this artifact is central to the practical use of this system since it generates spurious signals that can vary according to the degree of the poly(A) tails, giving rise to false differential signals. To control this particular problem, we spot on the membranes, in addition to the other colonies, clones containing different stretches of polyA tails. Of course, the measured signal on these control colonies must be null in each independent hybridization.

To standardize hybridization intensities obtained in several experiments, we use the *Arabidopsis thaliana* cytochrome c554 cDNA sequence (1 kb insert) that has no homology with mammalian DNA. The same amount of c554 RNA, transcribed in vitro from the corresponding cDNA clone, is added before labeling to the total RNA of each cell type or tissue to be tested. The quantification of corresponding colonies present on each filter (**Fig. 4A,B**) allows us to normalize each independent hybridization according to this value that corrects for differences in the labeling, washing, duration of exposure, and progressive degradation of the filters. These variations can be taken into account such that the differential expression levels for each clone can be compared with greater confidence.

2. Materials

2.1. Preparation of High Density Filters

1. LB: Bacto-Trypton 10 g/L, Bacto-yeast extract 5 g/L, NaCl 5 g/L adjusted to pH 7.0, and LB agar for plates: LB and bacto-agar 1.5% (w/v). Autoclaved.
2. 8 × 12 cm nylon filters HYBOND-N, Amersham (Amersham, UK).
3. 3 MM papers of 20 × 20 cm placed inside a 22 × 22 cm NEN plate.
4. Filters are prepared using BIOMEK 1000 (Beckman, Fullerton, CA) robotics workstation and a 96-pin tool (Various robots have recently been developed to make filters with tools of up to 384 pinsl adapted to the latest plate designs).

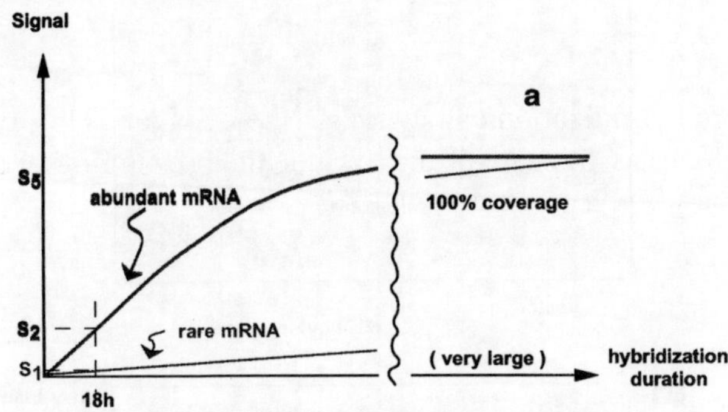

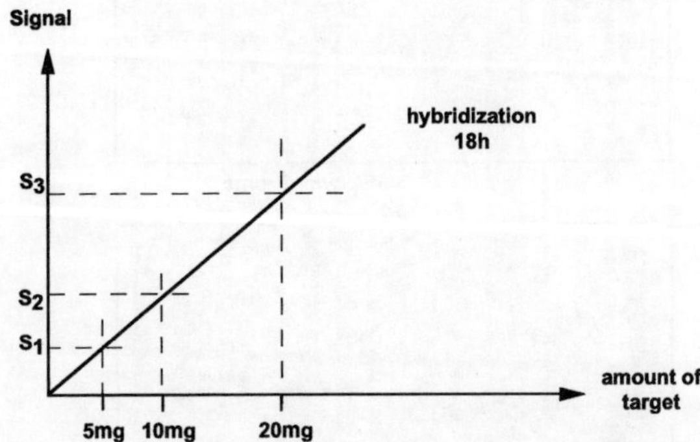

Fig. 2. Theoretical scheme of the hybridization conditions. (**A**) Hybridization with complex probe is performed in target excess. In usual experimental conditions, the hybridization reaction stays in the linear crescent phase of the kinetics curve and never reaches the plateau. Therefore the signal measured is proportional to the abundance of the corresponding messenger in the probe. (**B**) The hybridization with vector or a single probe is performed with a large excess of probe. In this case the signal is directly proportional to the amount of target fixed on the membrane. These two parameters must be taken into account when evaluating the expression levels.

5. Denaturing solution: 0.5 M NaOH, 1.5 M NaCl freshly prepared.
6. Neutralization solution: 1 M Tris-HCl, pH 7.4, 1.5 M NaCl.
7. Deproteinization buffer: 50 mM Tris-HCl, pH 7.4, 50 mM EDTA, 100 mM NaCl, 1% Na-lauryl-sarcosine (w/v) containing 250 µg/mL of Proteinase K freshly prepared.

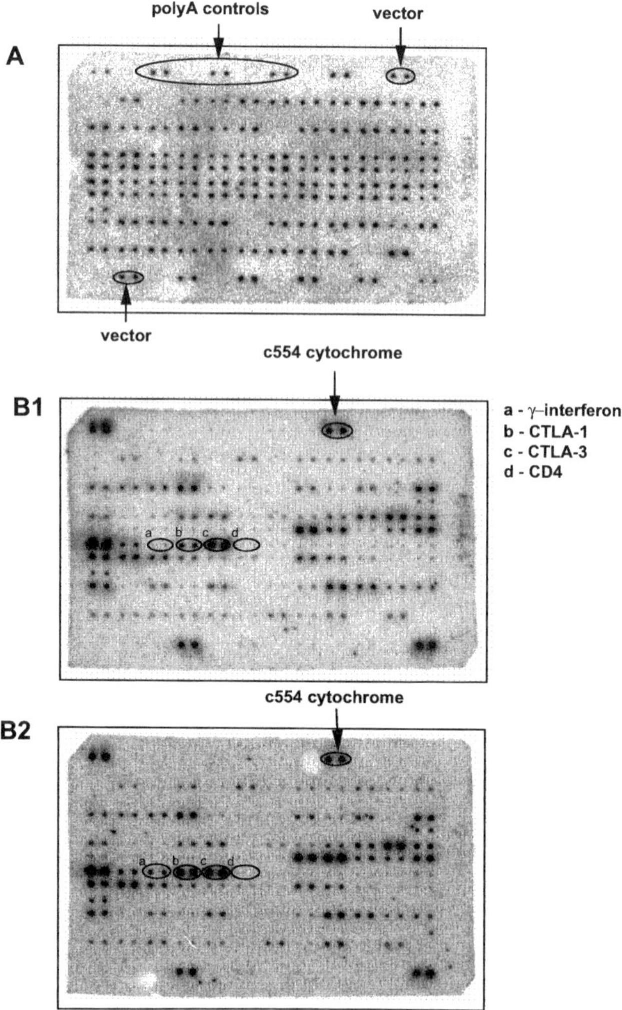

Fig. 3. **(A)** MMA colony filter hybridized with the vector oligonucleotide probe showing all of the clones that have grown and evaluation of the quality of growth. Each colony has been spotted in duplicate twice on two opposite symmetric areas of the filter. PolyA and vector control colonies are on the first line. **(B1)** Same filter hybridized with a complex probe made from 25 µg of total RNA of a resting cytotoxic T cell line, KB5.C20, **(B2)** and from the same T cell line after 3 h of stimulation by an anti-CD3 antibody. Here, some clones are clearly different between the two complex probes (γ-interferon, CTLA-1, CTLA-3). The signal shown on the spots corresponds to cytochrome c554 come from 0.5 ng of in vitro transcribed RNA added to the total RNA of cells before the labeling. The negative control polyA and vector present no signals with complex probes, as expected.

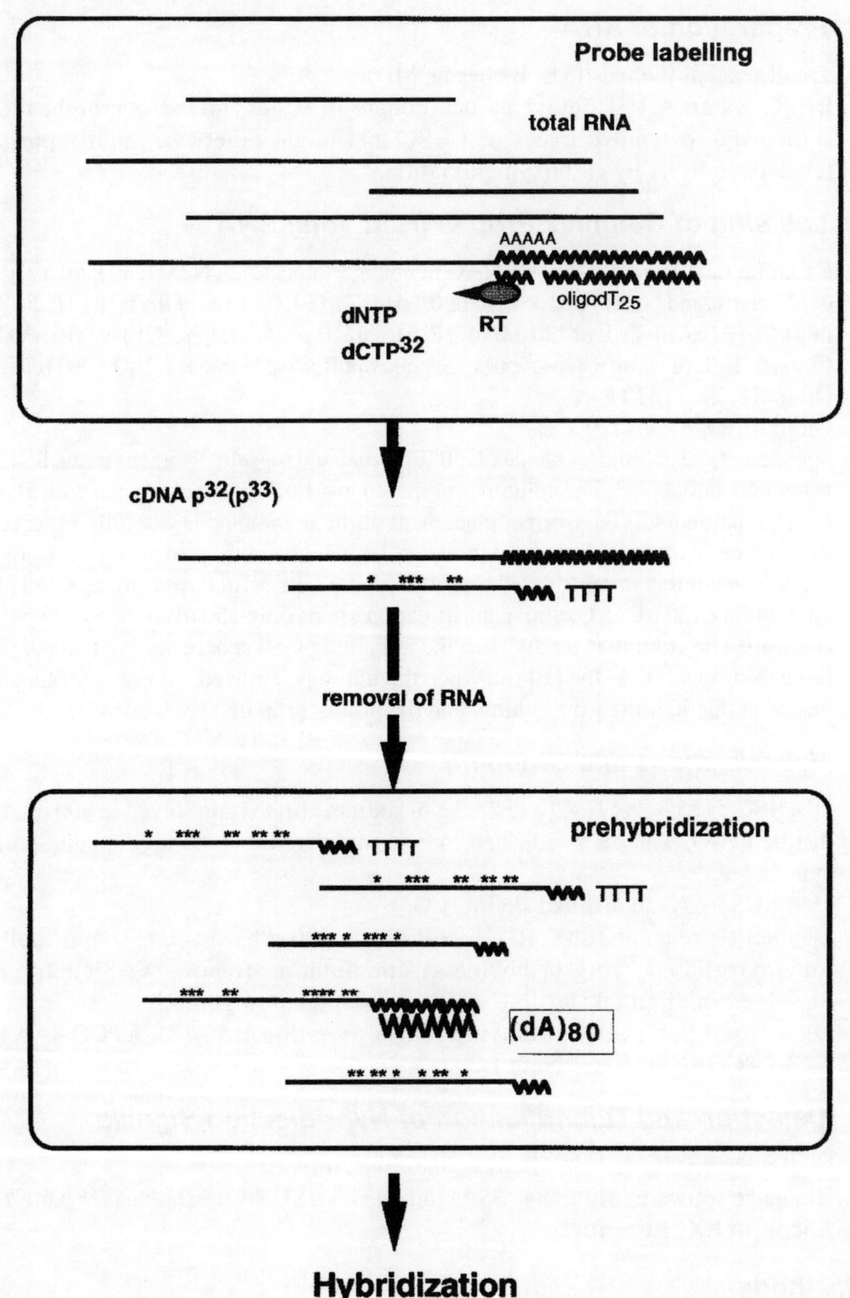

Fig. 4. Labeling scheme: The top square shows the first step for the labeling with the blocking of the polyA tails. The bottom square shows the second step to block the possible polyA tails left after the first treatment and before the hybridization of the filter.

2.2. Preparation of RNA

1. Trizol reagent (Gibco-BRL. Bethesda, MD).
2. DEPC water: 0.1% diethyl pyrocarbonate in water, mixed overnight then autoclaved to remove traces of DEPC that might otherwise modify purine residues in RNA by carboxymethylation.

2.3. Labeling of Complex Probes from Total RNA

1. RT buffer mix: 1 µL of RNasin (RNAse inhibitor, Promega, ref. N2511, 40 U/µL), 6 µL of 5X first strand buffer (BRL), 2 µL of 0.1 M DTT (BRL), 1 µL of dATP dTTP dGTP mix (20 mM each), 1 µL of 120 µM dCTP, 5 µL of 10 µCi/µL (alpha-32P) dCTP (>3000 Ci/mM), 1 µL of reverse transcriptase (Superscript RNAse H free RT, BRL, 200 µ/µL).
2. Oligo dT 25: $3'(dTTP)_{25}{}^{-5'}$.
3. Oligo dA80: $3'\text{-}(dATP)_{80}{}^{-5'}$.
4. Sephadex G50 column: sephadex G50 (Pharmacia, Uppsala, Sweden) is swelled in water and autoclaved. The column is prepared in a 1 mL syringe plugged with glass fiber (Whatman GF/B). Correct placement of the membrane is carefully observed to avoid recovering pieces of gel in the probe, which would provide hybridization spots. The column is centrifuged repeatedly for 2 min at 1000 rpm (Jouan GR 412) after adding 150 µL H_2O, until centrifugation yields only 150 µL of liquid (to pack column). The column is ready when the remaining G50 is between 0.8 and 0.9 µL (after 2–3 rounds). At the last run when the liquid is removed, an Ependorf tube is placed at the bottom of the column and the probes (150 µL) are loaded.

2.4. Hybridizations and Stripping

1. 20X SSC : 175.3 g of NaCl and 88.2 g of sodium citrate is dissolved in 800 mL of distilled H_2O. The pH is adjusted to 7.0, completed to 1 L and the solution is autoclaved.
2. 10% SDS (w/v) in distilled sterile H_2O.
3. Denhardt's reagent 100X:10 g Ficoll (Type 400, Pharmacia), 10 g of polyvinylpyrrolidone, 10 g of bovine serum albumin (fraction V; Sigma), are dissolved in distilled sterile H_2O, then completed to 500 mL.
4. Oligo used for pcDNAI (Invitrogen corporation): 5' CTTATCGAAAT-TAATACGACTC3' (*see* **Note 1**).

2.5. Detection and Quantification of Hybridization Signals

1. FUJIX BAS 1000 or 1500 (Fuji) system (*see* **Note 2**).
2. Bioimage software (Millipore, USA) running on a SUN workstation (*see* **Note 2**).
3. Microsoft EXCEL software.

3. Methods

3.1. High Density Filters Preparation

Most of the cDNA clones selected here were obtained from an adult mouse thymus cDNA library *(9)* by hybridization of filters containing part of the library with probes corresponding to known genes. Others were found among already sequenced clones from the same library. For some additional clones (including the control *A. thaliana* cytochrome *c554* gene), the cDNA insert was transferred from the original cloning vector to that used for the cDNA library (pcDNA1) and then transformed into MC1061 p3 bacteria to obtain a coherent set of clones in the same plasmid vector and bacteria. Three clones containing essentially polyA sequence (50, 60, 90 bp) were obtained by appropriate digests of the polyA tail of sequenced cDNAs, followed by cloning at the multiple cloning site of the pcDNA1 vector.

1. Colonies from freshly grown replica plates are spotted on to 8×12 cm filters *(9)*. Each colony is spotted in quadruplicate twice in two opposite symmetrical areas of the filter (**Fig. 3**). Filters are then placed with colony side up on the top of LB agar plates (containing antibiotic) and incubated at 37°C for approx 12 h (colony sizes are checked after 10 h of growth. Size should be 0.1–0.2 mm). Filters are subsequently treated by a modified protocol of Nizetic *(30)*.
2. Denaturation is performed by carefully placing the filters, colony side up, on 3 MM paper soaked with 50 mL of denaturing solution for 4 min at room temperature followed by a second treatment in the same buffer for 4 min at 80°C in a damp atmosphere. This step is repeated twice.
3. Membranes are then neutralized by placing them successively, on 3 MM papers soaked with 50 mL of neutralizing solution for 4 min each at room temperature. This step is repeated twice.
4. Protein is then removed by treating the filters with 50 mL of deproteinization buffer for at least 2 h.
5. Filters are rinsed by backing them one by one into 100–200 mL of 2X SSC, then air-dried on paper (never pile filters until they are completely dry, otherwise cDNA can stick to the back of the above paper loosing a part of the material).
6. The DNA is fixed by treatment at 80°C for 2 h followed by UV crosslinking (230 nm, 0.16 KJ/m^2) (*see* **Notes 3** and **4**).

3.2. Preparation of Total RNA

When working with RNA, one should not use any plasticware or glassware without first eliminating possible ribonuclease contamination (unless it is disposable and individually wrapped by the manufacturer). Only sterile, new pipet tips and microfuge tubes should be used, and clean microbiological aseptic techniques performed. For further information on controlling Rnase contamination (*see* **ref. 31**).

Total RNA is isolated from cell lines following the instruction manual provided with the Trizol kit (Gibco-BRL). Suspending RNA in DEPC water under standard conditions, we obtain 10 µg of total RNA per million cells (*see* **Note 5**).

3.3. Preparation of the A. thaliana Cytochrome c554 Messenger RNA

The messenger RNA of *A. thaliana* cytochrome c554 was obtained from cDNA cloned into Bluescript SK+ vector at the *Not*I restriction site, and was synthesized from the T3 promoter using the RiboMax large scale production system (Promega).

3.4. Labeling of Complex Probes from Total RNA

Reverse transcriptase (RT) simultaneously synthesizes and labels single-stranded DNA from the approx 500 ng of mRNA present in 25 µg of total RNA. To compare independent hybridizations precisely, the same amount of c554 RNA, in vitro transcribed with T3 polymerase from the corresponding cDNA clone, is added before labeling to the total RNA of each cell type or tissue to be tested. Complex probes are prepared from total RNA plus c554 RNA with an excess of oligo-dT *(25)* to saturate the polyA tails, and ensure that the reverse transcription will start near the beginning of the polyA tail, to avoid product containing long poly T stretches. Before hybridization the possible tails left are blocked by an excess of oligo-dA 80. The principle behind labeling the mRNA is shown in **Fig. 4**.

1. 25 µg total RNA in 11 µL DEPC water is mixed with 2 ng cytochrome RNA at 0.5 ng/µL (4 µL) and 8 µg of dT25 (1 µL at 8 µg/µL) in an ependorf tube. Sample is then placed for 8 min at 70°C in a water bath to remove secondary structure (*see* **Note 6**).
2. Progressively the mixture is cooled to reach 42°C. This is performed by placing the tube in a metal block preheated at 70°C then the block is backed into an oven set at 42°C. This step should take 30 min.
3. The RT buffer mix is then added to the tube kept at 42°C (in the block).
4. The reaction is incubated for 1 h at 42°C in the oven, then 1 µL of enzyme is added and incubated for an additional hour.
5. The RNA is removed by treatment at 68°C during 30 min with 1 µL of 10% SDS, 1 µL of 0.5 *M* EDTA, and 3 µL of 3 *M* NaOH, then the complex probe is equilibrated at room temperature for 15 min. This step degrades the mRNA and rRNA to obtain a single-stranded probe.
6. The probe is neutralized by adding 10 µL of 1 *M* Tris-HCl, pH 7.0, and 3 µL of 2 *N* HCl.
7. The unincorporated nucleotides are removed from the complex probe, (otherwise they increase background noise) by purification on a Sephadex G50 column. Probe (150 µL) is loaded on top of the column and then is spun for 4 min at 1000 rpm.
8. 1 µL out of the 150 µL recovered after spinning is counted. Normally the total radioactivity in the probe is around 30 million counts using Ready Cap scintillating capsules.
9. The possible polyT tail left during the first treatment is blocked by adding 2 µL dA80 solution at 1 µg/µL to the probe, then the whole probe is denatured for 5 min at 100°C.

10. After 1 mL of hybridization buffer (preheated to 65°C) is added to the probe, it is incubated for 2.5 h at 65°C then added to the 50 mL of hybridization buffer (*see* **Note 7**).

3.5. Hybridization Conditions with Complex Probes

1. Filters are prehybridized for at least 6 h at 68°C with 5X SSC, 5X Denhardt's, 0.5% SDS, and 100 µg/mL sheared denatured salmon sperm, then are hybridized with total probes with the same buffer for 48 h. Best results are obtained when no more than 4 filters are hybridized simultaneously per 50 mL. It is unnecessary to change buffer between prehybridization and hybridization. Both are performed in a water bath with shaking.
2. After hybridization, filters are washed three times at 68°C (1 h each) with 1 L of 0.1X SSC, 0.1% SDS. Washing buffer is warmed to 68°C before use.
3. Wrap filters in plastic bags before exposing to phosphor screens for 3 d or more. Plastic bags must be sealed to avoid drying otherwise a good stripping will be never be obtained.

3.6. Vector Oligo-Labeling and Hybridization

1. One µg of the oligonucleotide used for vector hybridization is labeled with [γ-^{32}P] ATP at the 5' end using standard methods *(31)*.
2. Colony filters are prehybridized for 3 h at 42°C with 6X SSC, 5X Denhardt's reagent, and 1% SDS, 100 µg/mL sheared denatured salmon sperm, and then hybridized with the oligonucleotide labelled (200,000 cpm/mL) and with unlabeled oligonucleotide (200 ng/mL) for at least 12 h at 42°C. Six filters of 8 × 12 cm can be hybridized at the same time in 50 mL of buffer.
3. Filters are washed once with 2X SSC 0.1% SDS at room temperature for 10 min, then with the same buffer once at 42°C for 10 min (*see* **Note 8**).

3.7. Stripping Conditions

1. Colony high-density filters hybridized with the pCDNAI oligonucleotide probe are stripped twice with 500 mL of 0.1% SDS, 1 m*M* EDTA from 80°C to room temperature (approx 1 h each).
2. Filters hybridized with the cDNA complex probes are stripped twice with the same buffer at 80°C for 3–5 h (*see* **Note 9**).

3.8. Detection and Quantification of Hybridization Signals

Quantitative data is obtained using an imaging plate device. The hybridized filter is exposed to an imaging plate for 65 h to 72 h and then scanned in a FUJIX BAS 1000 (Fuji) (**Figs. 2,4**) system. This system is far superior to methods based on autoradiography and should be useful in projects that involve the increasingly popular high density format. Autoradiography is still widely used because of its simplicity, familiarity, high resolution, and low equipment cost. For quantitative applications, autoradiography is very unsuitable because of its lack of linearity. Scanning of autoradiographs with subsequent processing has however been used with some success *(32)* in spite of its limitation. At this time, imaging plate systems provide the best answer. Their resolution (0.005–0.2 mm pixel size, depending on make and model) is adequate, and their range of linear response extends over 4–5 decades *(33–34)*. The standard software provided with these machines, however, is not adapted to quantitative analysis of high density filters. Hybridization signatures are determined by a modified version of the Bioimage software (Millipore) running on a UNIX workstation *(35)* (*see* **Notes 10–12**). This software is an adaptation of the existing and previous version designed for the analysis of two dimensional protein separations. The resulting quantified data were then analyzed on a microcomputer (Macintosh Centris 650) using EXCEL software with macrocommands that compute average values for each colony. This procedure is described by Granjeaud et al., 1996 *(36)*. The successive operations are:

1. Image acquisition is performed with a Fuji bas 1000 system. The data occupies a 2 MB file.
2. The resulting image files are imported to the quantification software and separated into images of individual filters.
3. Spots are detected without any assumption of their position. The "quantify" command then determines their shape and intensity individually, with local background subtraction.
4. The "compare" command then matches the quantified filter with the "template," a reference filter (vector hybridization) that has been previously edited to remove artifacts and displaying all spots.
5. The operator indicates (by clicking) a minimum of three corresponding spots on the two filters : this determines how the filters should be superimposed. The two images are then "matched," and the correspondence between colonies on the two filters are determined. The matching procedure eliminates essentially all artifactual spots, since they usually lie outside the expected positions.
6. The tables generated in the workstation are transferred over the network to a microcomputer. A set of Excel macro commands provide an easy conversion of text files into Excel tables in order to perform standard calculations, such as normalization of data, and produce a standard set of representations used to judge the quality of the data (**Fig. 5**).

4. Notes

1. For pT3T7pac: The oligonucleotides used for vector normalization are 5'TGTGGAATTGTGAGCGGATA3' or T7 5'TAATACGACTCACTATAGGGA3'.
2. Detection can be performed with a Phosphor Imager imaging plate system from Molecular Dynamics (Sunnyvale, CA). The resulting 16-bit images are then imported to a Sun workstation to perform the image analysis with the Xdotsreader software (Cose, Le Bourget, France) *(13)*. They can also be imported and analyzed in the Bioimage software.

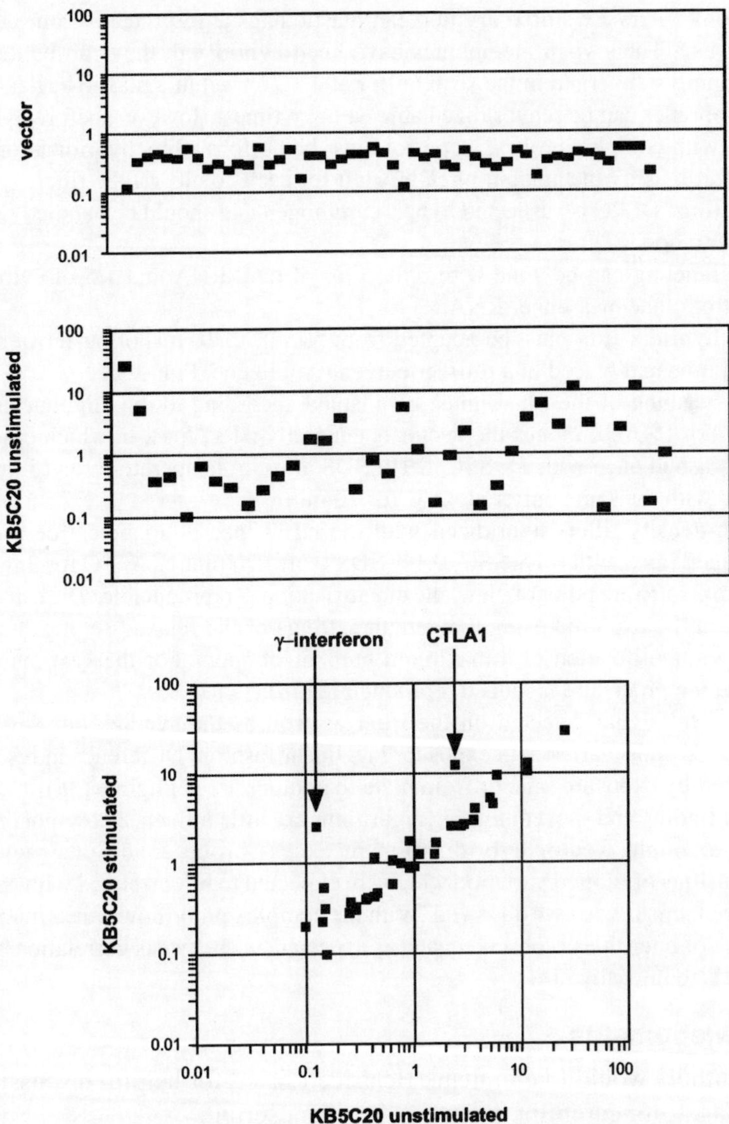

Fig. 5. Results for successfully quantified colonies. (**Top**) The intensities after vector hybridization corresponding to the average values of the four spots, and are plotted on a logarithmic scale. (**Middle**) the intensities corresponding to the average values of the four spots after hybridization using RNA of KB5C20 corrected by vector hybridization plotted on a logarithmic scale. (**Bottom**) the results of two independent hybridizations using RNA from the KB5C20 cell line unstimulated (abscissa) and after 3 h of stimulation by an anti-CD3 antibody (ordinate). The spots indicated by arrows were stimulated (γ-interferon 20 times, CTLA1 four times).

3. Colony filters are stored dry in clean plastic bags at room temperature until the first use. Then when membranes have been hybridized, they can be kept after stripping submerged in the strip buffer at 4°C, or wet in a plastic bag at –20°C.

4. Membranes can be rehybridized at least three times. However, before hybridization with complex probes, a control must be performed by hybridization with a vector to assay the amount of cDNA left for each colony on the filter.

5. **Caution:** DEPC is suspected to be a carcinogen and should be handled with care under a hood.

6. The labeling can be done with only 5 µg of total RNA and 1/5 of cytochrome control clone messenger RNA.

7. The hybridization must be adapted from 50 mL to 10 mL of buffer in a 15-cm long tube and placed in a rotisserie oven (Appligène, France).

8. The washing of the filters must be adapted according to the oligonucleotide in use. For IMAGE clones the vector is generally pT3T7pac, in which case filters are washed once with 2X SSC, 0.1% SDS at room temperature for 15 min, then once with the same buffer at 42°C for 10 min.

9. High-density filters hybridized with the pT3T7pac oligonucleotide probe are stripped once with 0.1X SSC, 0.1% SDS (soft stripping) at 68°C for 3 h.

10. From a software point of view, the quantification is reproducible. The same image file can be explored using the default settings or the relaxed settings chosen to allow quantification of a maximum number of spots. For the vast majority of spots the procedure is indeed reproducible *(36)*.

11. The total signal detected on the filter as well as the average intensity of the detected spots varies with exposure in a linear fashion. Difference in results was caused by exposure time or from plate to another are negligible *(36)*.

12. Spot finding and spot contouring algorithms are little influenced by spot intensity. For example, vector hybridization in excess probe conditions yields spot intensities of limited variation which are expected to be correlated with spot size. Indeed, this is what we observed. With the complex probe however, a much wider range of intensities is observed, and as expected, we see weak correlation between spot size intensity *(36)*.

Acknowledgments

The authors would like to thank Béatrice Loriod for helpful discussion and Becky Tagett for carefully reviewing the manuscript.

References

1. Adams, M. D., Kelley, J. M., Gocayne, J. D., Dubnick, M., Polymeropoulos, M. H., Xiao, H., Merril, C. R., Wu, A., Olde, B., Moreno, R. F., et al. (1991) Complementary DNA sequencing: expressed sequence tags and human genome project. *Science* **252,** 1651–1656.

2. Adams, M. D., Dubnick, M., Kerlavage, A. R., Moreno, R., Kelley, J. M., Utterback, T. R., Nagle, J. W., Fields, C., and Venter, J. C. (1992) Sequence identification of 2,375 human brain genes. *Nature* **355,** 632–634.

3. Okubo, K., Hori, N., Matoba, R., Niiyama, T., Fukushima, A., Kojima, Y., and Matsubara, K. (1992) Large scale cDNA sequencing for analysis of quantitative and qualitative aspects of gene expression. *Nat. Genet.* **2,** 173–179.
4. Adams, M. D., Soares, M. B., Kerlavage, A. R., Fields, C., and Venter, J. C. (1993) Rapid cDNA sequencing (expressed sequence tags) from a directionally cloned human infant brain cDNA library. *Nat. Genet.* **4,** 373–380.
5. Adams, M. D., Kerlavage, A. R., Fields, C., and Venter, J. C. (1993) Initial assessment of human gene diversity and expression patterns based upon 83 million nucleotides of cDNA sequence. *Nat. Genet.* **4,** 256–267.
6. Takeda, J., Yano, H., Eng, S., Zeng, Y., and Bell, G. I. (1993) Construction of a normalized directionally cloned cDNA library from adult heart and analysis of 3040 clones by partial sequencing. *Hum. Mol. Genet.* **2,** 1793–1798.
7. Sudo, K., Chinen, K., and Nakamura,Y. (1994) 2058 expressed sequence tags (ESTs) from a human fetal lung cDNA library. *Genomics* **24,** 276–279.
8. Gress, T. M., Hoheisel, J. D., Lennon, G. G., Zehetner, G., and Lehrach, H. (1992) Hybridization fingerprinting of high-density cDNA-library arrays with cDNA pools derived from whole tissues. *Mamm. Genome* **3,** 609–661.
9. Nguyen, C., Rocha, D., Granjeaud, S., Baldit, M., Bernard, K., Naquet, P., and Jordan, B. R. (1995) Differential gene expression in the murine thymus assayed by quantitative hybridization of arrayed cDNA clones. *Genomics* **29,** 207–215.
10. Velculescu, V. E., Zhang, L., Vogelstein, B., and Kinzler, K. W. (1995) Serial analysis of gene expression. *Science* **270,** 484–487.
11. Zhao, N., Hashida, H., Takahashi, N., Misumi, Y., and Sakaki, Y. (1995) High-density cDNA filter analysis: a novel approach for large-scale, quantitative analysis of gene expression. *Gene* **156,** 207–213.
12. Bernard, K., Auphan, N., Granjeaud, S., Victorero, G., Schmitt-Verhulst, A. M., Jordan, B. R., and Nguyen, C. (1996) Multiplex Messenger Assay: simultaneous, quantitative measurement of expression for many genes in the context of T cell activation. *Nucleic Acids Res.* **24,** 1435–1443.
13. Pietu, G., Alibert, O., Guichard, V., Lamy, B., Bois, F., Leroy E., Mariage-Samson, R., Houlgatte, R., Soularue, P., and Auffray, C. (1996) Novel gene transcripts preferentially expressed in human muscles revealed by quantitative hybridization of a high density cDNA array. *Genome Res.* **6,** 492–503.
14. Chee, M., Yang, R., Hubbell, E., Berno, A., Huang, X. C., Stern, D, Winkle, J., Lockhart, D. J., Morris, M. S., and Fodor, S. P. (1996) Accessing genetic information with high-density DNA arrays. *Science* **274,** 610–614.
15. Rocha, D., Carrier, A., Naspetti, M., Victorero, G., Anderson, E., Botcherby, M., Nguyen, C., Naquet. P., and Jordan, B. R. (1997) Modulation of mRNA levels in the presence of thymocytes and genome mapping for a set of genes expressed in mouse thymic epithelial cells. *Immunogenetics* **46,** 142–151.
16. http://www.ncbi.nlm.nih.gov/dbEST.
17. Bertrand, R. Jordan (1998) Large scale expression measurement by hybridization methods: From high-density membranes to "DNA chips". *Jap. J. Biochem.,* in press.

18. Schena, M., Shalon, D., Davis, R. W., and Brown, P. O. (1995) Quantitative monitoring of gene expression patterns with a complementary DNA microarray. *Science* **270,** 467–470.

19. Schena, M., Shalon, D., Heller, R., Chai, A., Brown, P. O., and Davis, R. W. (1996) Parallel human genome analysis: microarray-based expression monitoring of 1000 genes. *Proc. Natl. Acad. Sci. USA* **93,** 10,614–10,619.

20. Shalon, D., Smith, S. J., and Brown, P. O. A. (1996) DNA microarray system for analyzing complex DNA samples using two-color fluorescent probe hybridization. *Genome Res.* **6(7),** 639–645.

21. Derisi, J., Penland, L., Brown, P. O., Bittner, M. L., Meltzer, P. S., Ray, M., Chen, Y., Su, Y. A., and Trent, J. M. (1996) Use of a cDNA microarray to analyse gene expression patterns in human cancer. *Nature Gene.* **14,** 457–460.

22. Derisi, J. L., Iyer, V. R., and Brown, P. O. (1997) Exploring the metabolic and genetic control of gene expression on a genomic scale. *Science* **278,** 680–686.

23. Southern, E. M., Maskos, U., and Elder, J. K. (1992) Analyzing and comparing nucleic acid sequences by hybridization to arrays of oligonucleotides: evaluation using experimental models. *Genomics* **13,** 1008–1017.

24. Lockhart, D. J., Dong, H., Byrne, M. C., Follettie, M. T., Gallo, M. V., Chee, M. S., Mittmann, M., Wang C., Kobayashi, M., Horton, H. and Brown, E. L. (1996) Expression monitoring by hybridization to high-density oligonucleotide arrays. *Nature Biotechnol.* **14,** 1675–1680.

25. IMAGE consortium: http://www-bio.llnl.gov/bbrp/image/image.html.

26. Clontech "ATLAS array": http://www.clontech.com/clontech/Catalog/Hybridization/Atlas.html.

27. Genome Systems "Gene discovery array:" http://www.genomesystems.com/GDA/.

28. Weiss, A. and Imboden, J. B. (1987) Cell surface molecules and early events involved in human T lymphocyte activation. *Adv. Immunol.* **41,** 1–38.

29. Beltz, G. A., Jacobs, K. A., Eickbush, T. H., Cherbas, P. T., and Kafatos, F. C. (1983) Isolation of multigene families and determination of homologies by filter hybridization methods. *Methods Enzymol.* **100,** 266–285.

30. Nizetic, D., Dramanac, R. and Lehrach, H. (1991). An improved bacterial colony lysis procedure enables direct DNA hybridization using short (10, 11 bases) oligonucleotides to cosmids. *Nucleic Acids Res.* **19,** 182.

31. Sambrook, J., Fritsch, E. F., and Maniatis T. (1989) *Molecular Cloning: A Laboratory Manual*, 2nd ed. Cold Spring Harbor Laboratory Press, Cold Spring Harbor, NY, book 1, pp. 7.3–7.5.

32. Gress, T. M., Müller-Pillasch, F., Adler, G., Zehetner, G., and Lehrach, H. (1984) European pancreatic cancer reference library system, EPCRLS. *Eur. J. Cancer* **30A,** 1391–1394.

33. Johnston, R. F., Pickett, S. C. and Barker, D. L. (1990) Autroradiography using storage phosphor technology. *Electrophoresis* **11,** 355–360.

34. Mory, K. and Hmaoka, T. (1994) IP autoradiographiy system (BAS). *Protein Nucleic Acid Enzyme* **39,** 181–191.

35. Patterson, S. D. and Latte, G. I. (1993) Evaluation of storage phosphor imaging plating for quantitative analysis of 2-D gels using the Quest II system. *Biotechniques* **15,** 1076–1083.

36. Granjeaud, S., Nguyen, C., Rocha, D., Luton, R., and Jordan, B. R. (1996) From hybridization image to numerical values: a practical, high throughput quantification system for high density filter hybridizations. *Gene. Anal. Biomol. Engineer.* **12,** 151–162.

Index